IVUS A to Z

A Comprehensive Atlas of Intravascular Ultrasound

IVUS A to Z
A Comprehensive Atlas of Intravascular Ultrasound

Authors

Pankaj Manoria
MD DM (Cardiology) FACC (USA) FESC (Europe) FSCAI (USA) FICA (USA) FAPSIC (Asia) FIAMS FICC
Interventional Cardiologist and Director
Manoria Heart Care Centre
Bhopal, Madhya Pradesh, India

Prasant Kumar Sahoo
MD DM FRCP (London and Glasgow) FACC FSCAI FESC FCSI FICC
Senior Consultant and Director (Interventional Cardiology)
Apollo Hospitals
Bhubaneswar, Odisha, India

Forewords

Ashok Seth
AB Mehta

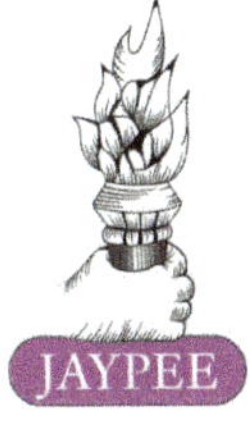

JAYPEE BROTHERS MEDICAL PUBLISHERS
The Health Sciences Publisher
New Delhi | London

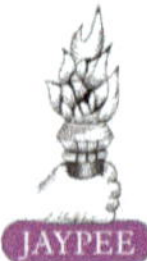

JAYPEE **Jaypee Brothers Medical Publishers (P) Ltd**

Headquarters
Jaypee Brothers Medical Publishers (P) Ltd
EMCA House, 23/23-B
Ansari Road, Daryaganj
New Delhi 110 002, India
Landline: +91-11-23272143, +91-11-23272703
+91-11-23282021, +91-11-23245672
Email: jaypee@jaypeebrothers.com

Corporate Office
Jaypee Brothers Medical Publishers (P) Ltd
4838/24, Ansari Road, Daryaganj
New Delhi 110 002, India
Phone: +91-11-43574357
Fax: +91-11-43574314
Email: jaypee@jaypeebrothers.com

Overseas Office
JP Medical Ltd.
83, Victoria Street, London
SW1H 0HW (UK)
Phone: +44 20 3170 8910
Email: info@jpmedpub.com

EU GPSR Authorised Representative
JP Medical Ltd.
83, Victoria Street, London
SW1H 0HW (UK)
Phone: +44 20 3170 8910
Fax: +44 (0)20 3008 6180
Email: info@jpmedpub.com

Website: www.jaypeebrothers.com
Website: www.jaypeedigital.com

Inquiries for bulk sales may be solicited at: jaypee@jaypeebrothers.com

IVUS A to Z: A Comprehensive Atlas of Intravascular Ultrasound

First Edition: **2025**

ISBN: 978-93-6616-652-0

Dedicated to

My parents
Professor PC Manoria and late Mrs Maya Manoria

Pankaj Manoria

My parents Late Dr Jaganath Sahoo, Late Mrs Sashimani Sahoo
My wife Dr Suneeta Sahoo
My children Dr Shyam Prasad Sahoo and Dr Pratyush Sahoo

Prasant Kumar Sahoo

Foreword

We are in an era where the complexity of coronary artery disease poses significant challenges to percutaneous coronary intervention (PCI) procedural planning and execution to achieve the best outcomes for our patients. Innovations in intravascular imaging and supporting scientific evidence have advanced our understanding of lesion morphology, thereby enabling appropriate device selection, technique modification, and result optimization. Intravascular imaging is now a guideline-recommended strategy to improve short- and long-term outcomes for our complex PCI patients.

IVUS A to Z: A Comprehensive Atlas of Intravascular Ultrasound by Pankaj Manoria and Prasant Kumar Sahoo offers a comprehensive, in-depth, and practice-based education on intravascular ultrasound (IVUS), a vital imaging modality that enabled the move from plain old balloon angioplasty to bare metal stents 30 years ago by demonstrating that IVUS-guided stent implantation could make metallic stents less thrombogenic and thereby safer, even with basic antiplatelet therapy in those days. Drawing upon their vast experience in the use of IVUS in their "real-world" PCI practice, the authors provide a detailed and 'step-by-step' guide for the use of IVUS in PCI. From the foundational concepts to its role in guiding PCI in complex scenarios, this book details image interpretation, stepwise decision-making, and meticulous execution.

Pankaj Manoria and Prasant Kumar Sahoo excel in bridging the gap between scientific knowledge and practical 'real-world PCI' application, thereby empowering readers to learn, interpret, and use IVUS with confidence and precision in daily PCI practice. This book aims to be informative for all generations of interventional cardiologists, from early career to more experienced ones.

This book is a must-read, must-understand, and must-possess educational resource for real-world PCI practice as we strive hard to improve outcomes for our complex CAD patients undergoing PCI.

Ashok Seth
FRCP (London, Edinburgh, Ireland) FACC FESC MSCAI FAPSIC FIMSA FCSI
DSc (BHU, AMU, Amity University, TMU, Shiv Nadar University) D Litt (Jamia Millia University)
Chairman, Fortis Escorts Heart Institute, New Delhi
'Padma Bhushan' and 'Padma Shri' Awardee
'BC Roy' National Award (2015) for Eminent Medical Person
Chairman, Fortis Healthcare Medical Council, New Delhi
Adjunct Professor, Department of Cardiology
JN Medical College, Aligarh Muslim University, Aligarh, Uttar Pradesh
Adjunct Professor, Department of Cardiology, National Board of Examinations
Director, Interventional Cardiology Foundation of India and "INDIA LIVE"
Director, Heart Valve Foundation of India and "INDIA VALVES"
Course Director, "AICT-AsiaPCR" and "CHIP-CTO INDIA"
Past President, Cardiological Society of India
Immediate Past President
Asian Pacific Society of Interventional Cardiology (APSIC), Hong Kong, China

Foreword

Coronary angiography, yesterday's gold standard, is no more a gold standard. It is simply a shadow of the passage of the dye going through the vessels and inferences are made from the deformation of that shadow. This has left behind many lacunae. When the vessels are examined from inside, they reveal startling facts and have impacted the preciseness of interventional treatments.

Today, intravascular ultrasound of coronary arteries is an indispensable investigation. Surprisingly, there is not a single book or atlas by any Indian author or on Indian patients. Our coronary arteries are different in several ways as compared to Westerners. There was a long-standing need of having an atlas on intravascular ultrasound based on our patients. This need has been completely satisfied by "IVUS A to Z".

The illustrations are of immense clarity and have been successfully driving message at home. The book has successfully served its purpose and I would strongly recommend that every interventional cardiologist should possess it. The authors are extremely well qualified and have a special knack of transmitting knowledge through their atlas.

I compliment both the authors for coming out with what is most needed in every library.

AB Mehta
Director
Department of Cardiology
Jaslok Hospital and Research Centre, Mumbai
Mentor in Cardiology
Sir HN Reliance Foundation Hospital and
Research Centre
Mumbai, Maharashtra, India
Padma Bhushan Awardee

Preface

Intravascular ultrasound (IVUS) has become like a third eye for an interventional cardiologist. It has revolutionized how we diagnose, treat, and conceptualize coronary artery disease.

IVUS A to Z: A Comprehensive Atlas of Intravascular Ultrasound is our in-depth exploration into this advanced imaging technology (IVUS). This book serves as an essential guide for interventional cardiologists (both seasoned cardiologists and new trainees) involved in complex procedures.

Over the years, as a practitioner and researcher, we have witnessed firsthand the power of this technology to unveil the hidden narratives within vascular walls—narratives that have significant implications for patient care and outcomes. The genesis of this book lies in our desire to share these insights, demystifying the techniques and interpretations that IVUS demands.

The synopsis highlights the book's step-by-step approach to understanding IVUS, from basic principles to detailed application techniques. Through meticulously detailed illustrations, high-resolution images, and clear medical insights, it bridges the gap between theory and practice, offering readers a visual and textual grasp of how IVUS operates and its immense value in diagnosing and treating cardiovascular diseases.

The book is a valuable and high-quality reference for interventionalists, trainees, and catheterization laboratory staff. It is both practical and sophisticated, filling a gap in the market for IVUS resources.

All the images included in the Atlas were taken from Boston HD 60 MHz IVUS.

IVUS A to Z: A Comprehensive Atlas of Intravascular Ultrasound is more than a book; it is a compass for navigating the dynamic and often challenging terrain of intravascular imaging. It is our hope that the clarity and depth offered within these pages will empower you, the reader, to harness IVUS with greater confidence and precision, ultimately advancing the care you provide to your patients.

Notably, it is one of the few IVUS atlases available from an Indian author, making it a solid and user-friendly contribution to the field.

In closing, we extend our deepest gratitude to all those who have contributed to the development and evolution of IVUS technology. Their innovation and dedication have been the guiding lights in the creation of this Atlas. To the readers embarking on this journey, may this Atlas be your trusted companion in the pursuit of cardiovascular excellence.

Warm regards

Pankaj Manoria
Prasant Kumar Sahoo

Acknowledgments

We would like to express our deepest gratitude to everyone who supported the creation of *IVUS A to Z: A Comprehensive Atlas of Intravascular Ultrasound.*

We are particularly grateful to Professor Gary Minz, Akiko Mehra, Dr Ashok Seth, Dr AB Mehta, Dr Sanjog Kalra and Dr Kirti Punamia for their expert advice and encouragement, which have greatly enriched the quality of this Atlas.

We are deeply indebted to Boston Scientific for providing a high-quality IVUS machine, ensuring that the images in this atlas meet the highest standards of excellence.

To our family, thank you for your unwavering understanding and support, especially during the times our focus was solely on this project.

Our sincere appreciation goes out to M/s Jaypee Brothers Medical Publishers (P) Ltd, New Delhi, India, for their dedication in bringing this book to publication. Your professionalism and commitment are unmatched.

Above all, we owe special thanks to our patients. Your trust and cooperation have not only allowed this work to flourish but also inspired us daily.

We are also immensely thankful to all the PCI Imagers WhatsApp group members, especially our admin, Dr Nishith Chandra and Dr Arun Mohanti, for their invaluable insights and camaraderie throughout this journey. Your shared wisdom and support have been instrumental.

Lastly, We acknowledge the hospital staff whose tireless work in the background provides the foundation for excellence in patient care.

Thank you all for your incredible support.

Contents

Assessment of procedural risks and post-procedural outcomes

Intracoronary imaging guidance by IVUS or OCT is recommended when performing PCI on anatomically complex lesions, in particular left main stem, true bifurcations, and long lesions	I	A

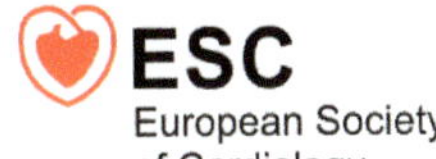

European Heat Journal (2024) **00**, 1–123
https://doi.org/10.1093/eurheart/ehae177

ESC GUIDELINES

2024 ESC Guidelines for the management of chronic coronary syndromes

Developed by the task force for the management of chronic coronary syndromes of the European Society of Cardiology (ESC)

Endorsed by the European Association for Cardio-Thoracic Surgery (EACTS)

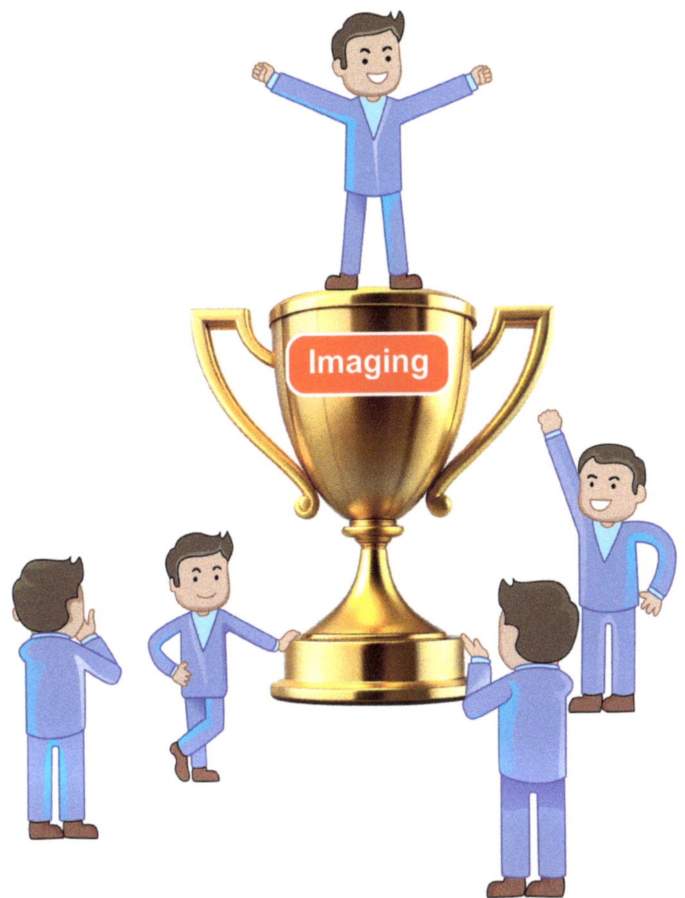

Class I a Recommendation for Imaging in complex lesions

CHAPTER 1

Basics of Intravascular Ultrasound

Intravascular ultrasound (IVUS) is a reflection technique **(Fig. 1)**.

The IVUS transducer emits sound waves. These sound waves reach the structure and are reflected back. After reflection from tissue, part of the ultrasound energy returns to the transducer and is converted into the image.

The strength of the echo signal depends upon the acoustic impedance and density of the structure being traversed.

For example, when imaging a calcified structure whose density is high, the entire ultrasound waves are reflected back, so you get an echo-dense image, whereas when imaging a lipidic structure whose density is low, most of these ultrasound waves are absorbed and very few are reflected back, so you get an echo-lucent image. If the ultrasound waves are not able to penetrate the object there will be signal attenuation beyond that object on IVUS. Since the IVUS cannot penetrate both calcium and lipid there is signal attenuation and we see nothing beyond them **(Fig. 2)**.

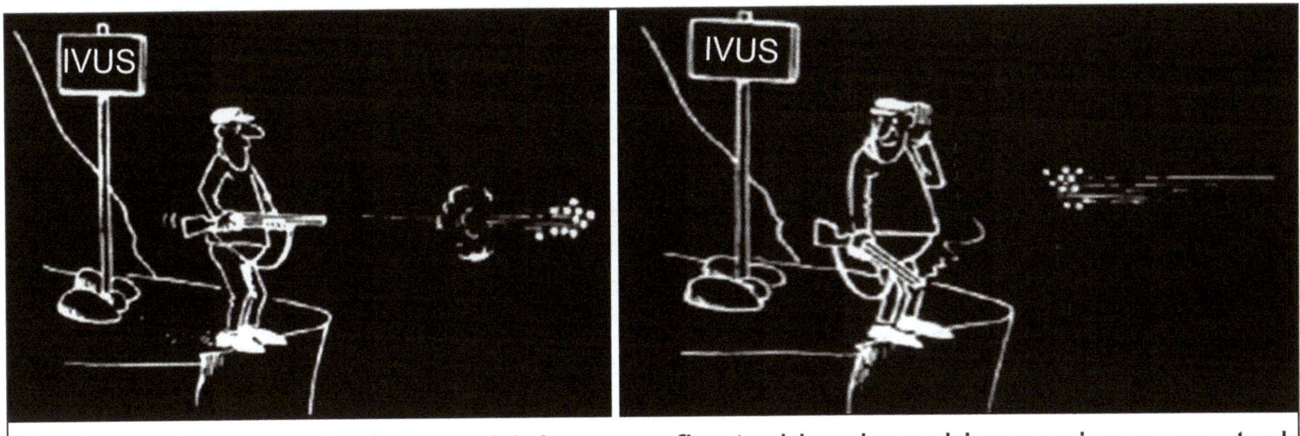

Fig. 1: Intravascular ultrasound (IVUS) is a reflection technique.

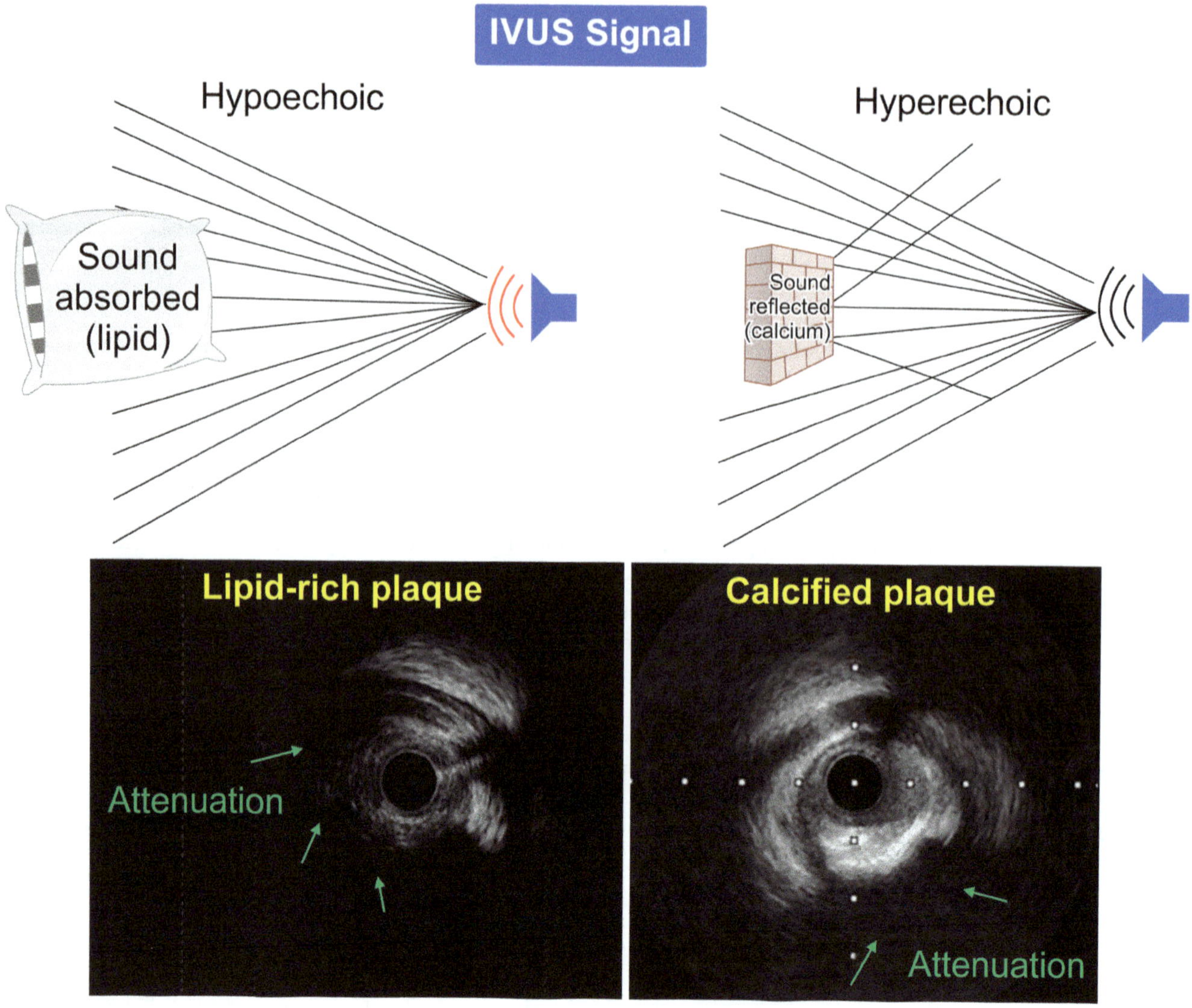
IVUS Signal
Hypoechoic
Sound absorbed (lipid)
Hyperechoic
Sound reflected (calcium)
Lipid-rich plaque
Attenuation
Calcified plaque
Attenuation

Fig. 2: The echogenicity of intravascular ultrasound (IVUS) image is directly proportional to the intensity of reflection where as signal attenuation is inversely proportional to the penetrating power of the ultrasound waves.

My perspective on imaging
The Old (Angio)
The Gold standard (imaging)

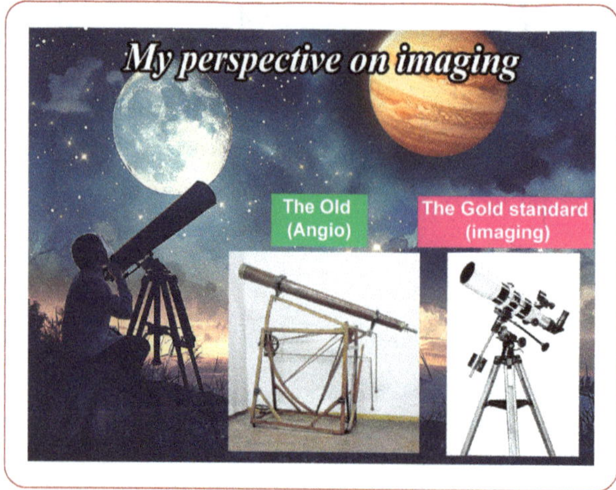

CHAPTER 2

Intravascular Ultrasound Equipment

EQUIPMENT FOR INTRAVASCULAR ULTRASOUND EXAMINATION

The intravascular ultrasound (IVUS) acquisition system consists of a catheter, a pullback device, and a scanning console **(Figs. 1A to C)**.

Intravascular Ultrasound Catheter

They are usually 150 cm long and have a tip size of 3.2–3.5 F and can easily go through a 5–6 F guiding catheter. These catheters are monorail designs to facilitate rapid exchange. The catheter is visible in angiographic images and is advanced along with a guidewire. The ultrasound transducer is mounted at the tip of the catheter.

Intravascular Ultrasound Transducer

Currently available transducers have a frequency ranging from 20 to 60 MHz, which can provide an axial resolution of 40–200 µm and a penetration of 5–10 mm. Higher the frequency, greater will be the resolution but lesser will be the penetration. Similarly, the lesser the frequency, the greater will be the penetration but less will be the resolution. So, a high-frequency transducer will have better near-field resolution as compared to a lower frequency catheter, which has high far-field resolution. Two different transducer designs are commonly used: Mechanically rotated devices and electronically switched multielement array systems **(Fig. 2)**.

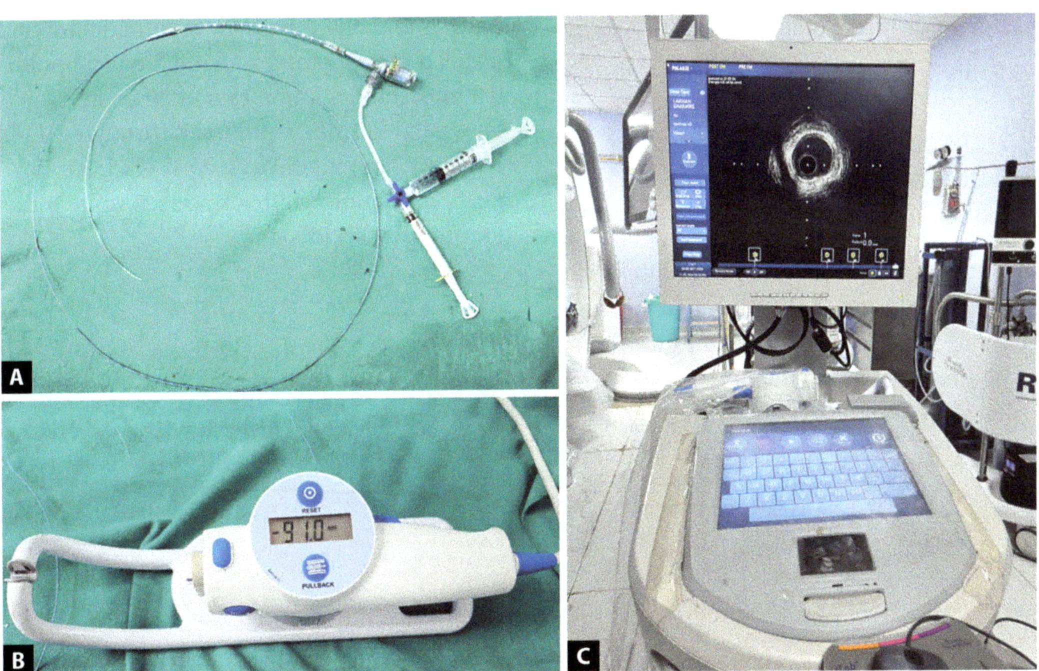

Figs. 1A to C: Intravascular ultrasound (IVUS) equipment [IVUS catheter with ultrasound transducer (A), a motorized pullback device (B), and the IVUS console (C)].

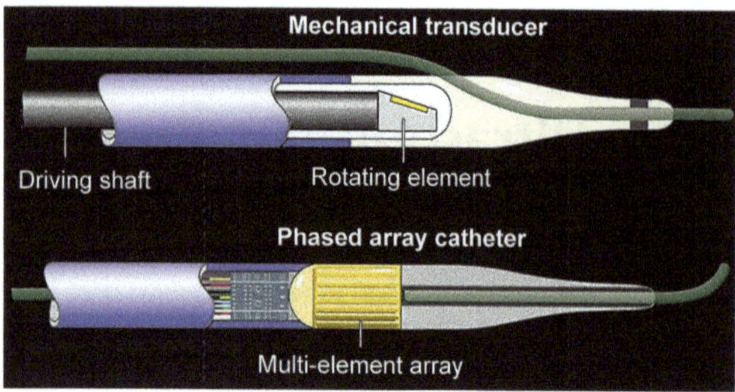

Fig. 2: Mechanical transducer catheters use rotating ultrasound sources, while phased array catheters use sequentially flashing ultrasound sources.

TABLE 1: Difference between mechanical and electronic system.

Mechanical transducer (Boston Sci) (single rotating transducer)	***Phased array (Volcano) (64 circumferential transducers)***
Short monorail 2 cm	Long monorail 24 cm
Wire artifact	No wire artifact
Less pushability	More pushability
Sleeve over the catheter (need adequate flushing to remove air artifacts)	No sleeve (less air artifacts)
Higher resolution 40–60 MHz	Lower resolution 20 MHz
Brighter blood speckles	Less blood stasis artifact
No Chromaflo	+Chromaflo and HV
Nonuniform rotational distortion (NURD) artifact in tortuous vessel preventing rotation	Ring down artifact

Mechanical transducers: Mechanical probes use a drive cable to rotate a single transducer at 1,800 rpm (30 revolutions per second), sweeping an ultrasound beam perpendicular to the catheter. The transducer sends and receives ultrasound signals at 1° increments, providing 256 individual radial scan lines for each image. In mechanical catheter systems, the imaging transducer is inside a protective sheath, which is advanced through the lesion or into the segment of interest. During the examination, the transducer is moved within the sheath, facilitating smooth and uniform pullback. Flushing with saline is required to provide a fluid pathway for the ultrasound beam, as small air bubbles can degrade image quality.

Currently available mechanical IVUS systems in India are:

- Opticross (40–60 MHz) from Boston
- Kodama (40–60 MHz) from ACIST
- Refinity 45 MHz from Philips

Electronic systems: In electronic systems, multiple transducer elements (currently up to 64) arranged in an annular array are activated sequentially to generate the image. The array can be programmed so that one set of elements transmits while a second set receives simultaneously. 5 F compatible Eagle Eye catheter (Volcano Corporation) is commercially available. The difference between the two transducers is highlighted in **Table 1**.

Catheter Pullback Device

The catheter is manually advanced to the distal end of the lesion of interest in the coronary artery and is then pulled back, manually or with an automatic pullback system, at a speed of 0.5–1 mm/s. Using a typical pullback speed of 0.5 mm/s and a frame rate of 30 images/s, 60 images will be available from a pullback through a 1-mm segment. Recently launched AVVIGO IVUS from Boston includes faster automatic pullback speeds up to 8 mm/s allowing for quick vessel imaging.

Intravascular Ultrasound Scanning Consoles

A scanning console carries a computer that is used for postprocessing and storage of recorded IVUS data. A cable from the end of the pullback device is connected with a computer for data processing.

"Interventional cardiologists: Making the invisible visible with a touch of IVUS."

CHAPTER 3

Intravascular Ultrasound Examination Technique/Imaging Controls

- **Guide support:** A stable guiding catheter position with good support is very desirable, since current ultrasound catheters have less trackability due to short monorail. The majority of modern intravascular ultrasound (IVUS) catheters are 5F compatible.
- **Guidewire:** Routine workhorse 0.014 mm wire.
- **Anticoagulation:** To prevent risk of thrombosis in the catheter, always give 2,500–5,000 IU heparin.
- **Nitroglycerin (NTG):** Intracoronary NTG 100 µg should always be given to overcome spasm induced by the wire or IVUS catheter.
- **Pullback:** Motorized pullback is recommended for detailed quantitative and qualitative analysis. The speed of pullback varies with different companies ranging from 0.5 to 8.0 mm/s. Lesser speed will give you more number of frames per second. For example, 0.5 mm pullback will give you 60 frames/second whereas 1 mm pullback will give you 30 frames/second. So if you want just the overview of the vessel go for high speed but if you want to analyze each segment in detail go for lowest speed of 0.5 mm/s. The total pullback length is 100 mm.
- **Preparation of the catheter and flushing in vitro prior to imaging:** Mechanical transducers have a protective plastic sheath over it and if it is not flushed properly, there is a high likelihood of air getting trapped between the transducer and sheath. It is recommended to flush the IVUS catheter twice with 3 cc saline before inserting **(Fig. 1)**. This is how a well-flushed IVUS catheter image looks like in vivo, which is now ready for imaging the coronaries **(Fig. 2)**.
- **Gain:** Gain amplifies the returned signal, but increasing it can lead to more noise and less grayscale information in the image. Higher overall gain results in increased image brightness. Setting the overall gain too low affects the detection of low-amplitude signals.

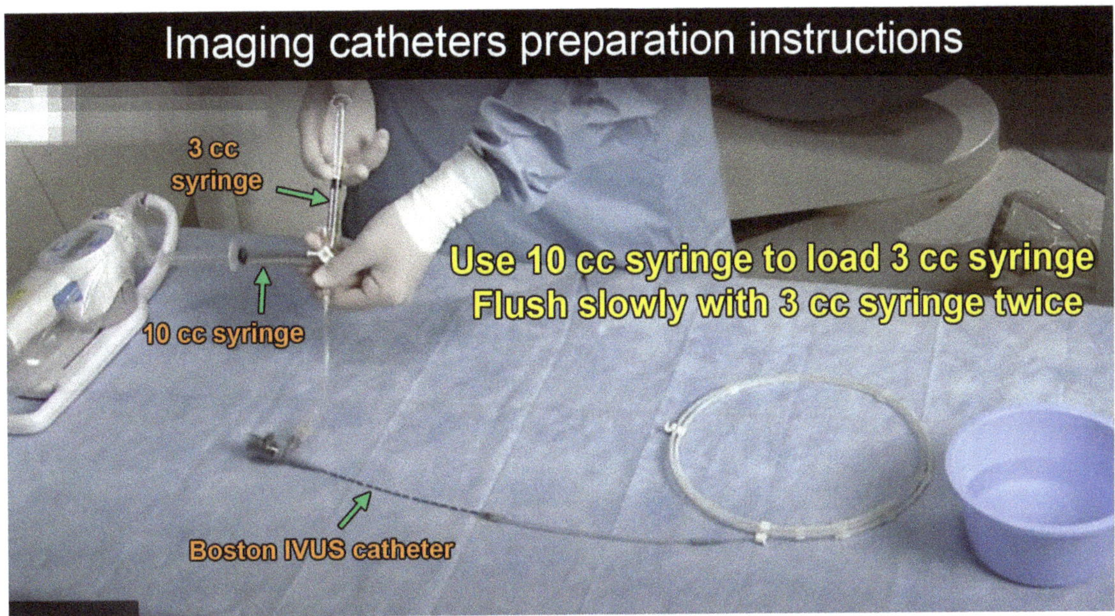

Fig. 1: Preparation of the catheter and flushing in vitro prior to imaging. (IVUS: intravascular ultrasound)

Conversely, setting the overall gain too high compresses the grayscale and causes tissue to appear overly bright **(Fig. 3)**. Overall, the balance of gain is crucial in achieving optimal image quality.

- **Depth:** The depth or scale setting adjusts the depth of the outer boundary of the image. It should be set so that the entire external elastic membrane is on the screen throughout the length of the vessel. When imaging a big vessel, the depth scale can be increased to accommodate the full image. In a small vessel, the depth can be decreased to get a magnified image of the vessel **(Fig. 4)**.

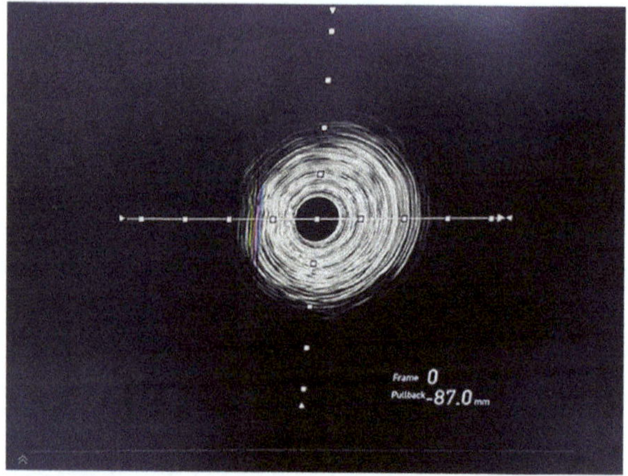

Fig. 2: Ideal image one should aim for before imaging.

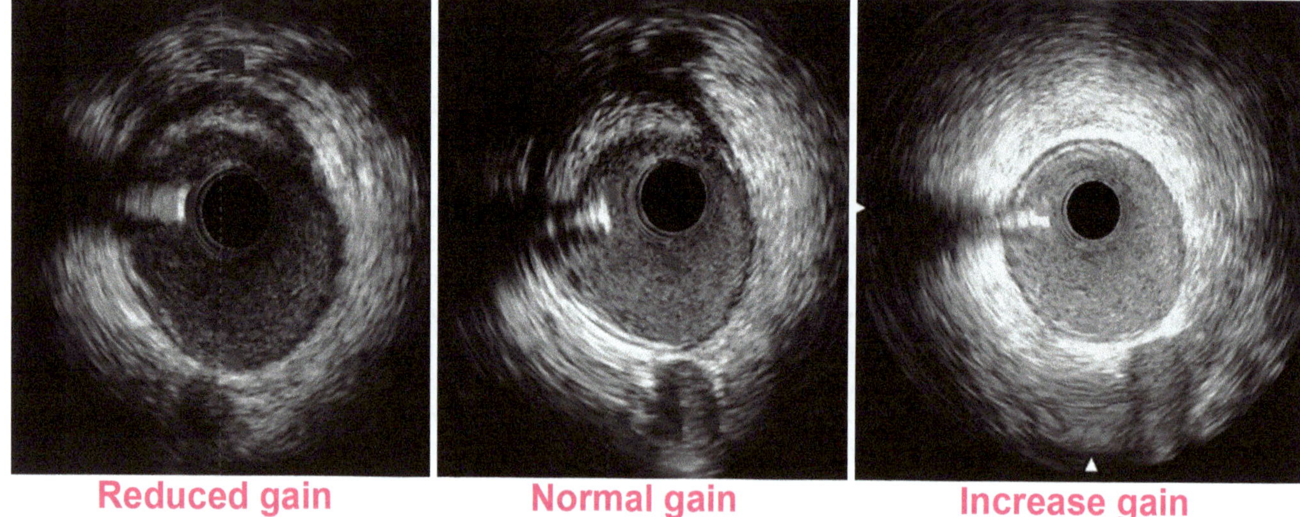

Fig. 3: Effect of gain setting. Reducing gain augments the grayscale but reduces the brightness. Increasing gain will increase the brightness but at the cost of compression of grayscale.

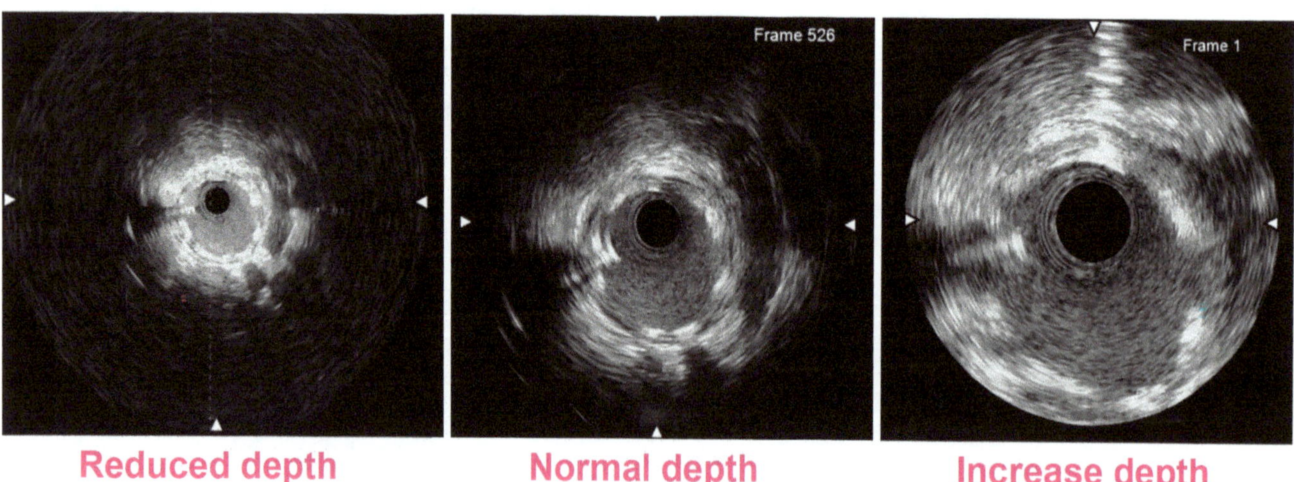

Fig. 4: Effect of depth scale setting: Increasing depth reduces the size of the image whereas reducing depth magnifies the image.

CHAPTER 4

Orientation of Intravascular Ultrasound Images

- Intravascular ultrasound (IVUS) images are analogous to histological sections.
- They are oriented from the ostium of the coronary artery **(Fig. 1)**.
- There is no absolute anterior versus posterior and left versus right orientation to the images.
- Side branches and perivascular landmarks (the pericardium, muscle, and the venous system) are used to orient the images.
- The image is described as if viewing the face of a clock.

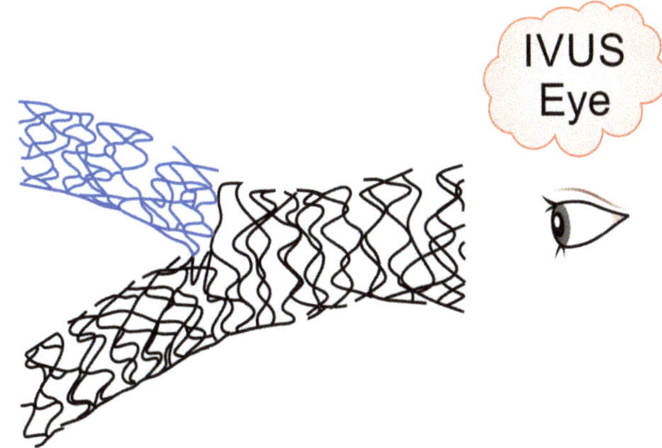

Fig. 1: Orientation of intravascular ultrasound (IVUS) from the ostium of coronary artery.

"Before you see IVUS, always imagine what you expect"

CHAPTER 5

Cross-sectional and Longitudinal Images

Intravascular ultrasound (IVUS) provides a series of tomographic and cross-sectional images of the vessel. Using a typical pullback speed of 0.5 mm/s and a frame rate of 30 images/s, 60 images will be available from a pullback through a 1-mm segment. IVUS usually provides cross-sectional images. However, motorized transducer pullback and digital storage of cross-sectional images can be used to create longitudinal imaging (L-mode).

*Usage of **L-mode**:*

- Length measurements **(Fig. 1)**
- Identifying reference segments of the vessels **(Fig. 1)**
- Look for the carina **(Fig. 2)**

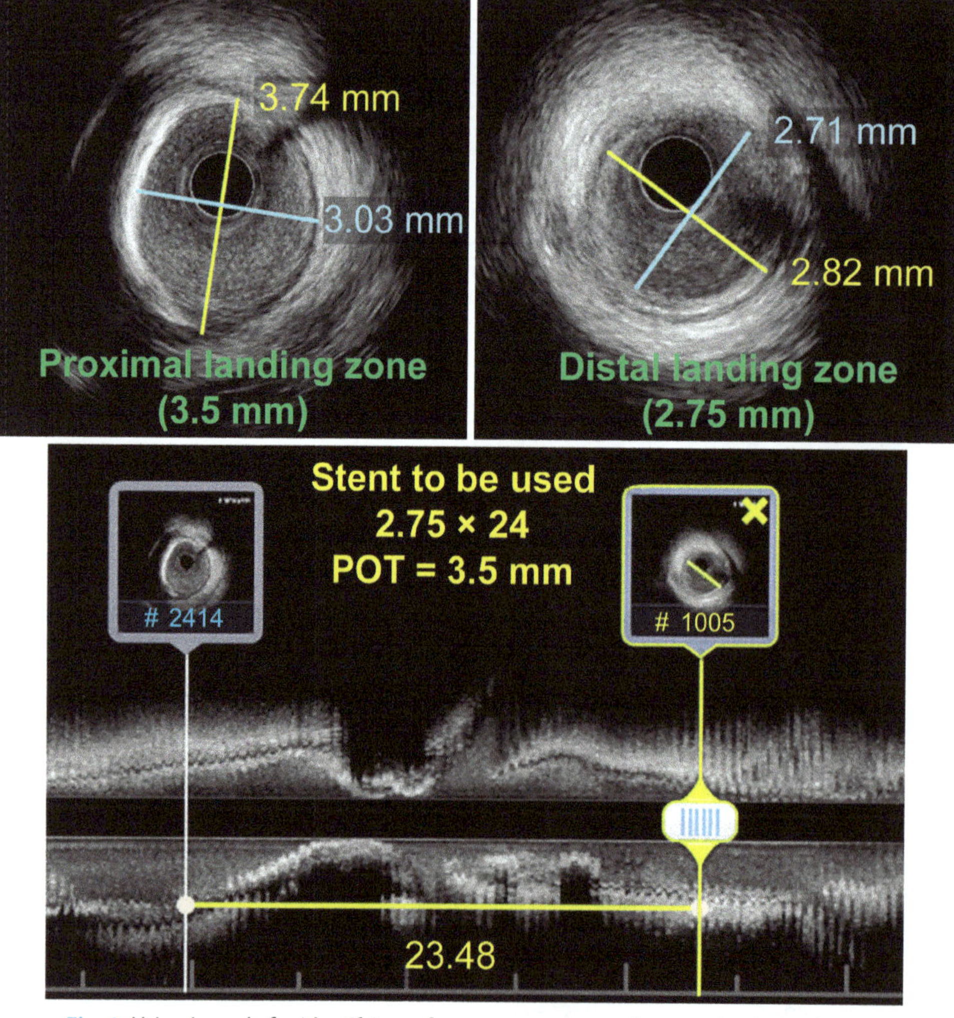

Fig. 1: Using L-mode for identifying reference segments and measuring lesion length.

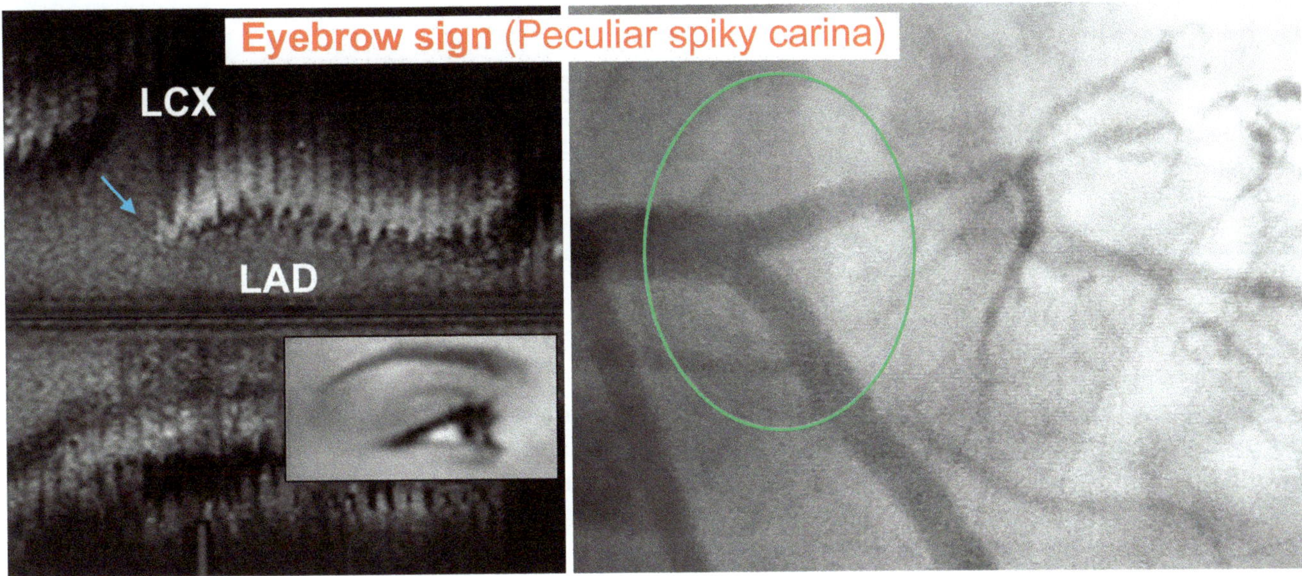

Fig. 2: Identifying hairy spiky carina on L-mode (eyebrow sign).

Limitation of ***L-mode****:*

- Obligate straight reconstruction of the artery
- Display of only a single cut plane
- Changes of vessel size during the cardiac cycle result in a characteristic "saw-tooth" appearance artifact

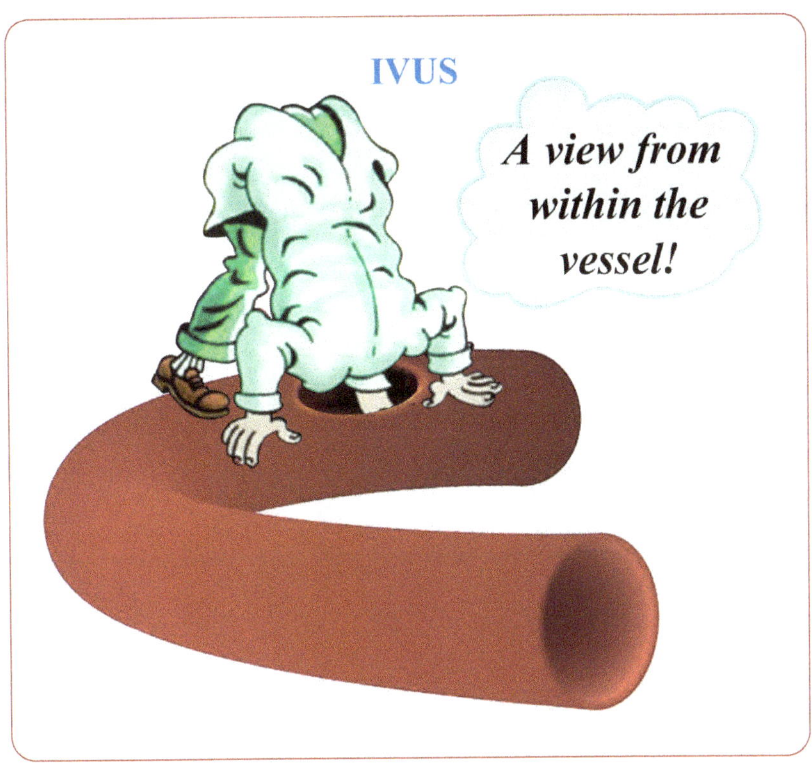

CHAPTER 6

Normal Arterial Morphology on Intravascular Ultrasound

A normal artery seen on intravascular ultrasound (IVUS) typically shows a three-layered appearance **(Fig. 1)**. Now, the first thing one should do when seeing the IVUS is to identify the echolucent black ring, which is the media.

The inner layer to media is the echodense layer, which is the intima (the intima is nothing but the plaque).

The outer layer to media is a more echogenic mesh-like structure that blends with the surrounding tissue, called the adventitia.

The outer border of media is called external elastic lamina (EEL) and the inner border is called internal elastic lamina (IEL).

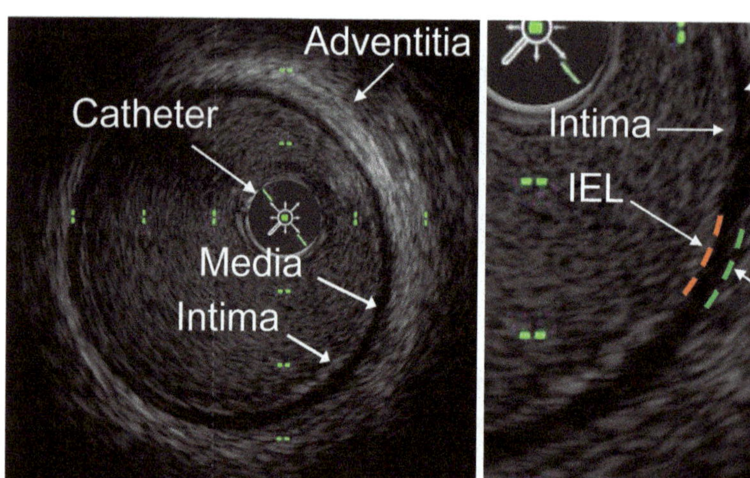

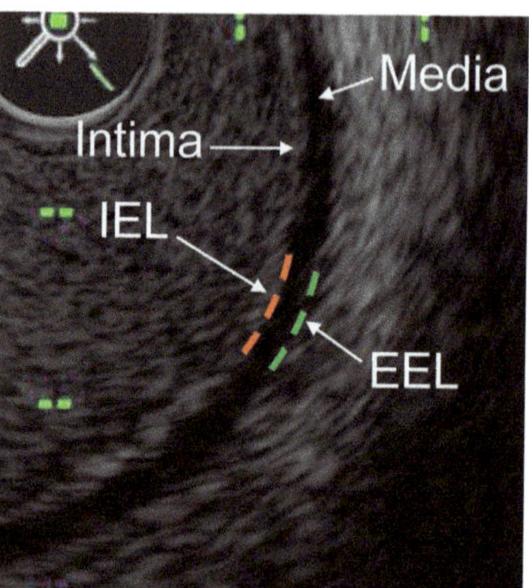

1. Intima = scouring pad
2. IEL = rubber band
3. Media = dense sponge
4. EEL = rubber band
5. Adventitia = mesh

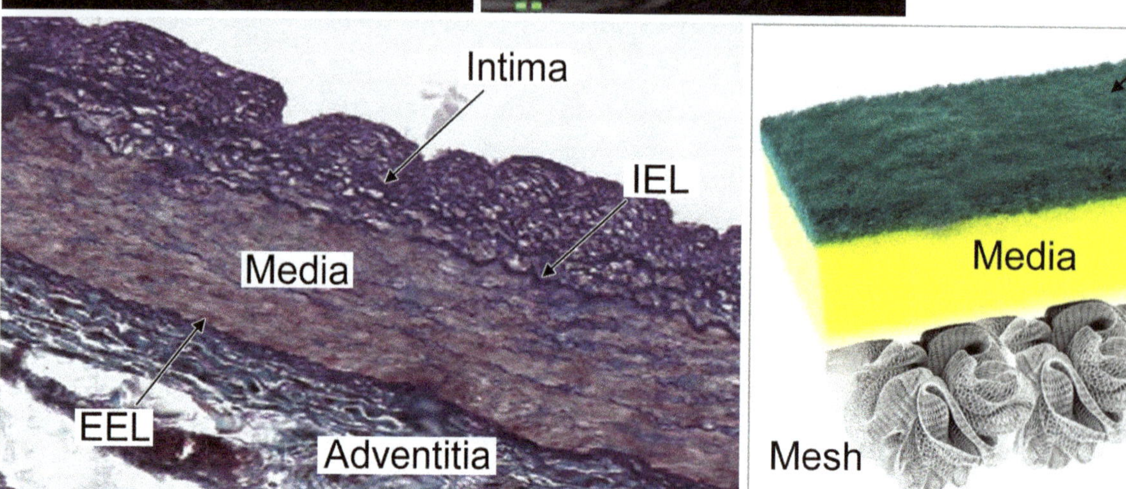

Fig. 1: Normal arterial morphology on IVUS. (EEL: external elastic lamina; IEL: internal elastic lamina; IVUS: intravascular ultrasound)

CHAPTER 7

Intravascular Ultrasound Measurements

MINIMUM LUMEN AREA

Identify the intimal luminal (plaque-lumen) interface and encircle it completely. The area occupied by this circle is the minimum lumen area (MLA) **(Figs. 1 and 2)**.

For identifying intima-luminal interface, we need to appreciate the blood speckles on intravascular ultrasound (IVUS), which appear as finely textured echoes moving in a swirling pattern. The point of separation of these blood speckles with intima is the intima-luminal interface.

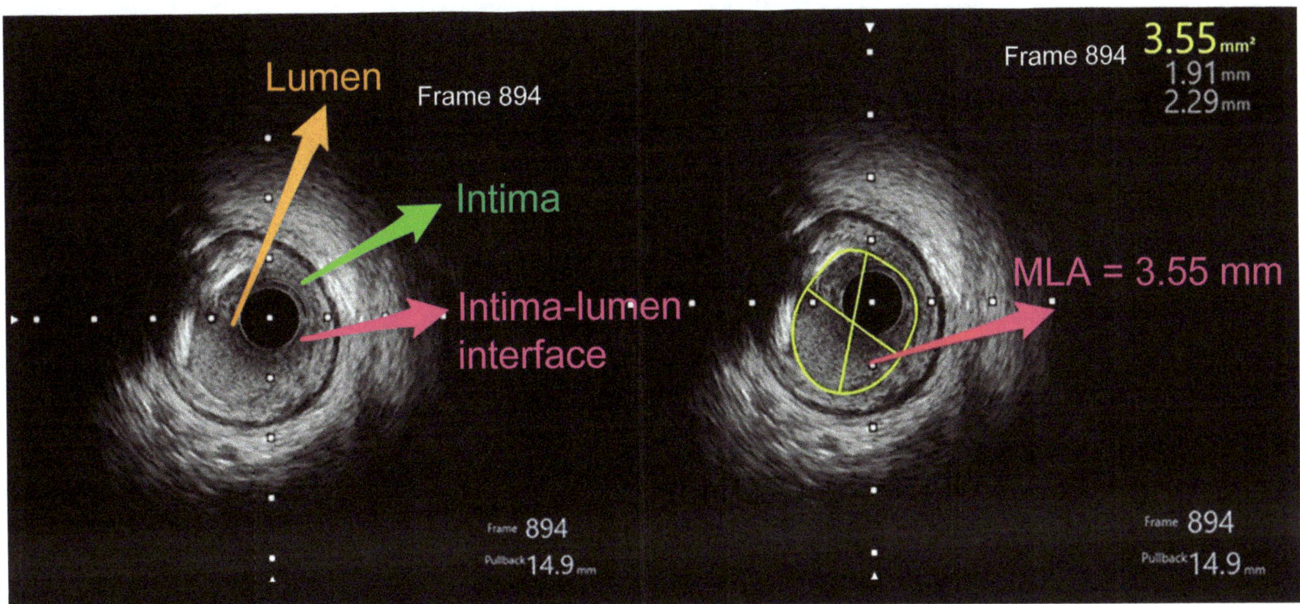

Fig. 1: Measuring minimum lumen area.

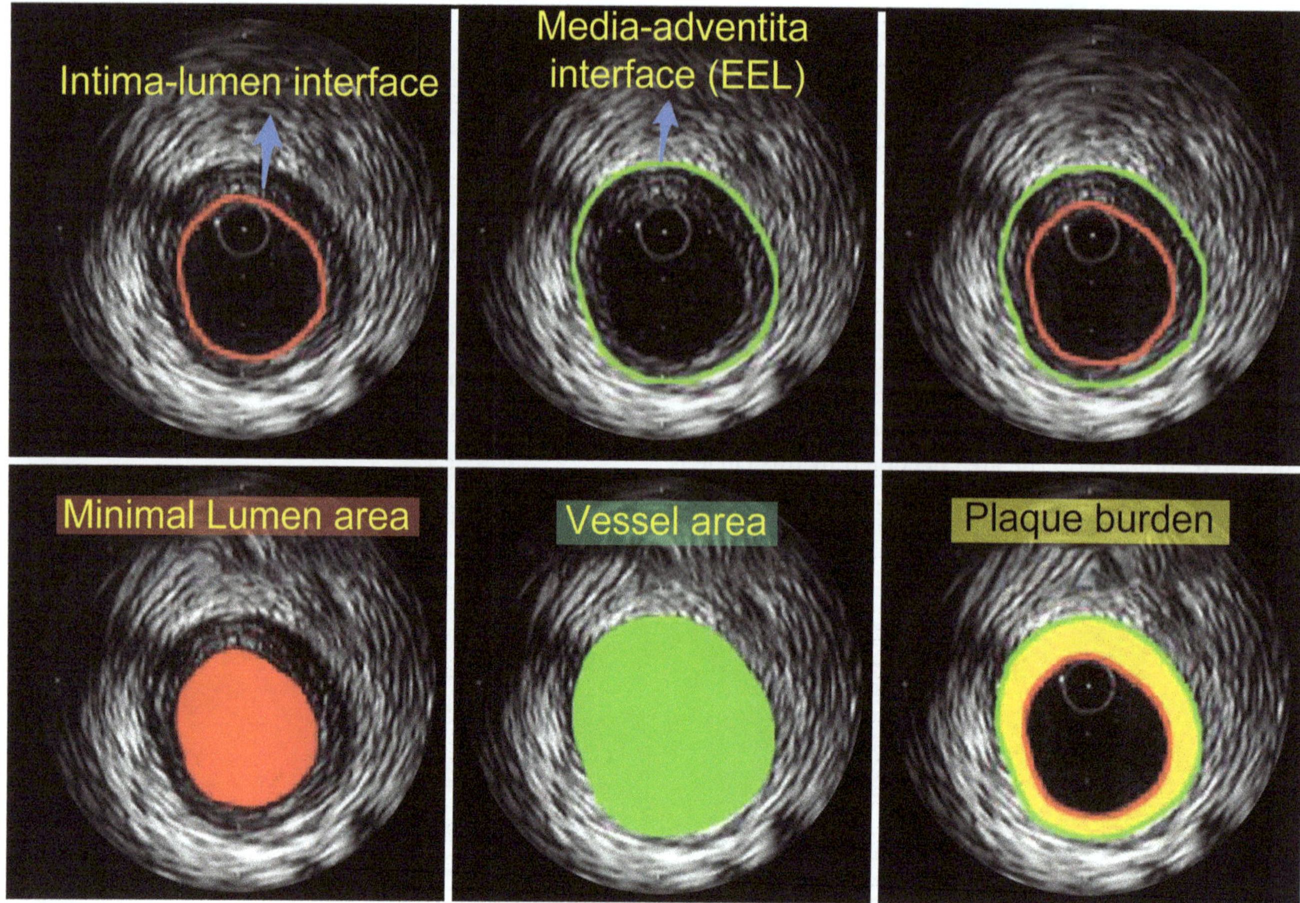

Fig. 2: Intravascular ultrasound (IVUS) measurement involving minimum lumen area (MLA), plaque burden (PB), and vessel area (VA).

VESSEL AREA

Trace the external elastic lamina (EEL) (EEL is nothing but the media-adventitita interface). The area occupied by the EEL is the vessel area (VA) **(Figs. 2 and 3)**. The measurement of EEL border should be avoided at the sites where large side branches originate or with extensive calcification and acoustic shadowing. If acoustic shadowing involves a relatively small arc (<90°), planimetry of the circumference can be performed by estimation from the closest identifiable EEL borders, although the accuracy and reproducibility will be reduced. If calcification is more extensive than 90° of arc, EEL measurements should not be reported.

Note: IVUS measurements should be performed at the leading edge of each interface never the trailing edge. These measurements should be performed relative to the center of the mass of the lumen and not center of the IVUS catheter.

PLAQUE BURDEN

The area occupied by the plaque can be estimated by subtracting the lumen area from the VA **(Figs. 2 and 4)**.

Note: Plaque burden (PB) is not the same as percentage stenosis. Blood flow is determined by lumen area and not by how much plaque is present.

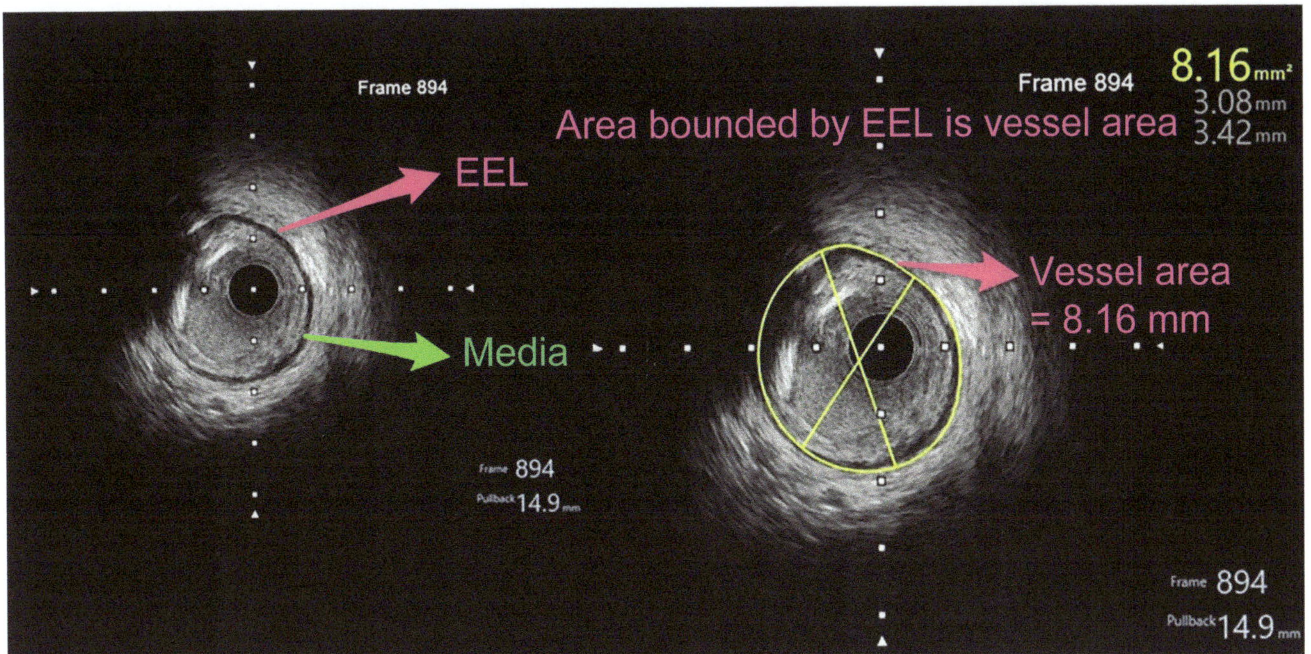

Fig. 3: Measuring vessel area. (EEL: external elastic lamina)

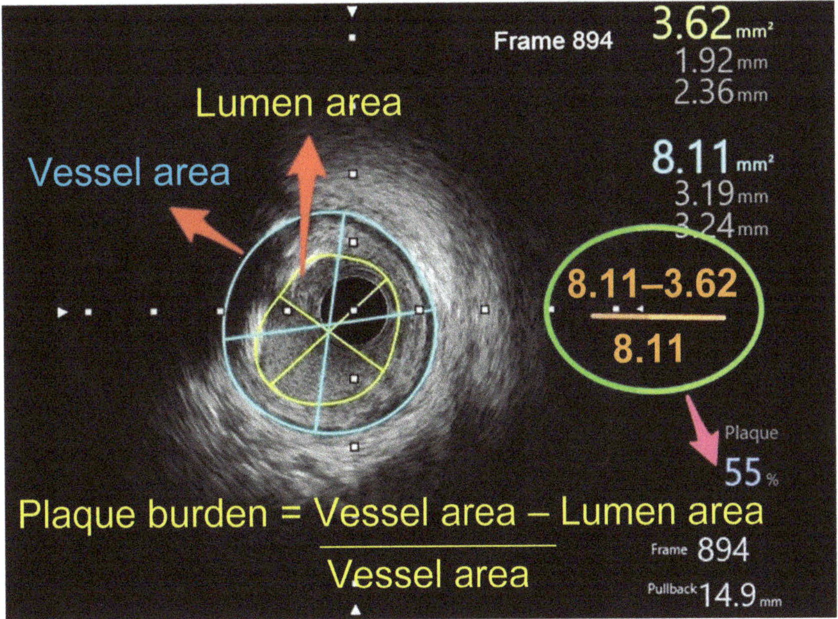

Fig. 4: Measuring plaque burden.

MEASUREMENT OF LENGTH OF LESION

There are three simple steps to measure lesion/stent length **(Figs. 5A and B)**:

1. *Bookmark the proximal landing zone:* It is the biggest area nearest to the lesion site which has a PB of <50% and has no calcium or muscle bridge or lipidic plaque.
2. Similarly, bookmark the distal landing zone.
3. Measure the distance between the two bookmarks on L view. This will give you the lesion length.

Note: If we are using a pullback device with a speed of 0.5 mm/s, then the distance or length measured in mm = measured sec × 0.5. However, we do not have to do these measurements, the AI automatically does it.

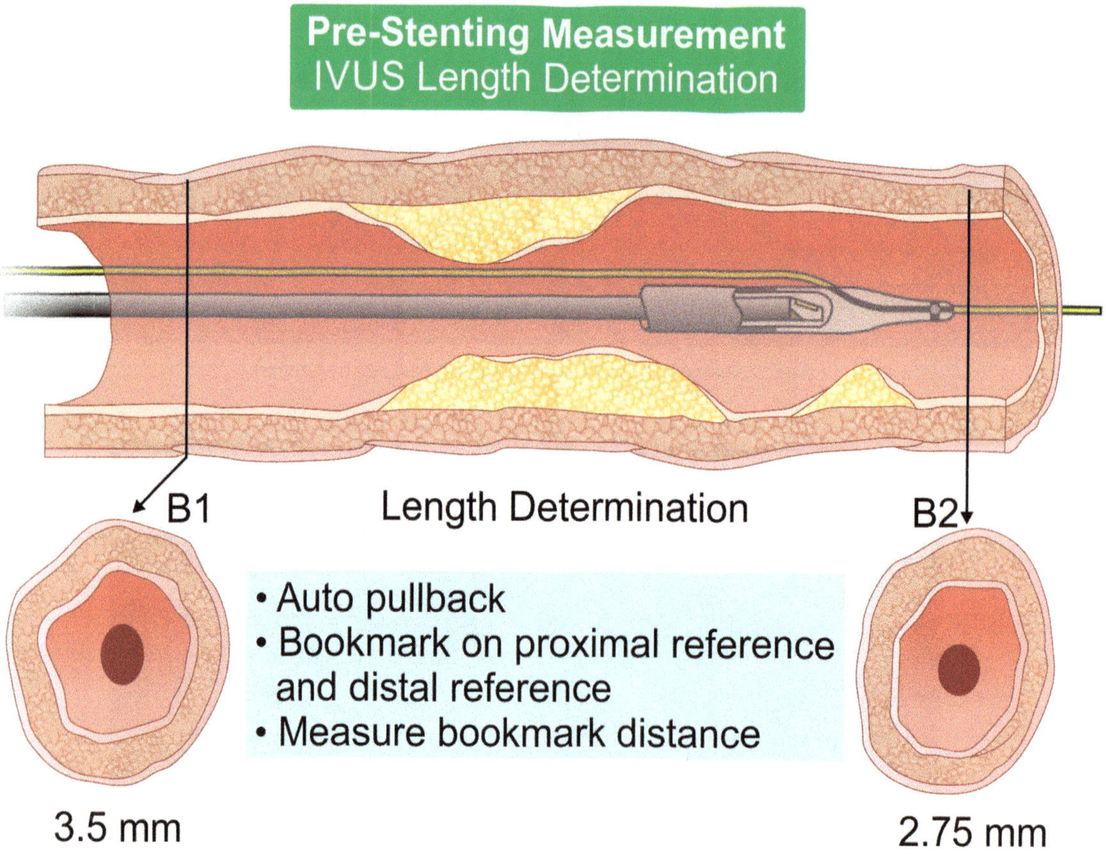

Fig. 5A

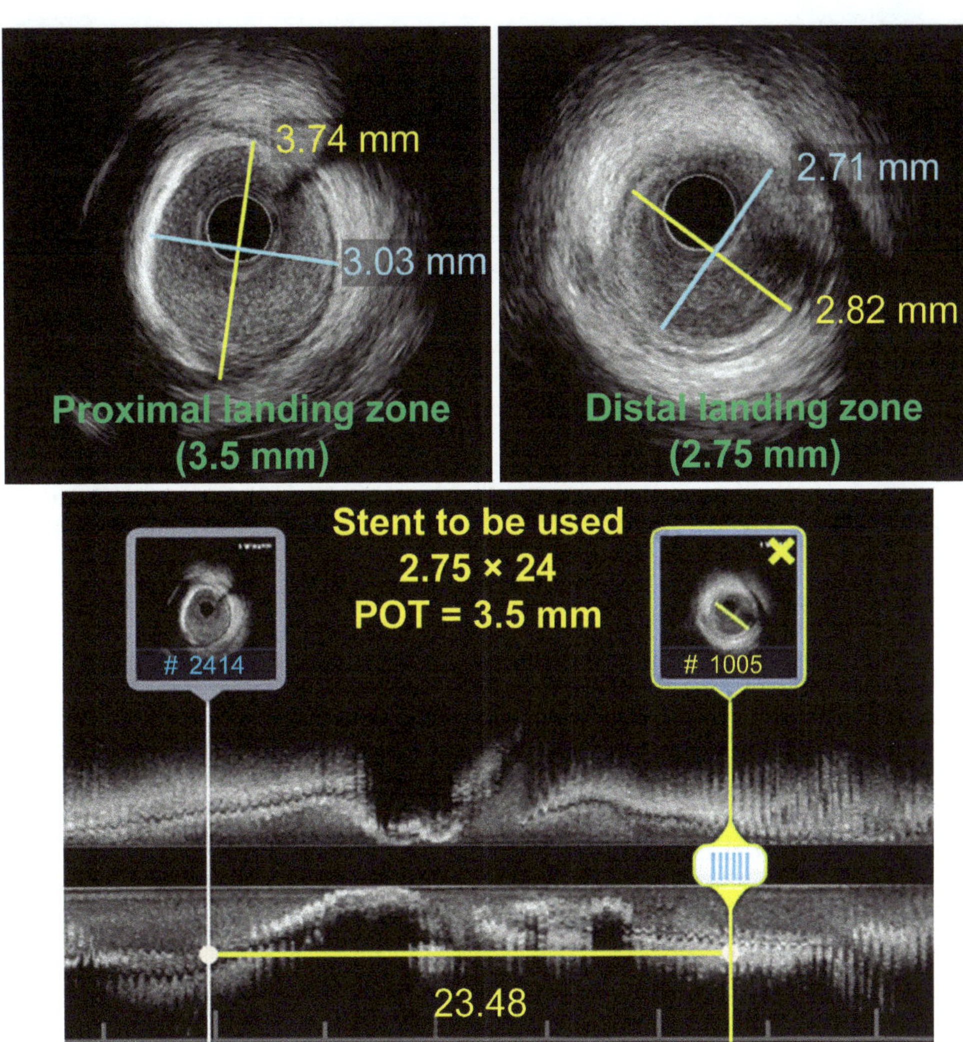

Fig. 5B

Figs. 5A and B: Schematic diagram measuring lesion length on intravascular ultrasound (IVUS).

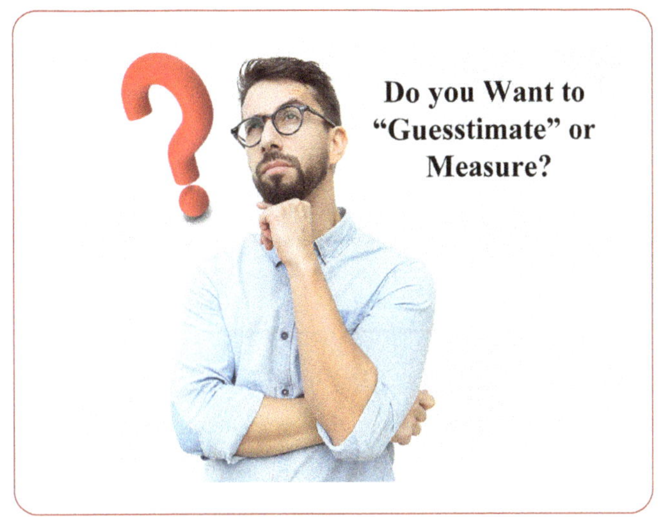

CHAPTER 8

Looking Beyond the Coronaries

For better axial and spatial orientation during intravascular ultrasound (IVUS) imaging, one should identify these perivascular structures such as:

- Pericardium
- Arterial Branches
- Veins

PERICARDIUM

It is usually seen as a bright and relatively thick structure with varying degrees of spoke-like reverberations **(Fig. 1)**.

If the pericardial side is imagined at 12 o'clock, the myocardial side is 6 o'clock, diagonal branches usually at 9 o'clock, a circumflex artery at 7–8 o'clock, and the septal branches at 4–5 o'clock **(Fig. 2)**.

Since the pericardium lies on the anterior surface of the left anterior descending (LAD), diagonals and septals can be easily differentiated from each other.

- The septal branches emerge directly opposite to the pericardium toward the myocardium side, whereas diagonals emerge in the same direction or 90° to the pericardium **(Fig. 3)**.
- Since diagonals are parallel to the LAD, they follow and merge into LAD gradually, while septals, being vertical, disappear quickly after merging with LAD.
- Finally, diagonals are in the same direction as left circumflex (LCX), whereas septals are in the opposite direction **(Fig. 4)**.

Besides pericardium and arterial branches, other structures which are commonly seen are the veins **(Fig. 5)**.

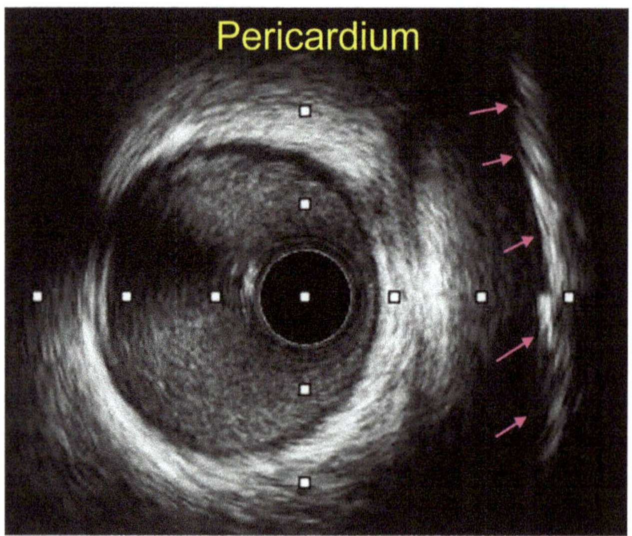

Fig. 1: Pericardium as seen on intravascular ultrasound (IVUS).

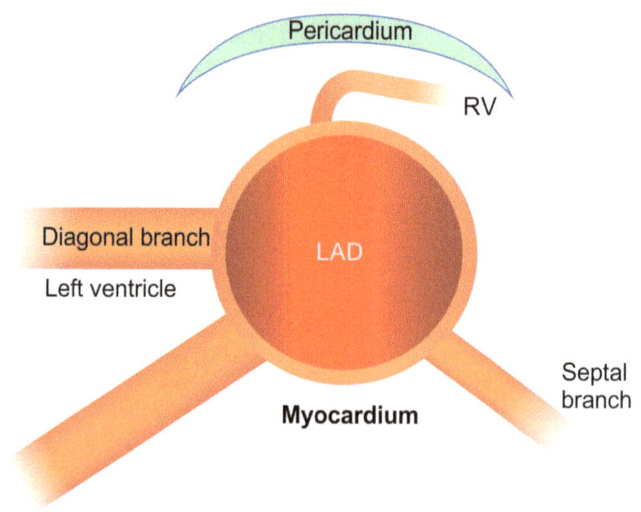

Fig. 2: Orientation of septals and diagonals using pericardium as landmark. (LAD: left anterior descending; RV: right ventricular)

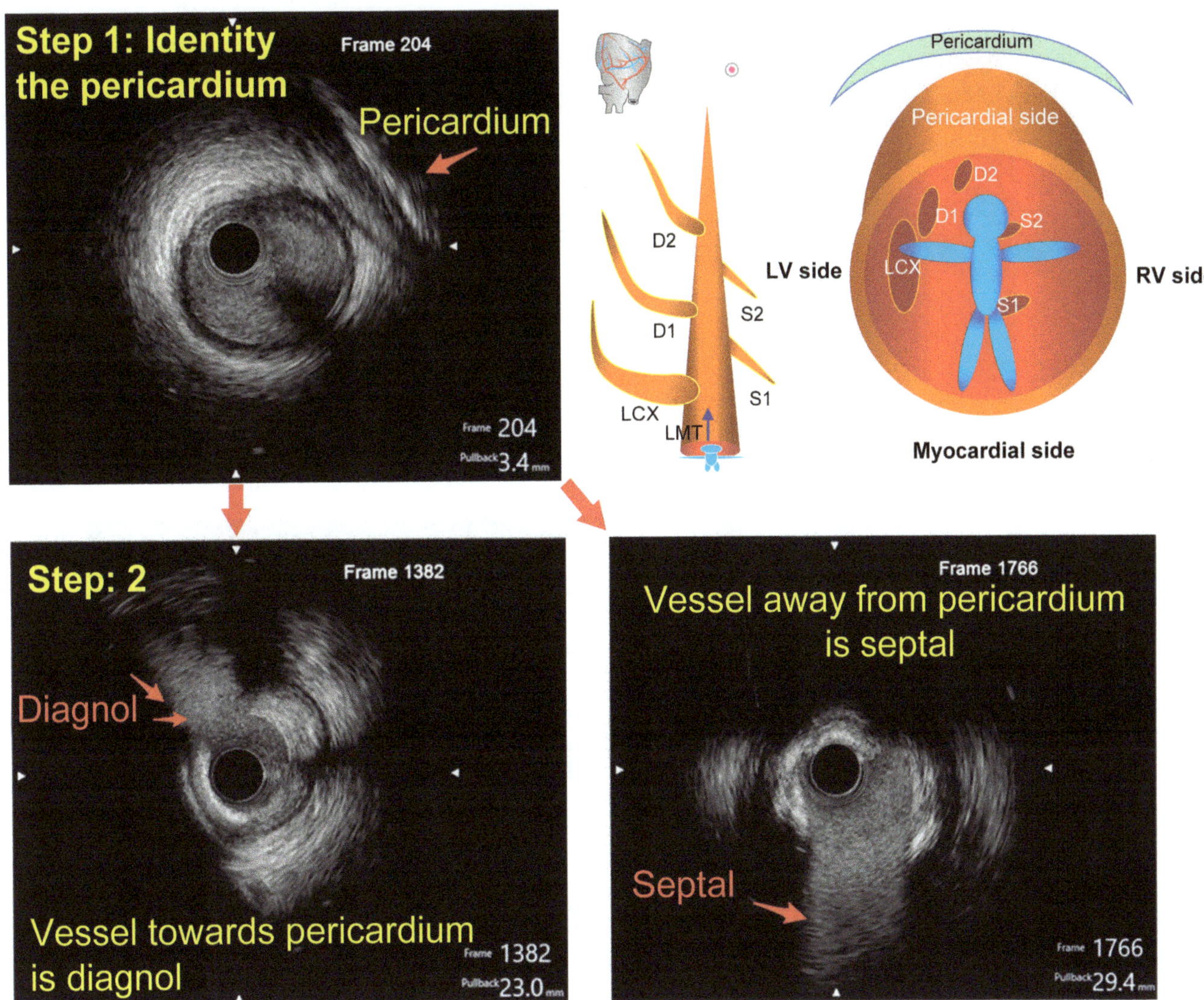

Fig. 3: Differentiating septals from diagonals using pericardium as landmark. (LV: left ventricular; RV: right ventricular)

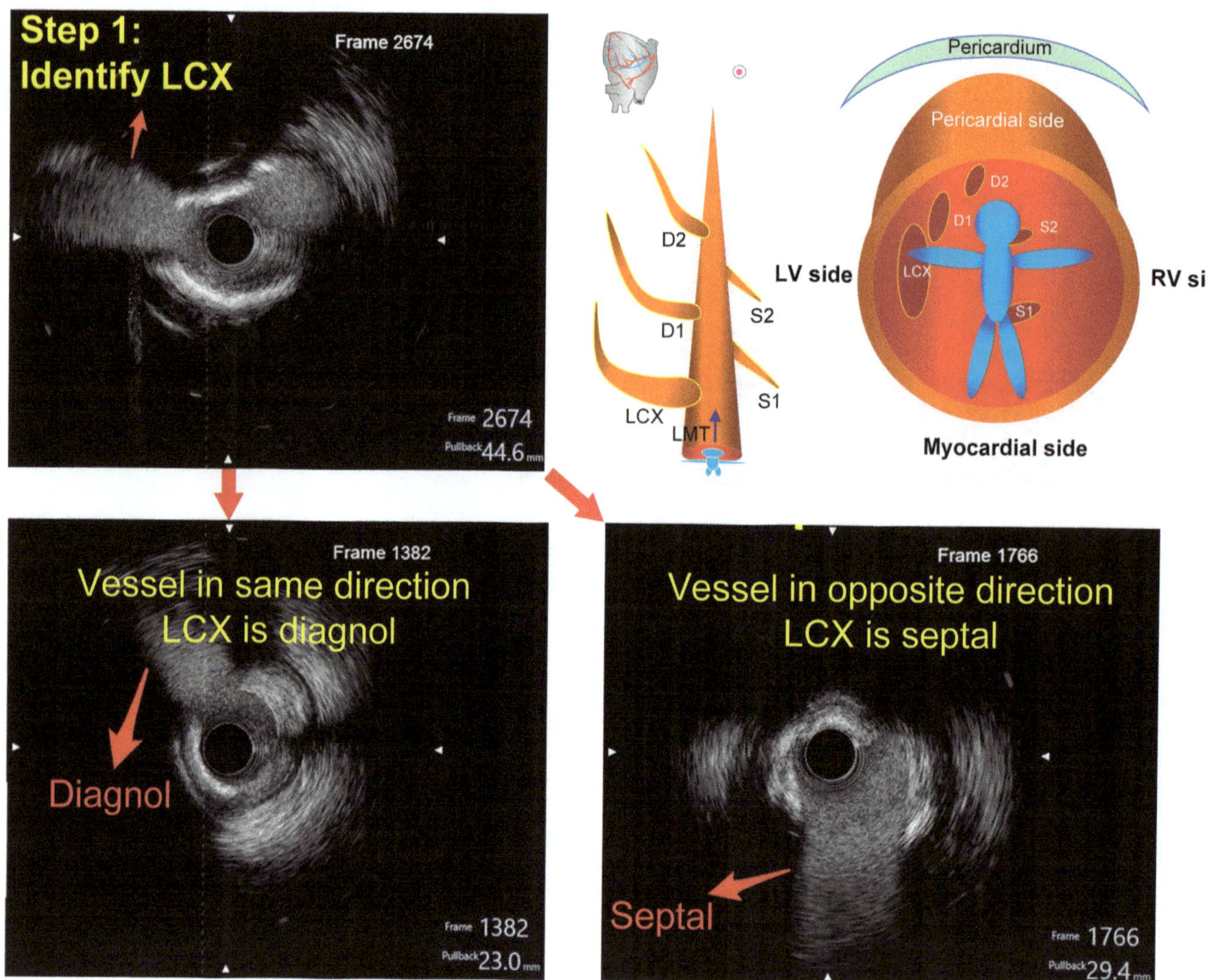

Fig. 4: Differentiating septals from diagonals using LCX as landmark.
(LCX: left circumflex; (LV: left ventricular; RV: right ventricular)

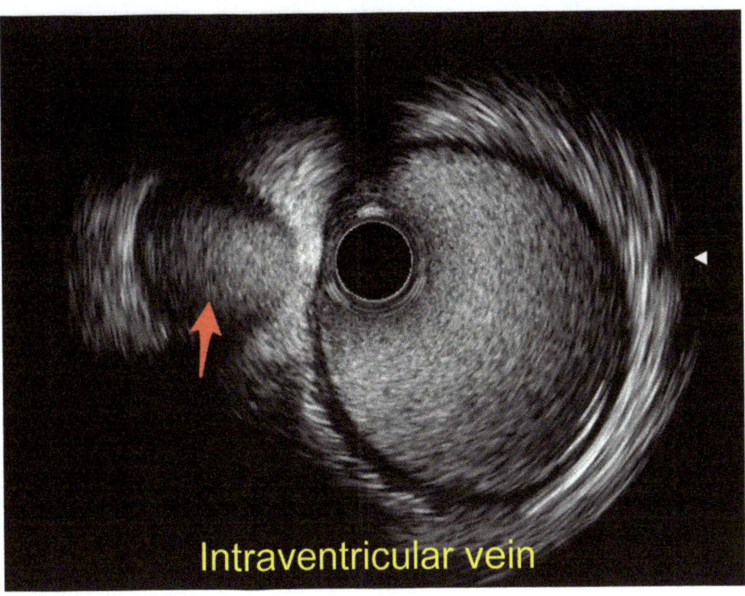

Fig. 5: Intraventricular veins.

POINTS DIFFERENTIATING VEINS FROM ARTERIAL BRANCHES

- Do not merge with the main vessel
- Usually oval in shape except right coronary artery (RCA) where it can be horseshoe shape
- Systolic compression seen
- No media visible
- Different echogenic (since they have low-velocity flow)

The main identifying feature of LCX on IVUS is the presence of a large echolucent structure alongside which is the great cardiac vein (GCV) **(Fig. 6)**.

The main identifying feature of RCA on IVUS is the presence of a large echolucent horseshoe-shaped structure alongside which is the right ventricular vein **(Fig. 7)**.

Note: Usually veins are parallel to coronary arteries, so they are seen as a circular structure. But in RCA, they are perpendicular, so they appear horseshoe-shaped.

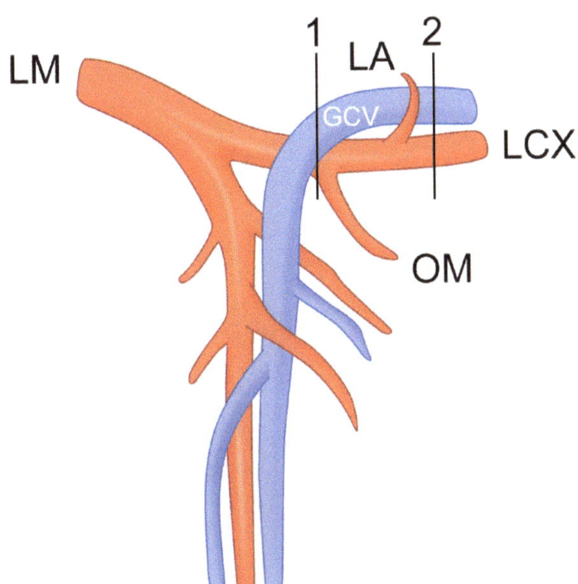

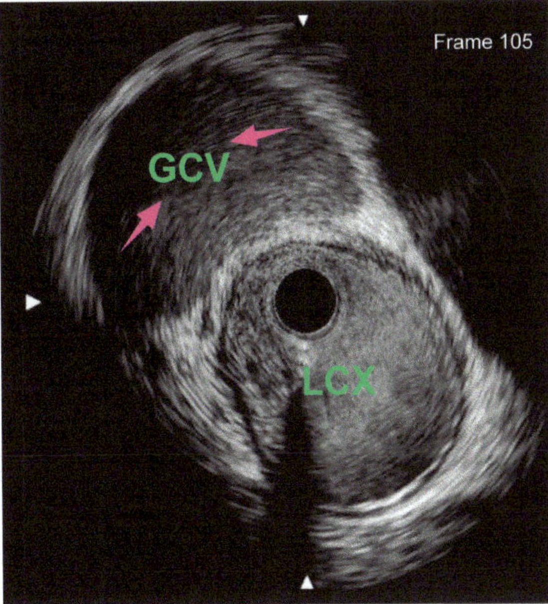

Fig. 6: Left circumflex (LCX) along with great cardiac vein (GCV).

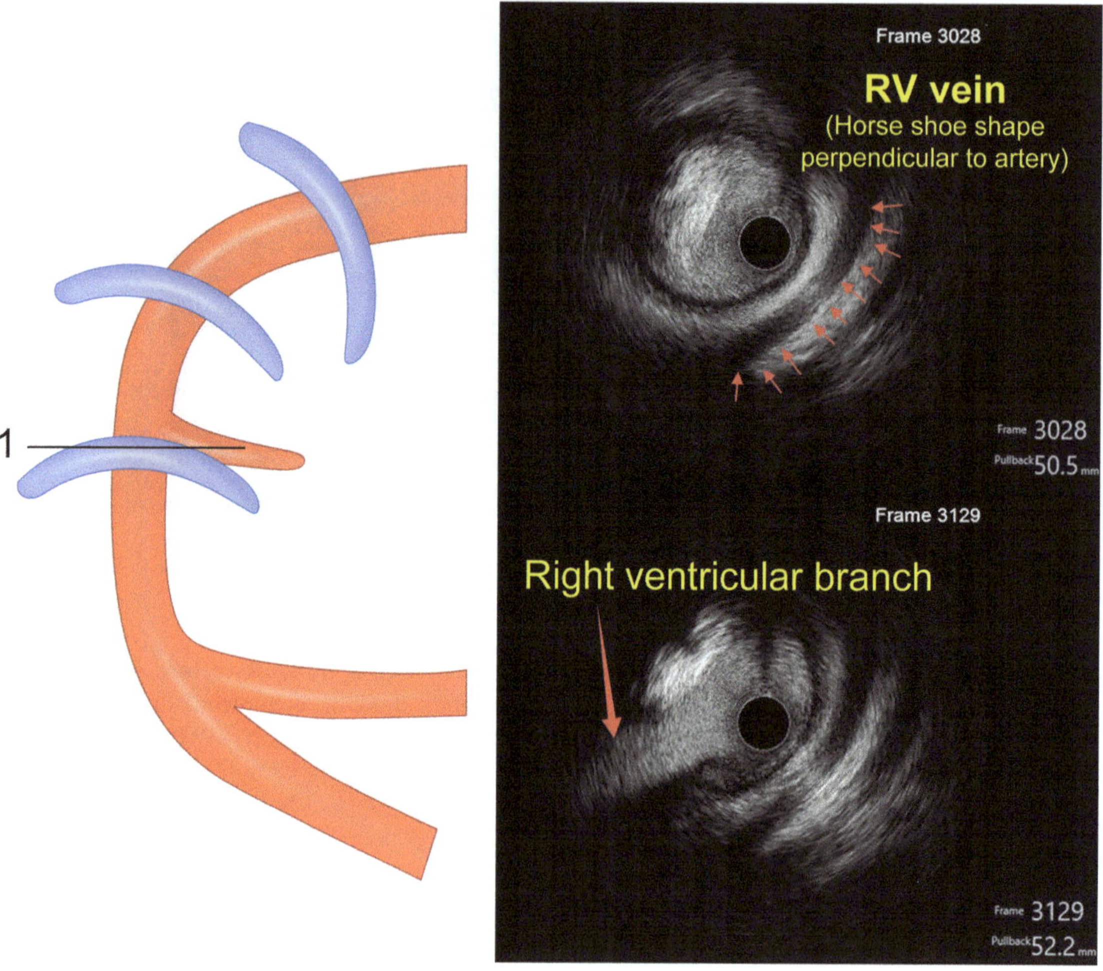

Fig. 7: RCA along with horse shoe shape right ventricular vein. (RCA: right coronary artery; RV: right ventricular)

TRIANGLE OF BROCQ-MOUCHET

It is a triangular anechoic area that may be seen outside the proximal LAD near the confluence of LCX. It is a physiological pericardial effusion surrounded by the LAD, the LCX, and the transition between the anterior interventricular vein and GCV **(Fig. 8)**. The triangle is roofed by pericardium, and its floor is myocardium.

It serves as a distinct landmark during imaging.

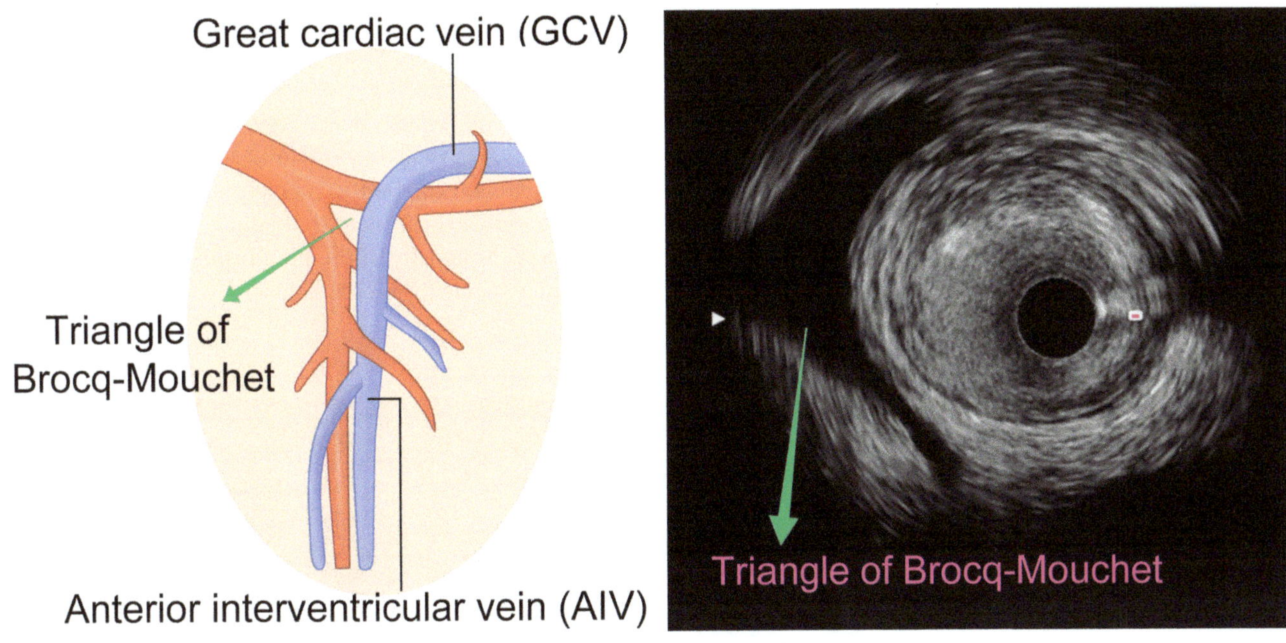

Fig. 8: Triangle of Brocq-Mouchet.

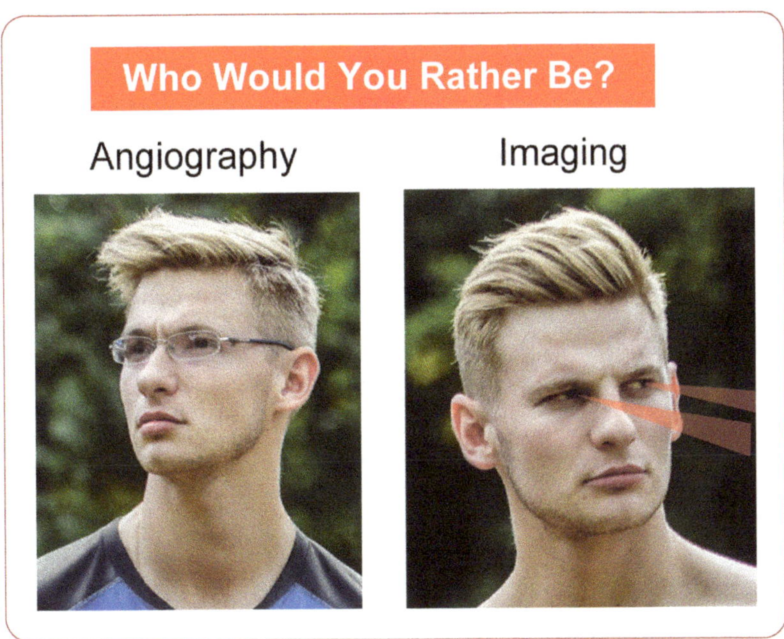

CHAPTER 9

Plaque Morphology on Intravascular Ultrasound

Three types of plaque morphology can be identified on intravascular ultrasound (IVUS) **(Figs. 1A to C)**:

1. Fibrofatty
2. Lipid-rich
3. Calcified

A simple way to identify the morphology of plaque is to just compare the appearance of plaque with the adventitia. If it is less white (echolucent), then it is lipid-rich. If it has the same echodensity, then it is fibrous, and if it is more echodense (white), then it is calcified.

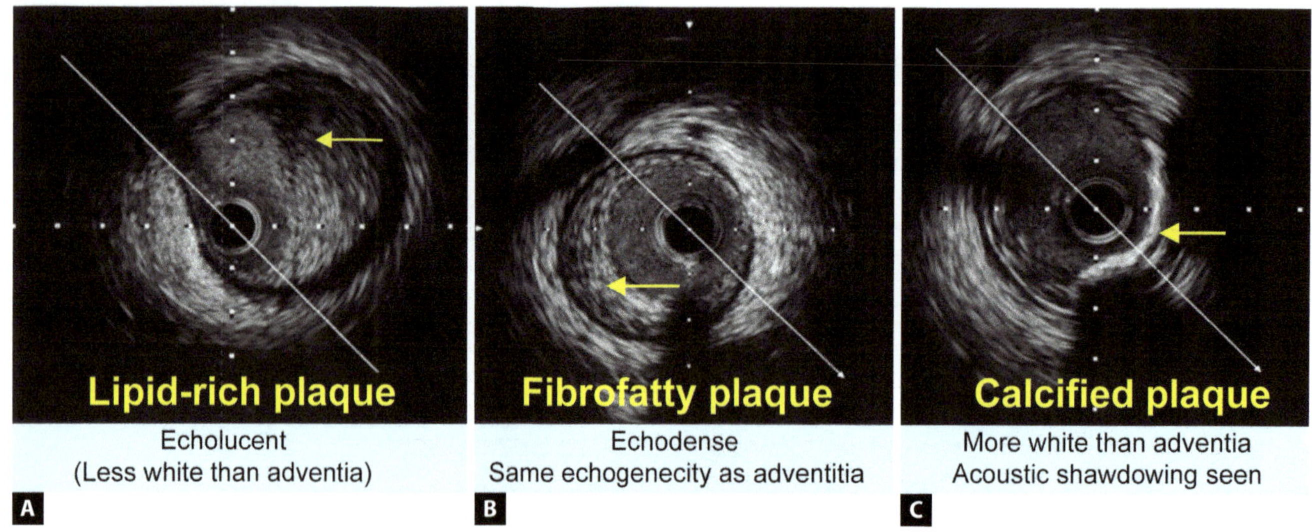

Figs. 1A to C: Different morphology of plaque on high-definition intravascular ultrasound (HD-IVUS).

HOW DOES LIPID LOOK ON INTRAVASCULAR ULTRASOUND?

Lipids do not reflect ultrasound waves, so we get hypoechoic (black image). Also, IVUS does not penetrate lipid, so we do not see the vessel beyond the lipid plaque. This leads to acoustic shadowing or attenuation **(Fig. 2)**.

Importance of identifying lipid-rich plaque:

- Predictor of slow flow during stent implantation or ballooning.
- Predictor of future events (if the stent lands on lipid-rich plaque, it can lead to edge restenosis).
- It is one of the main components of vulnerable plaque.

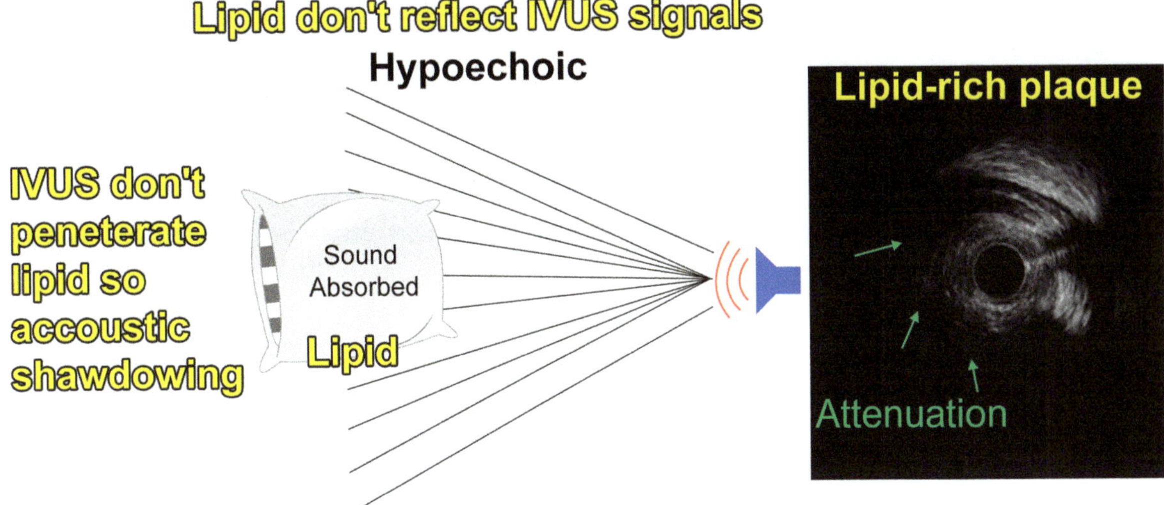

Fig. 2: Lipid-rich plaque on intravascular ultrasound (IVUS).

HOW DOES CALCIUM LOOK ON INTRAVASCULAR ULTRASOUND?

Ultrasound waves reflect calcium strongly, so we get an echodense (bright white image). Also IVUS does not penetrate calcium, so we get acoustic shadowing (do not see anything beyond) **(Fig. 3)**.

Acoustic shadowing will be seen in both calcium and lipidic plaque, but calcium will appear bright whereas lipid will appear as dark image on IVUS.

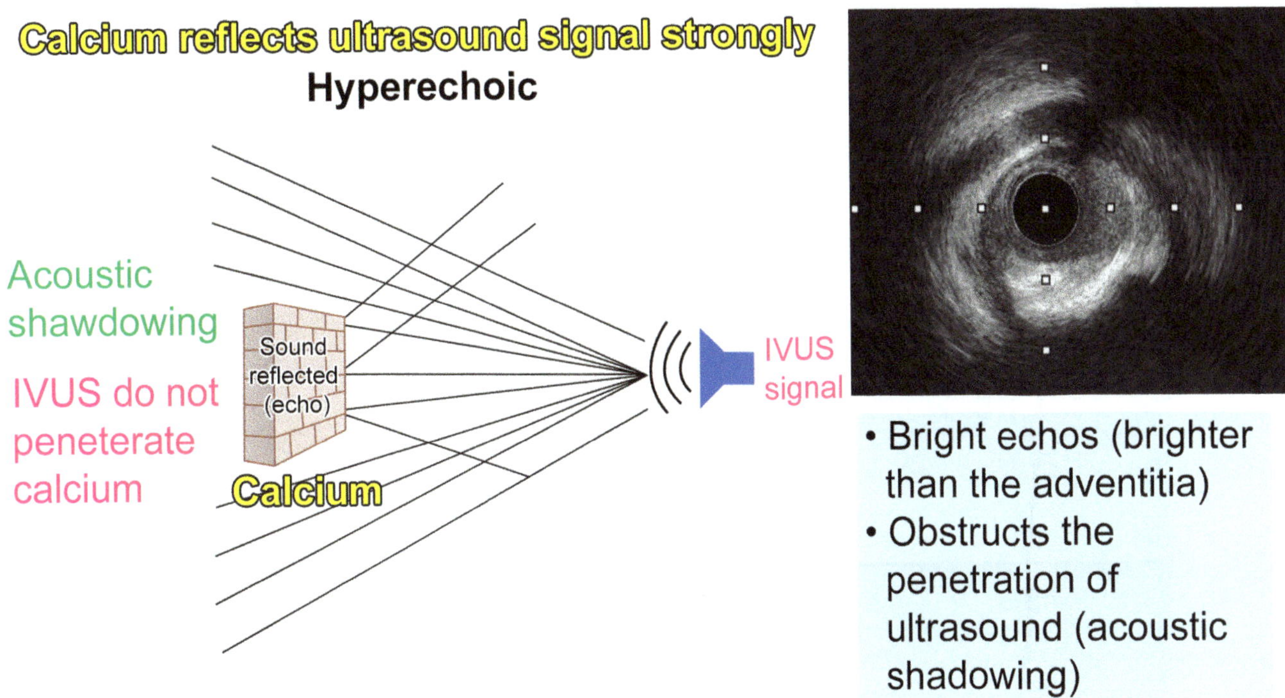

Fig. 3: Calcium on intravascular ultrasound (IVUS).

CHAPTER 10

Image Artifacts

Like any imaging techniques, intravascular ultrasound (IVUS) images can sometimes have artifacts that may affect the quality of images and interpretation of results. Some common artifacts are discussed here.

AIR ARTIFACTS

Air bubbles produce a variety of image artifacts ranging from blurred images, concentric ring, reverberations to complete loss of image. Infact air bubble is the most common cause of weak image by IVUS **(Fig. 1)**.

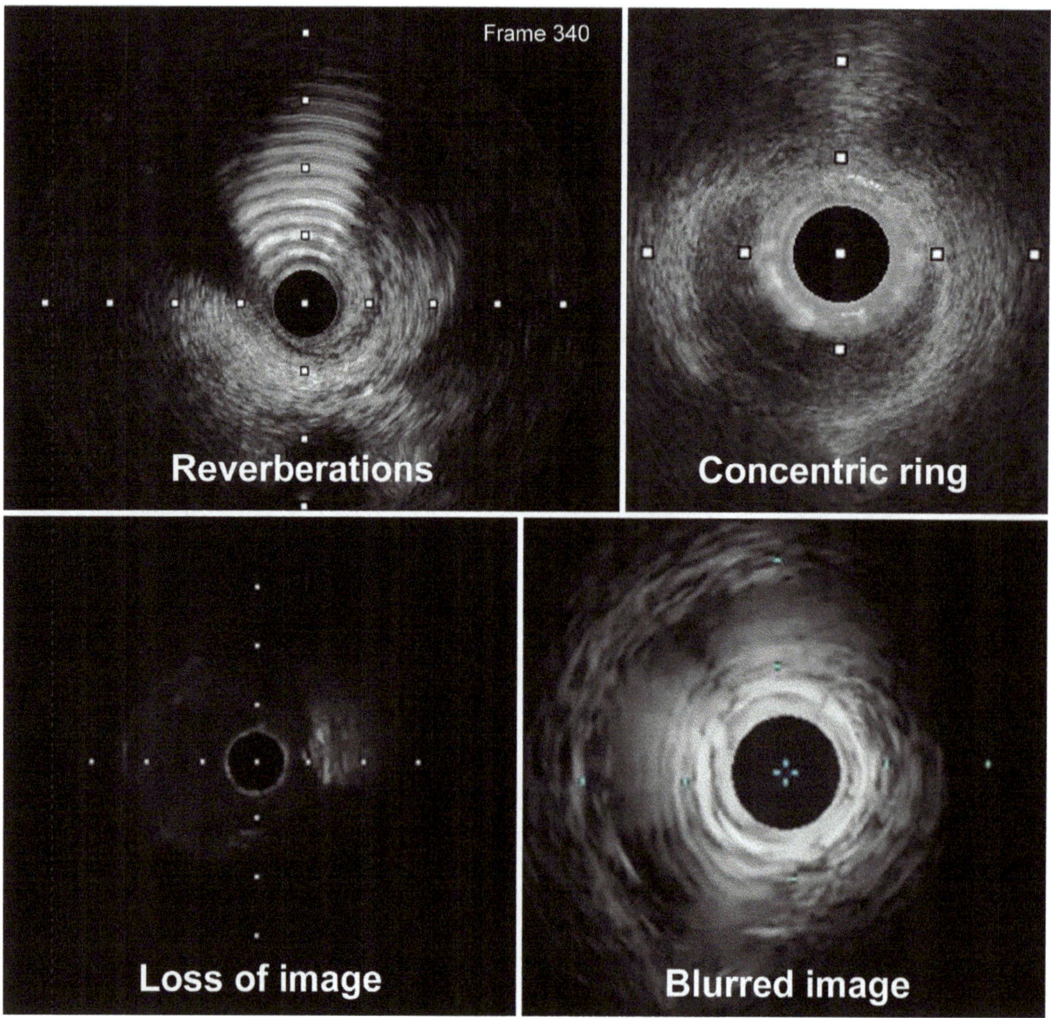

Fig. 1: Various types of air bubble artifacts.

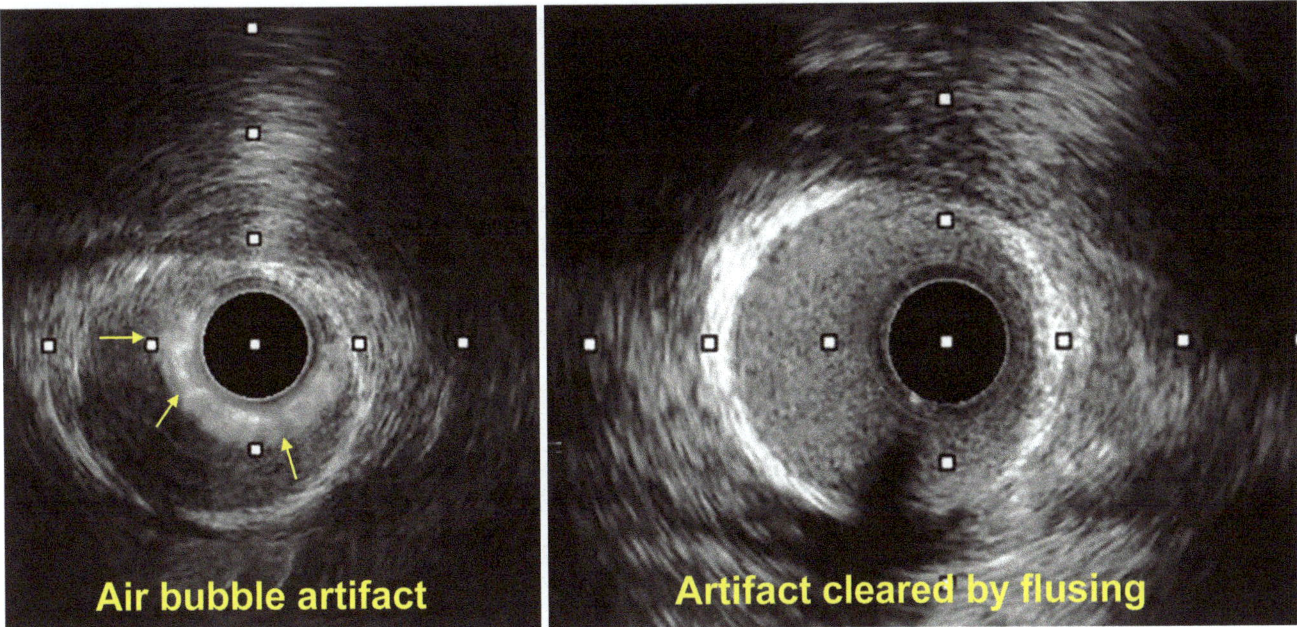

Fig. 2: Flushing clear air bubble artifacts.

The main reason for these is air trapping in the sheath of IVUS catheter, which can be easily rectified by flushing of the IVUS catheter **(Fig. 2)**.

GUIDEWIRE ARTIFACTS

The guidewire, a strong echo-reflective object, creates a narrow angle acoustic shadow, impacting lumen and vessel observation **(Fig. 3)**. It is often visible with short monorail catheters, as the guidewire is outside the transducer. It is crucial to differentiate the guidewire artifact from a stent strut, as both are metallic reflectors. At times, guidewire artifacts can obscure a significant portion of the image.

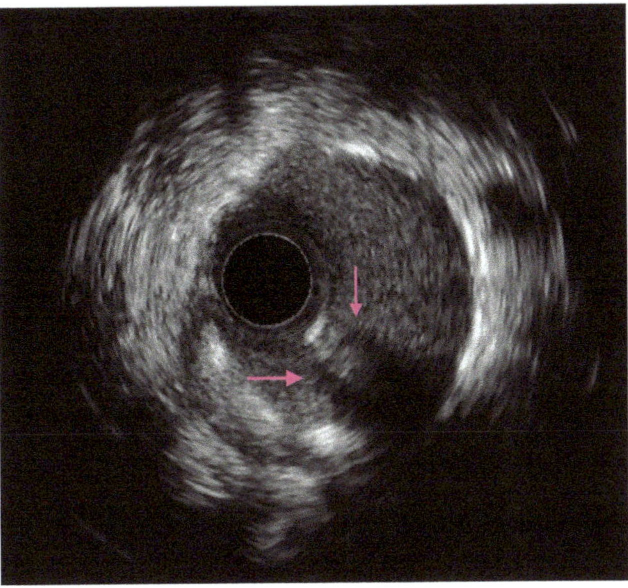

Fig. 3: Guidewire artifact.

NONUNIFORM ROTATIONAL DISTORTION

For optimal imaging, there must be a constant rotational velocity of the mechanical transducer. Nonuniform rotational distortion (NURD) is the consequence of asymmetric friction (or drag) along any part of the drive-shaft mechanism, causing the transducer to lag during one part of its rotation and whip through the other part of its 360° course, resulting in circumferential distortion of the image, which sometimes makes image interpretation difficult **(Fig. 4)**. It is unique to mechanical catheter systems and not seen with solid state systems.

Causes:

- Tightening of hemostatic valve
- Tortuous course of arteries
- Kinking of imaging catheter

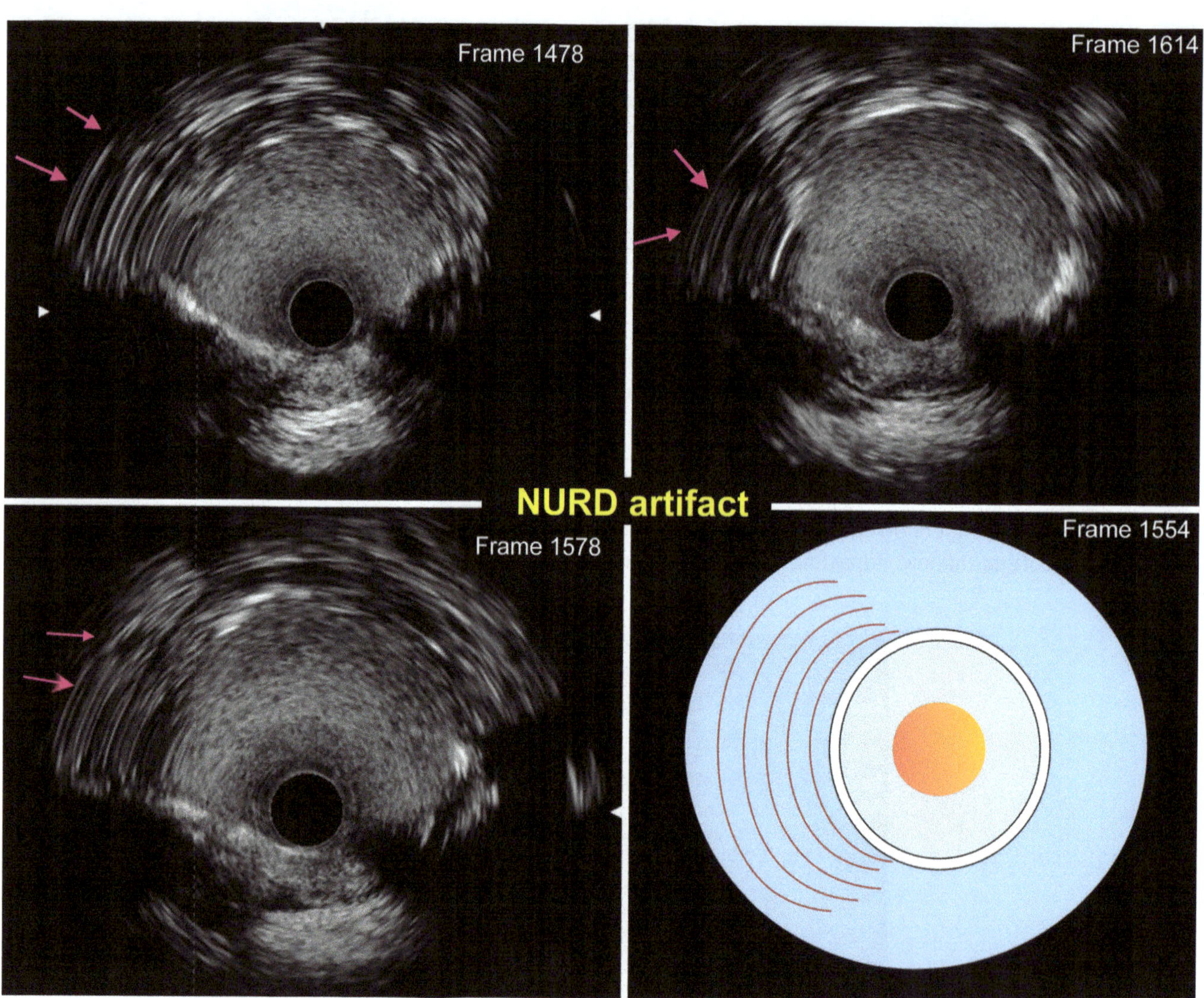

Fig. 4: Nonuniform rotational distortion (NURD).

REVERBERATION

These are repeated reflections or false echoes of the same structure. Reverberations are false, repetitive echoes of the same structure that give the impression of second, third, etc., interfaces at fixed-multiple distances from the transducer **(Fig. 5)**.

Causes:

- Calcium (especially after rotablation)
- Metal (stent)
- Plastic (guidelines/transducer)
- Guidewire

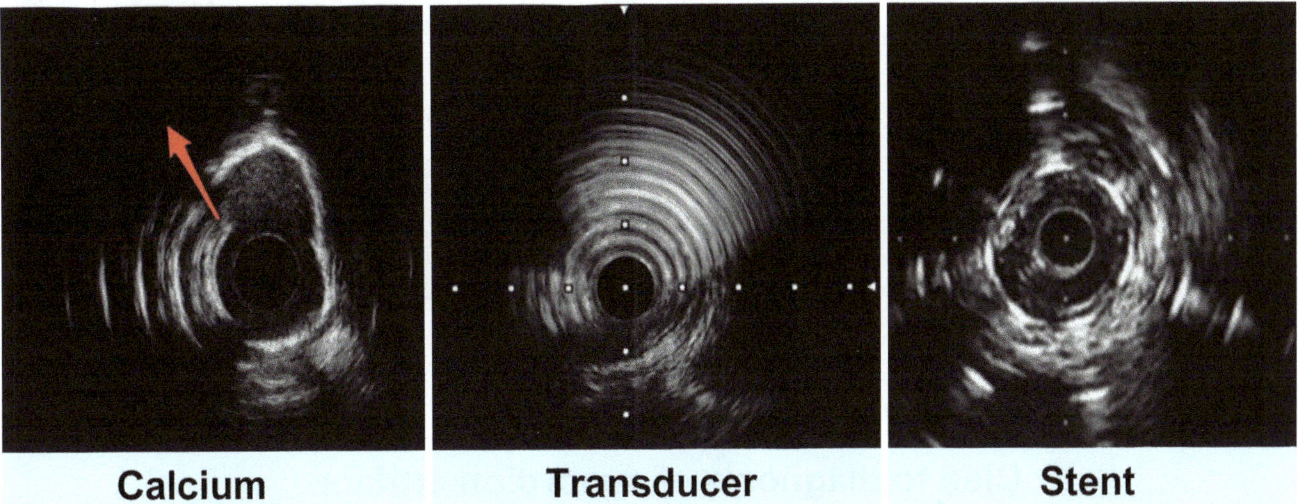

Fig. 5: Different causes of reverberation.

STENT GHOST

Stent ghosts are reflections from the stent metal on the opposite side of the true structure **(Fig. 6)**. It makes it difficult to distinguish from the true stent or malapposition. Just scrolling the IVUS films forward and backward will help in differentiating the true stent from the stent ghost.

Ghost artifacts can be decreased by reducing the overall gain.

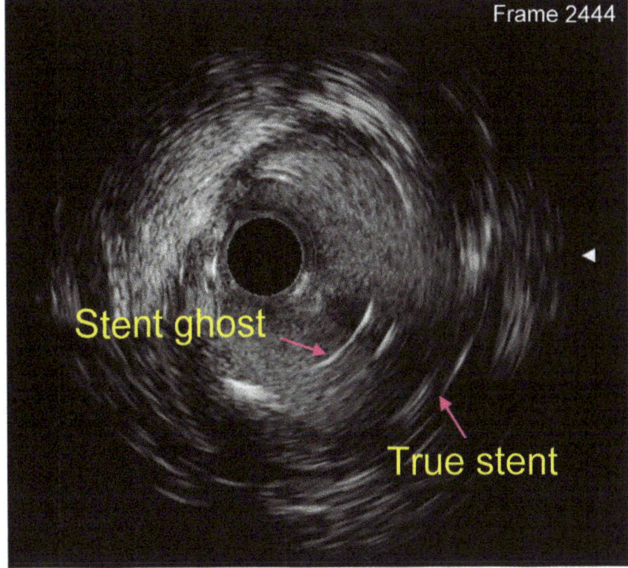

Fig. 6: Stent ghost.

DYE/SALINE ARTIFACTS

Super echolucent structure which appears suddenly and disappears after flushing in most cases due to contrast or saline that has dribbled out during pullback **(Fig. 7)**.

ACCORDION/WRINKLING ARTIFACT

It is the appearance of a pseudo lesion due to straightening of tortuous arteries by a guidewire **(Fig. 8)**. It can be mistaken for a lipid-rich plaque, or intramural hematoma (IMH), or a dissection.

Clues to a diagnosis of accordion **(Fig. 9)** are:

- Circumferential blackout
- Abrupt change from adjacent site
- Double layer of vessel wall
- Media in the middle of vessel wall

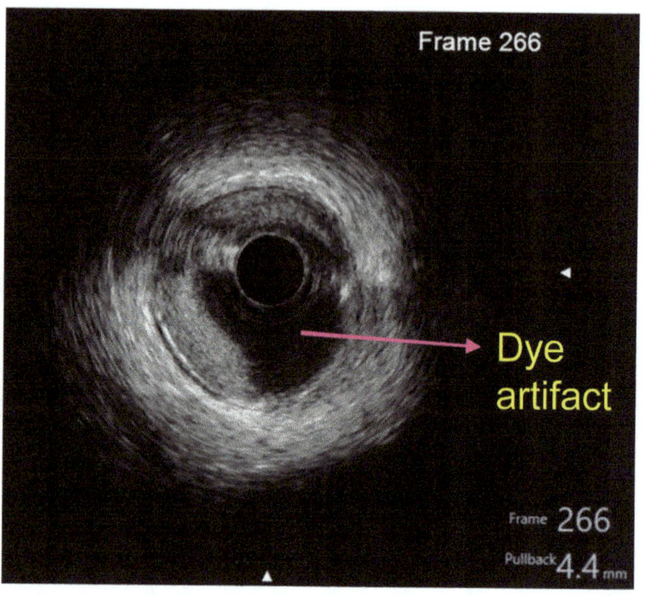

Fig. 7: Dye artifact.

Clue to diagnosis of accordion artifact

- Sudden change from adjacent area
- Outside BLACKOUT
- Double layer of vessel wall
- Media in the middle of vessel wall

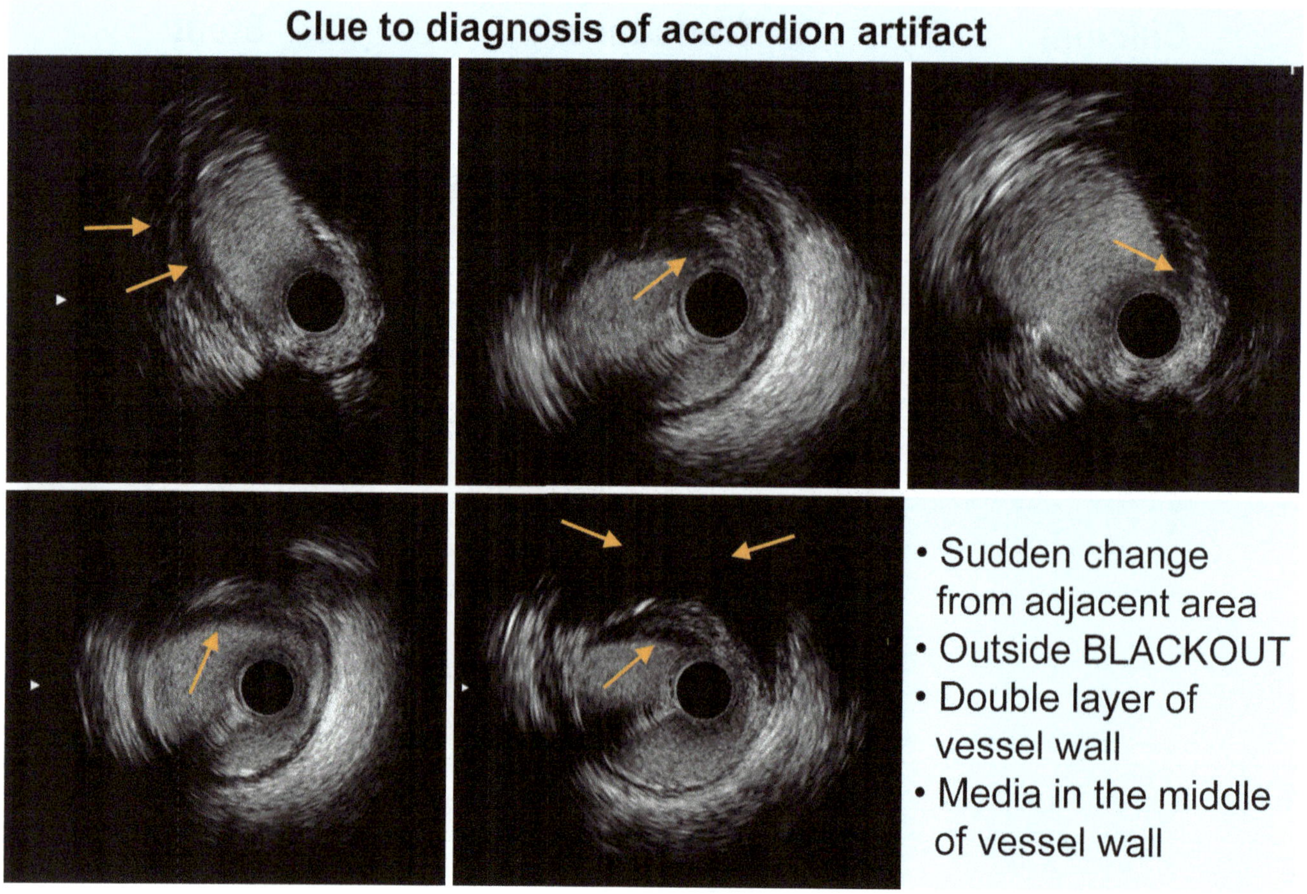

Fig. 8: Accordion artifacts.

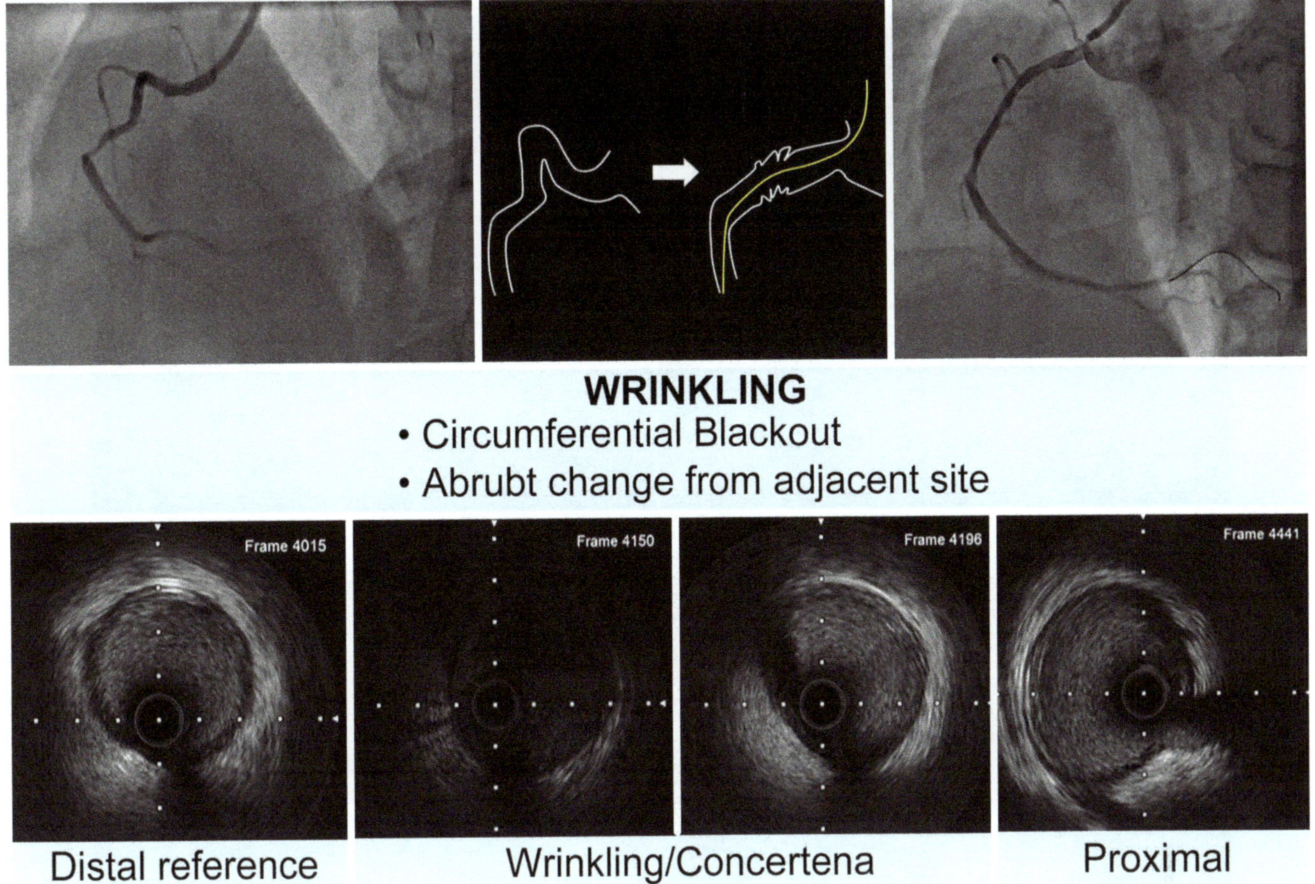

Fig. 9: Clues to a diagnosis of accordion artifacts.

SPASM

If the vessel diameter at the segment appears smaller than the distal reference segment, then the vessel could be in spasm.

During spasm, the smooth muscle cells contract, which leads to thickening of the media, which is an indicator of spasm **(Fig. 10)**. The spasm can be cleared by giving intracoronary nitroglycerin (NTG) **(Fig. 11)**.

"Good image interpretation can only be done by recognizing image artifacts"

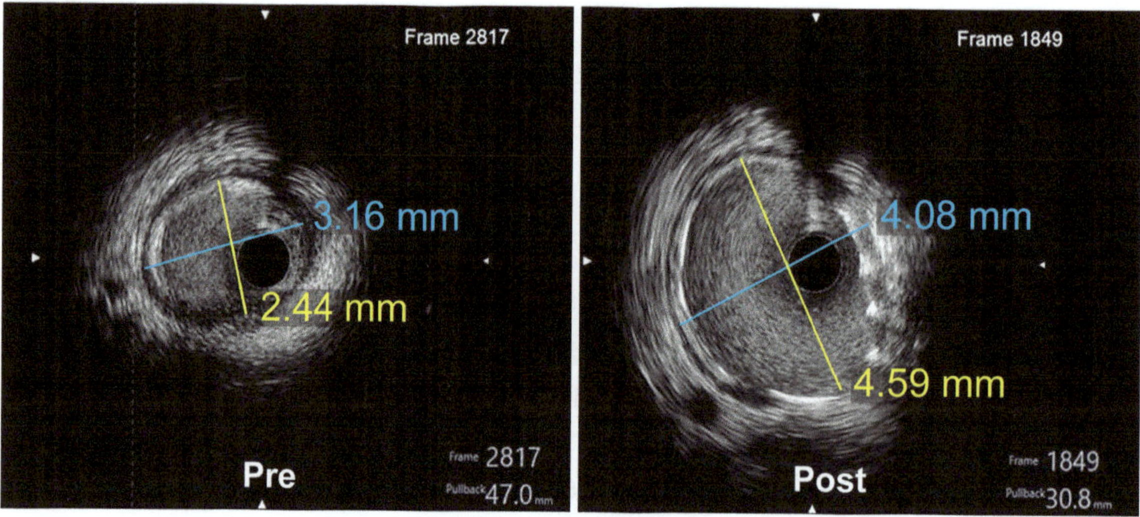

Fig. 10: Left main coronary artery (LMCA) spasm.

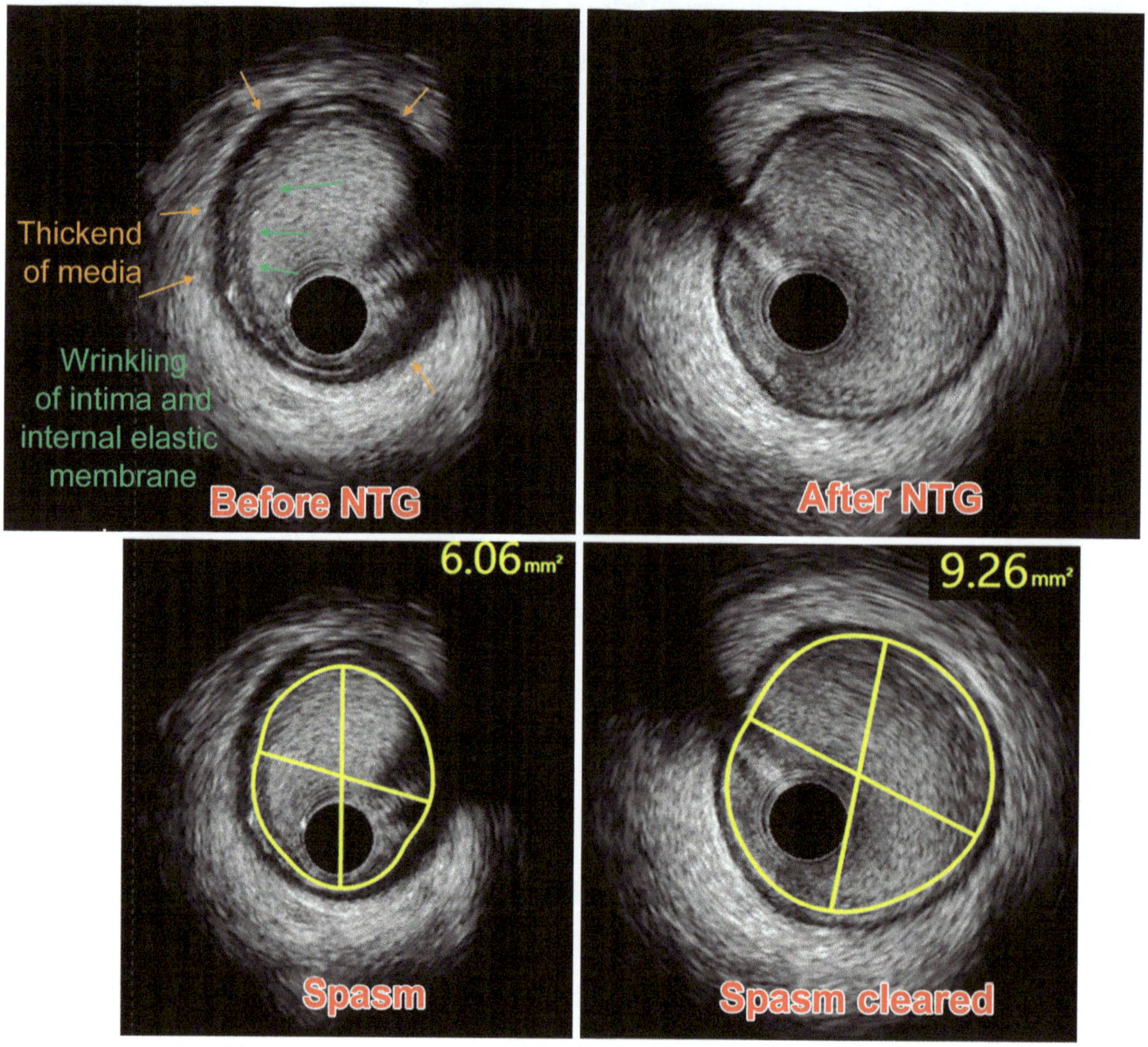

Fig. 11: Spasm seen which got relieved with intracoronary. (NTG: nitroglycerin)

GUIDING CATHETER ARTIFACT

The material of the guiding catheter, such as calcium and metal, is highly echogenic. Deep insertion of the guiding catheter may cause a concentric, high-echo intensity structure at the ostium, and sometimes reverberations. This can result in inadequate observation of the lumen area and possibly missing stenosis or injury at the entrance. It can also be mistaken for circumferential calcium at the aorta-ostial junction **(Fig. 12)**.

To correct it, unhook the catheter and do the imaging again.

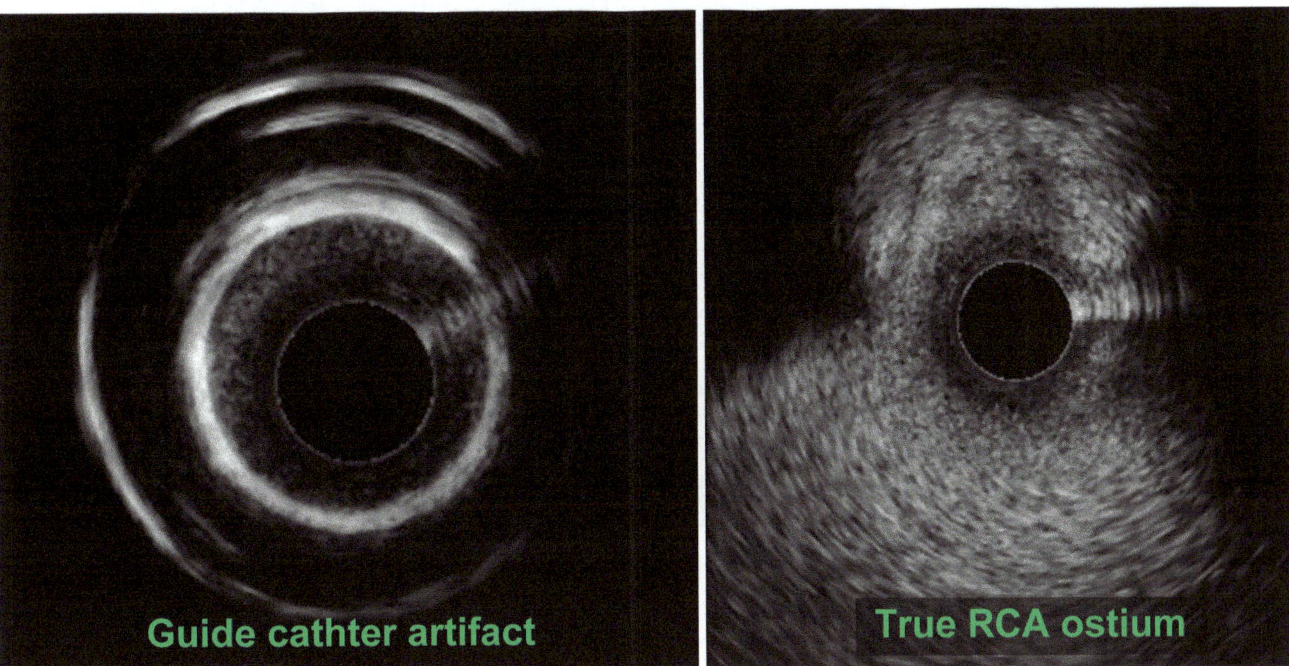

Fig. 12: Guiding catheter artifact seen on the left image. Unhooking the catheter revealed the true RCA ostium (right image).

"If there is a discrepancy between angio and IVUS, make sure that it is not an artifact"

SAWTOOTH ARTIFACT

This artifact is caused by excessive swinging of the transducer during the pullback period. This results in a "sawtooth" appearance on the longitudinal reconstructed image (L mode) **(Fig. 13)**. It commonly occurs in tortuous vessels, rapid beating hearts, and fast-moving coronary arteries, e.g., right coronary artery (RCA).

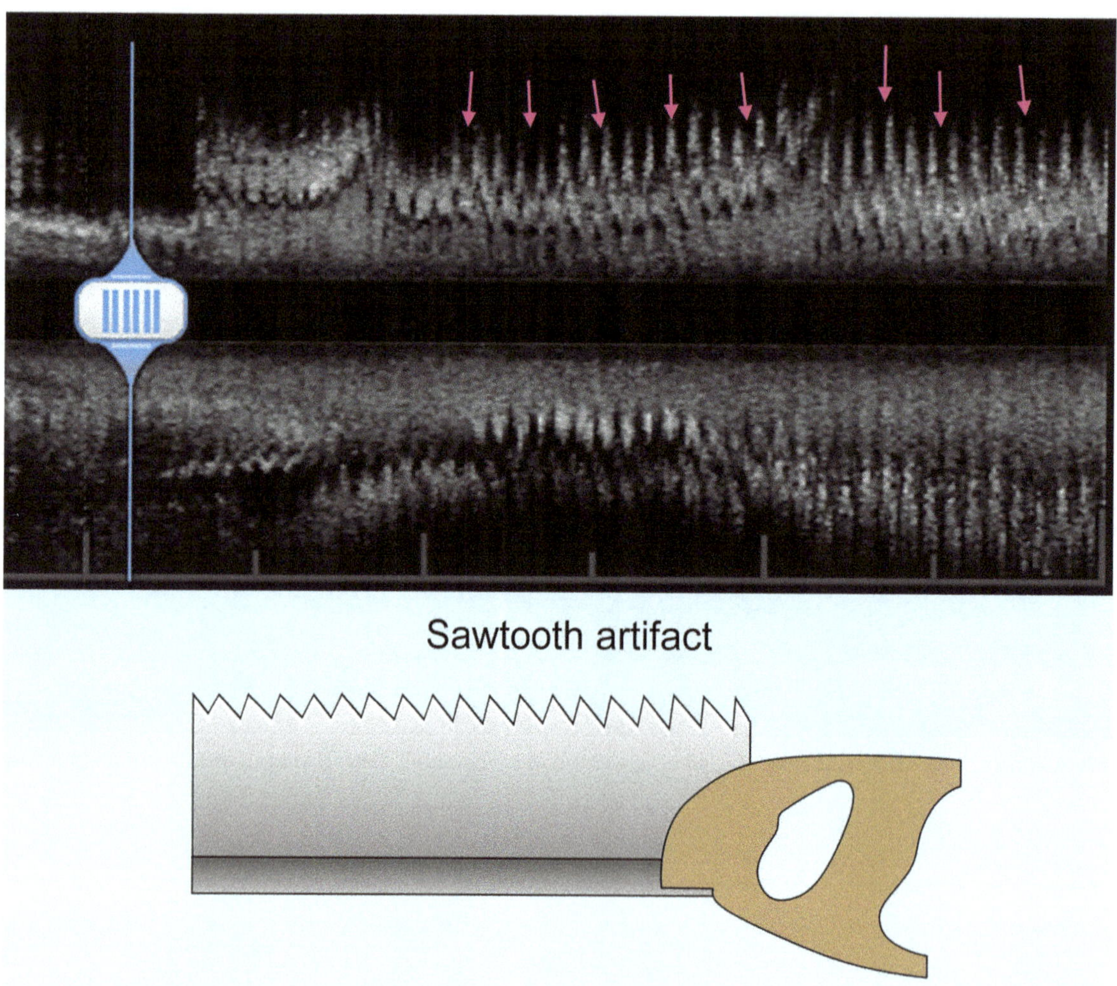

Fig. 13: Sawtooth artifact as seen on reconstructed image on L mode due to a rapid swinging right coronary artery (RCA).

"Know what to expect, know what is not real"

FAR FIELD ELECTRICAL INTERFERENCE ARTIFACT

Intravascular ultrasound is sensitive to ambient radiofrequency noise or ultrasound signal, causing alternating spokes or random white dots in the image **(Fig. 14)**. This is known as far field electrical interference artifact. There are various ambient sources of energy that can cause this, such as an activated Doppler flow wire in the same artery or performing a transthoracic echocardiography (TTE) or a transesophageal echocardiography (TEE). These factors can lead to interference and affect the quality of the IVUS image. If the source of the noise can be identified, it can be avoided by switching off or moving the devices.

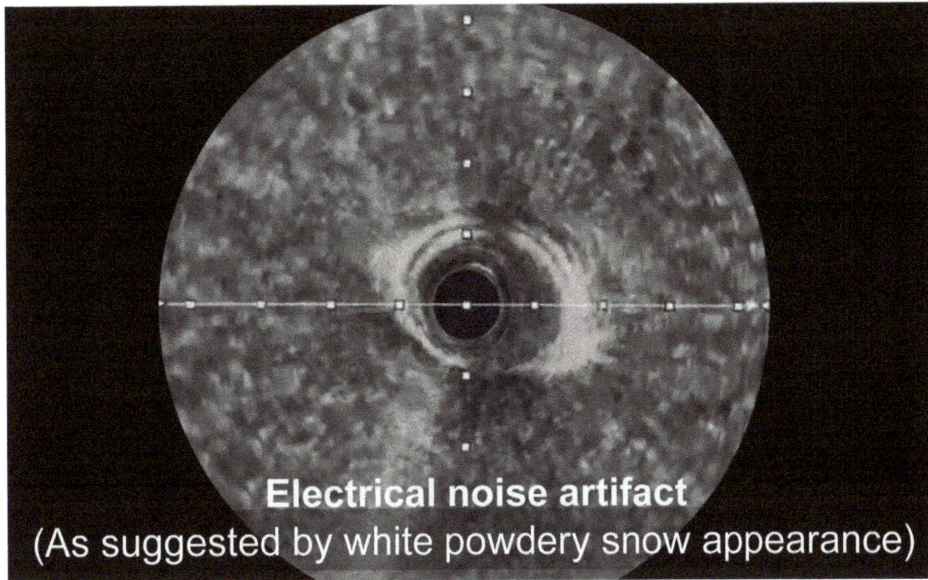

Fig. 14: Far field electrical interference artifact.

PSEUDOHYPERTROPHY OF THE MEDIA

This medial hypertrophy is an artifact caused by signal attenuation of the ultrasound waves as it passes through the hyperechoic plaque **(Fig. 15)**. In reality, the media becomes thinner with increasing atherosclerosis. One more clue of a false or exaggerated medial thickness is that the media appears to be thicker under a thicker plaque layer than under a thinner plaque layer.

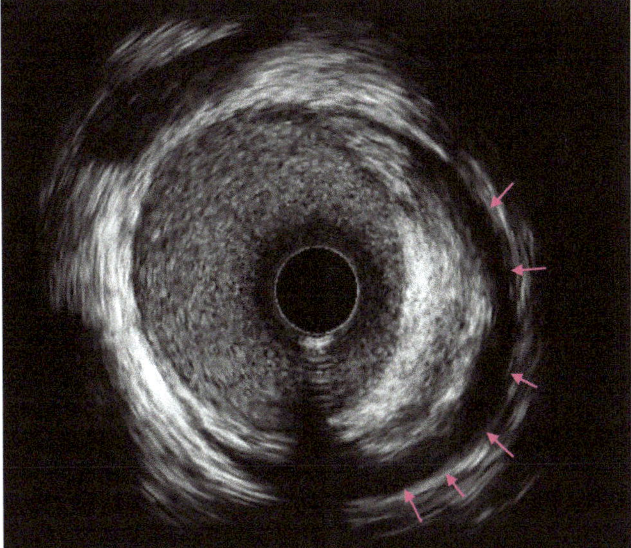

Fig. 15: Media appears hypertrophic here. This medial thickness is an artifact caused by signal attenuation of the ultrasound waves as it passes through the hyperechoic plaque.

CHAPTER 11

Vessel Remodeling

Vessel remodeling refers to the change in the vessel area [external elastic membrane (EEM)-EEM] that occurs during the development of atherosclerosis **(Fig. 1)**.

Lumen reduction may not occur until the plaque occupies >40% of the total vessel area (vessel expansion = positive remodeling).

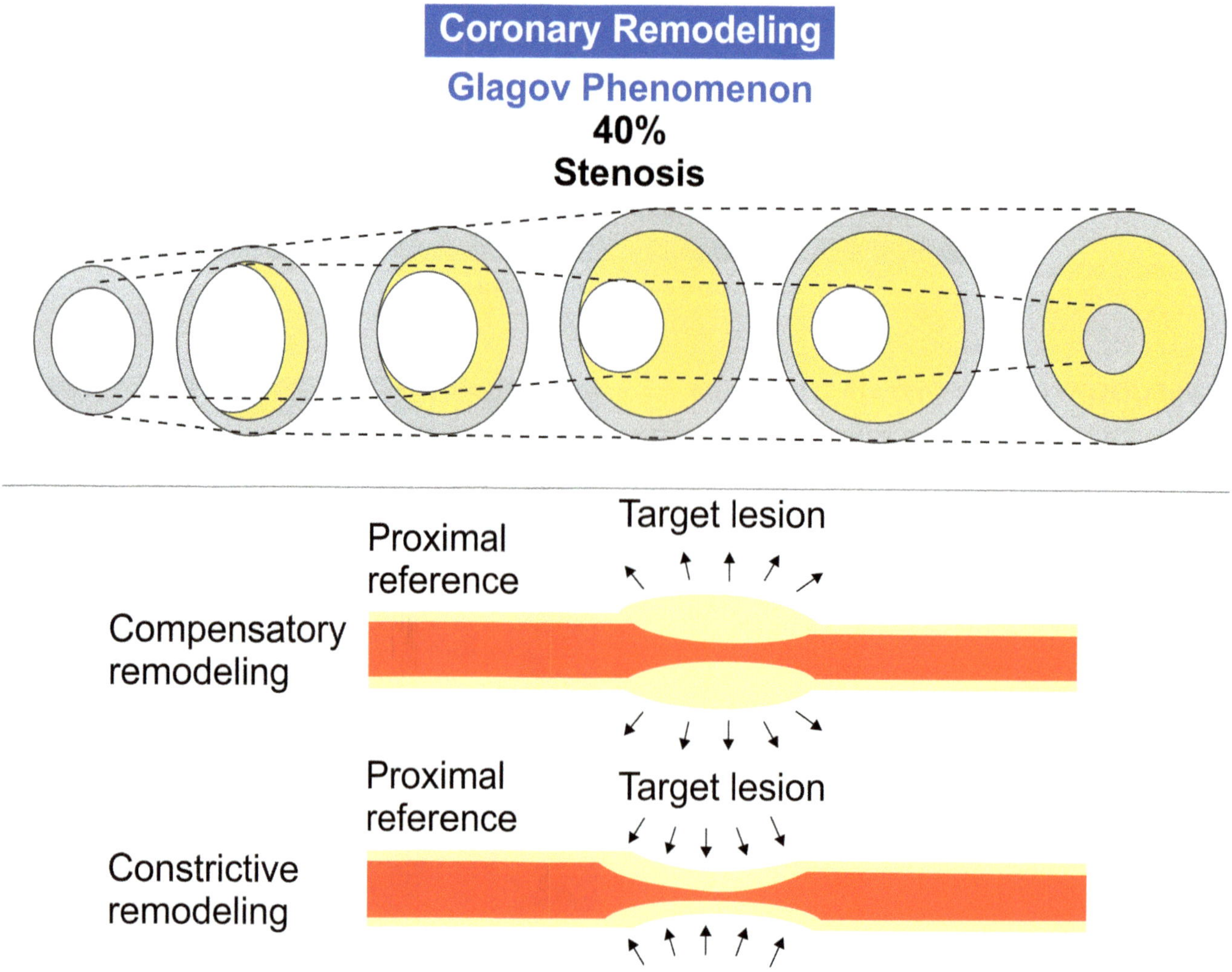

Coronary Remodeling
Glagov Phenomenon
40%
Stenosis

Proximal reference
Target lesion
Compensatory remodeling

Proximal reference
Target lesion
Constrictive remodeling

Fig. 1: Vessel remodeling concept.

In other words, if the vessel diameter at the lesion site is more than the proximal reference vessel diameter, it is called positive remodeling **(Fig. 2)**.

We may also have negative remodeling, which means the vessel constricts in response to plaque development.

In other words, if the vessel diameter at the lesion site is less than the distal reference vessel diameter, it is called negative remodeling **(Fig. 2)**.

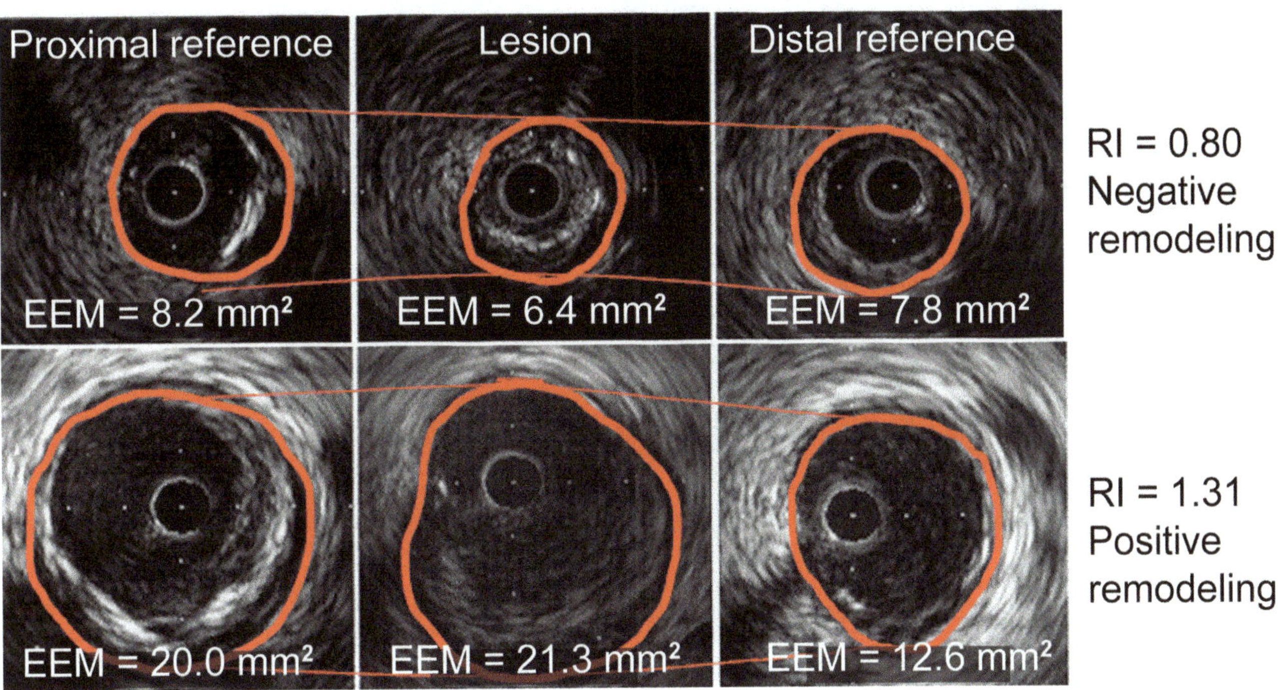

Fig. 2: Positive and negative remodeling. (EEM: external elastic membrane; RI: remodeling index)

The magnitude of remodeling can be expressed by the remodeling index (RI).

Remodeling index = EEM at lesion/EEM at reference vessel **(Fig. 3)**

If RI is > 1.1 = +ve remodeling

If RI is < 0.95 = –ve remodeling

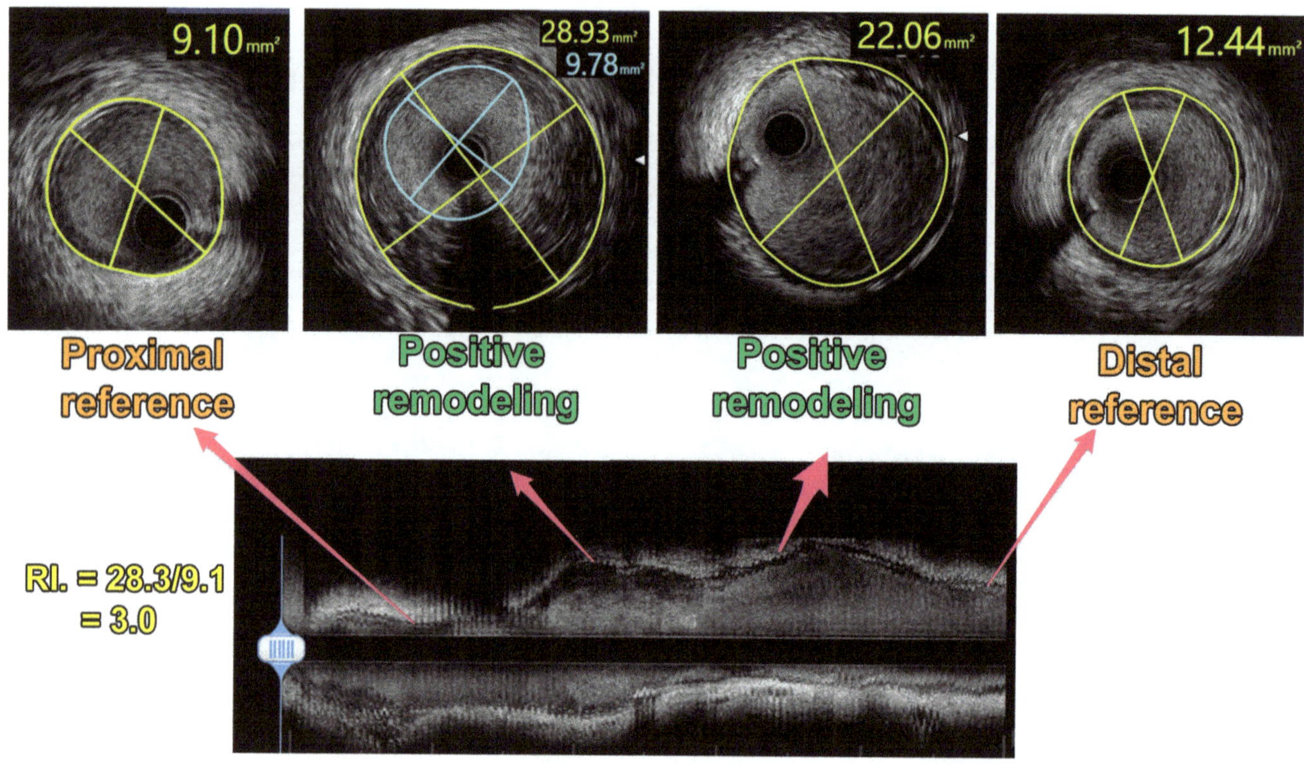

Fig. 3: Remodeling index (RI) calculation.

Clinical implications of remodeling: Positively remodeled vessels are more biologically active than negatively or intermediately remodeled vessels. Positive remodeling has been shown to be a predictor of no flow during interventions, recurrent MACE, TLR, neointimal hyperplasia, and also in-hospital complications.

Never chase the vessel area in a positively remodeled vessel. Always set your target MSAs in reference to the distal reference lumen area.

Any negative remodeling, if missed during post-stent optimization, can lead to fatal perforations.

"IVUS: Proof that you don't need a magic mirror to see what's inside."

CHAPTER 12

Vessel Tapering

There is a tendency of coronaries to taper in size as they advance downward. The tapering is more seen in left anterior descending (LAD) than left circumflex (LCX) and right coronary artery (RCA). On average, LAD tapers by 0.33 mm for every 10 mm length **(Fig. 1)**.

Also, one should keep in mind that after every major branch, there is a sudden decrease in the size of the vessel **(Fig. 2)**.

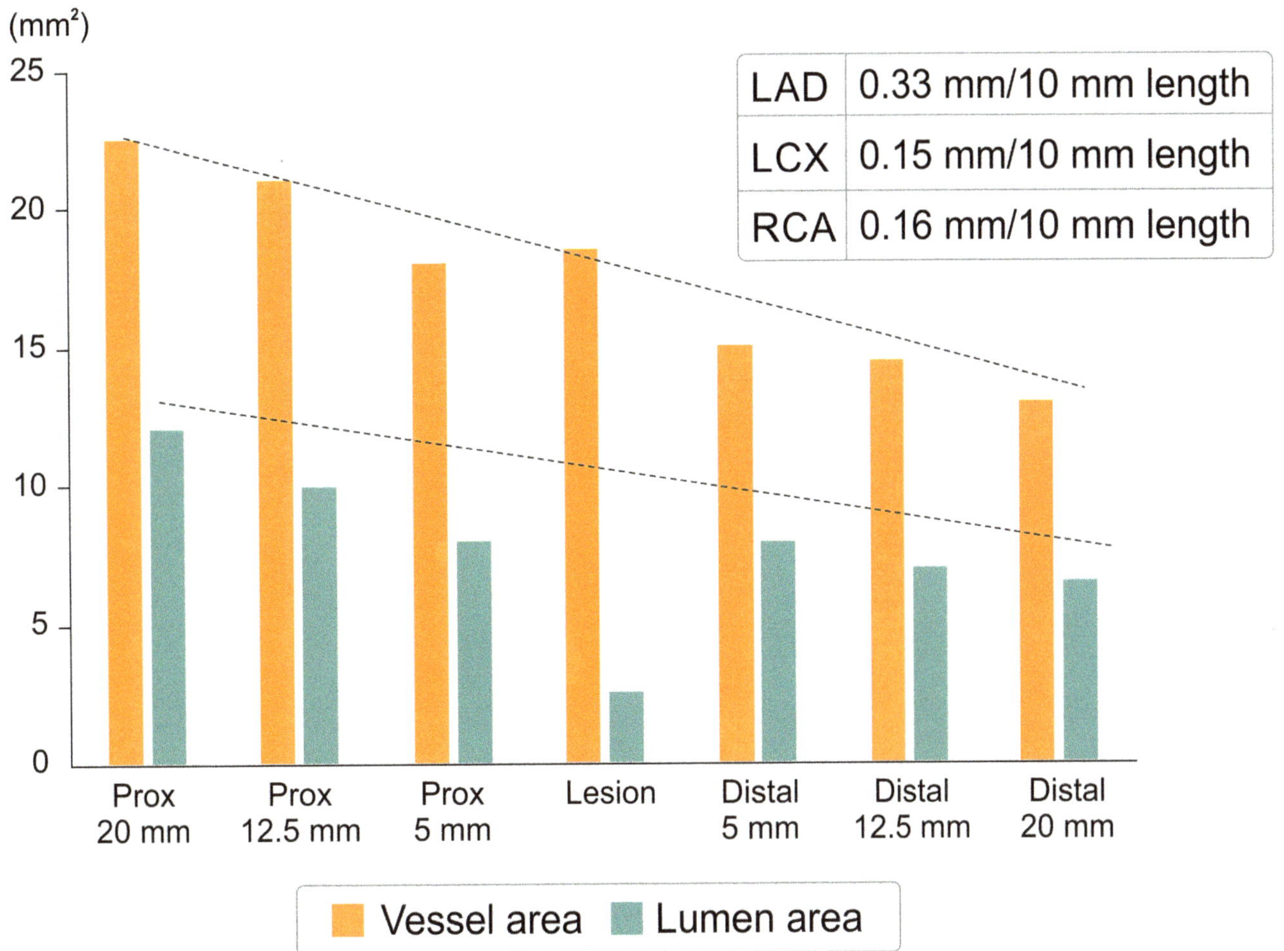

Fig. 1: Vessel tapering phenomenon. (LAD: left anterior descending; LCX: left circumflex; RCA: right coronary artery)

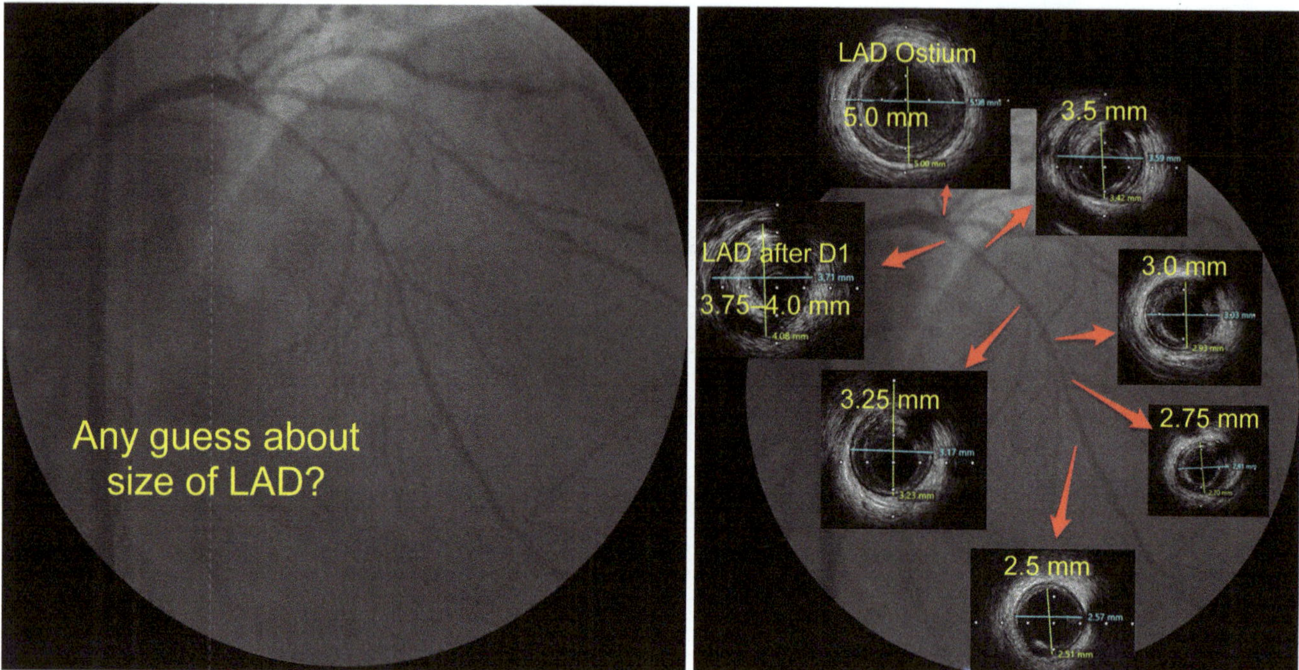

Fig. 2: How left anterior descending (LAD) tapers in size from 5.0 to 2.5 mm. Because of this vessel tapering phenomenon it is very important to use IVUS to ascertain vessel size in particularly diffuse long lesions.

Because of this vessel tapering phenomenon, it is very important to use IVUS to ascertain vessel size in particularly diffuse long lesions.

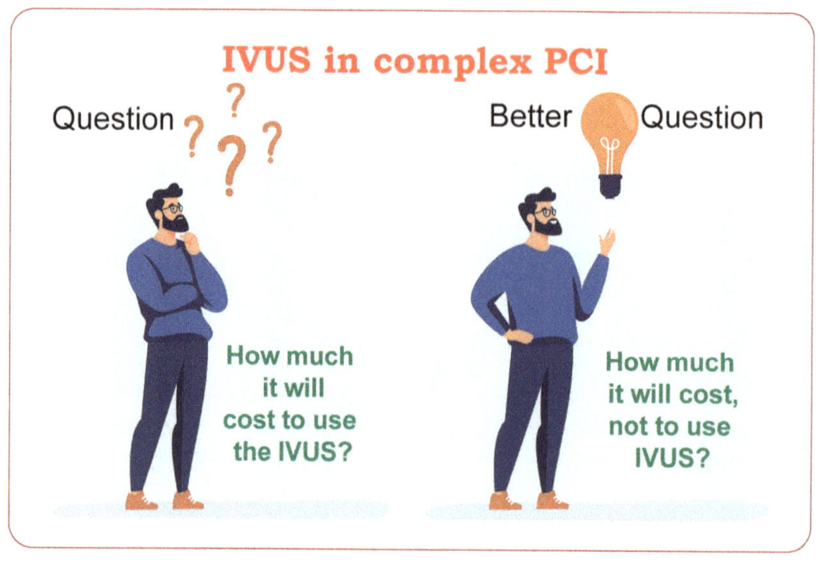

CHAPTER 13

Thrombus on Intravascular Ultrasound

Diagnosis of a thrombus was a challenge with 20 MHz intravascular ultrasound (IVUS). But with high-definition (HD) IVUS, we can not only detect thrombus easily but can also differentiate between acute and chronic thrombus **(Fig. 1)**.

Thrombus usually appears as a relatively echolucent or variable gray-scale image with a layered or lobulated appearance with speckling **(Fig. 2)**.

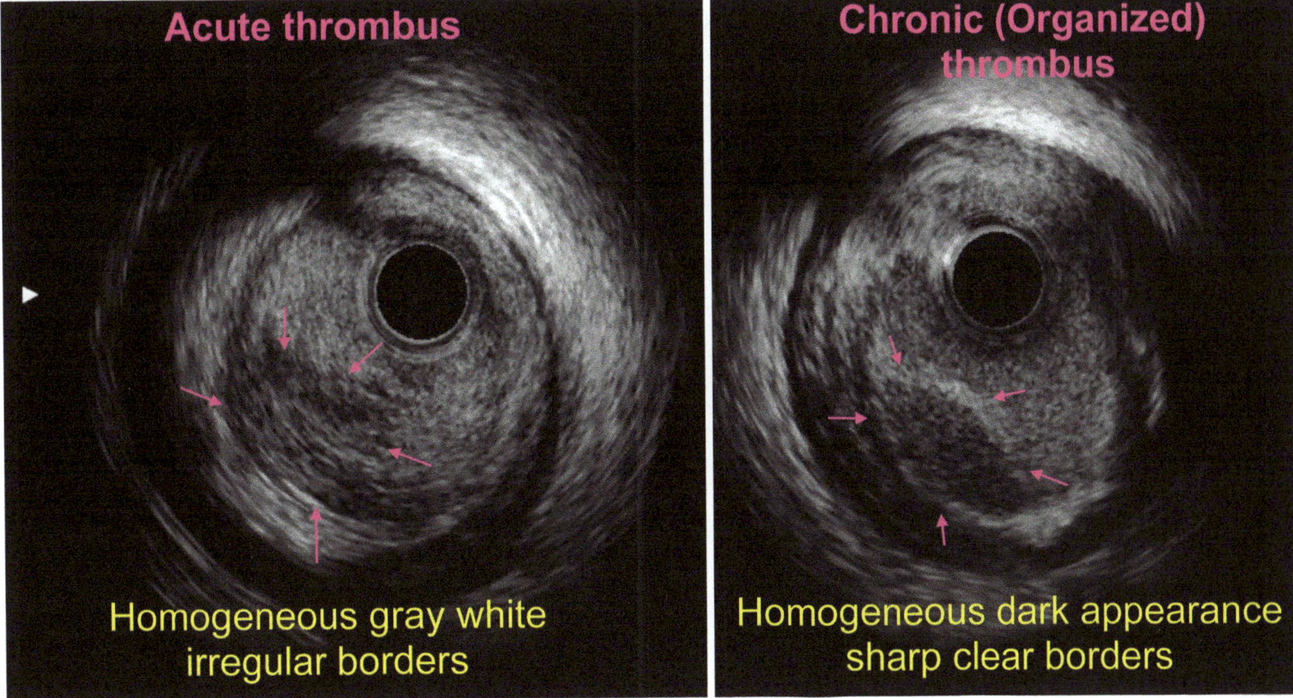

Fig. 1: Acute versus chronic thrombus.

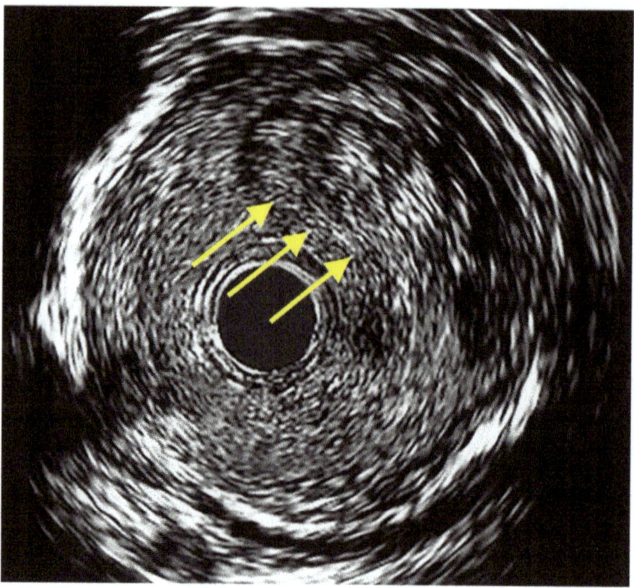

Fig. 2: Thrombus shown by arrows.

DISTINCTIVE FEATURES OF THROMBUS ON INTRAVASCULAR ULTRASOUND

- Sparkling or scintillating appearance
- Lobulated mass projecting into the lumen
- Lumen-thrombus interface is not well defined
- Identification of blood speckle indicating micro-channels
- Mobility

Acute thrombus usually has irregular borders with gray white appearance whereas organized thrombus usually has dark appearance with regular borders **(Fig. 1)**.

Thrombus attached to the vessel wall (mural thrombus) is hard to distinguish from plaque, but its sparkling appearance and blood speckles help differentiate them **(Fig. 3)**.

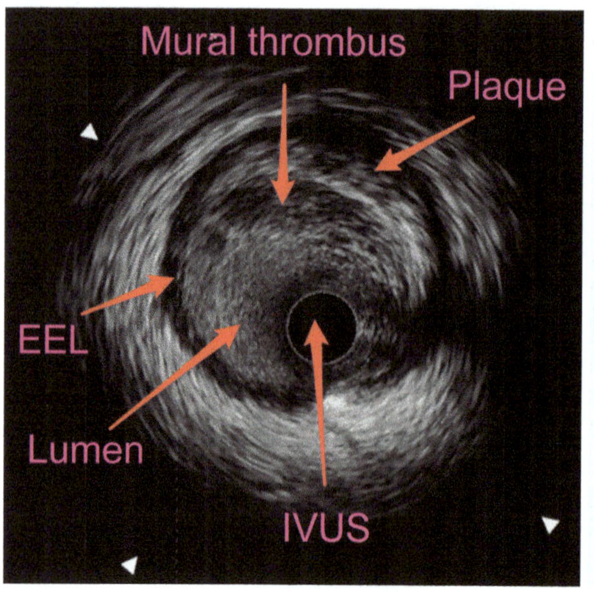

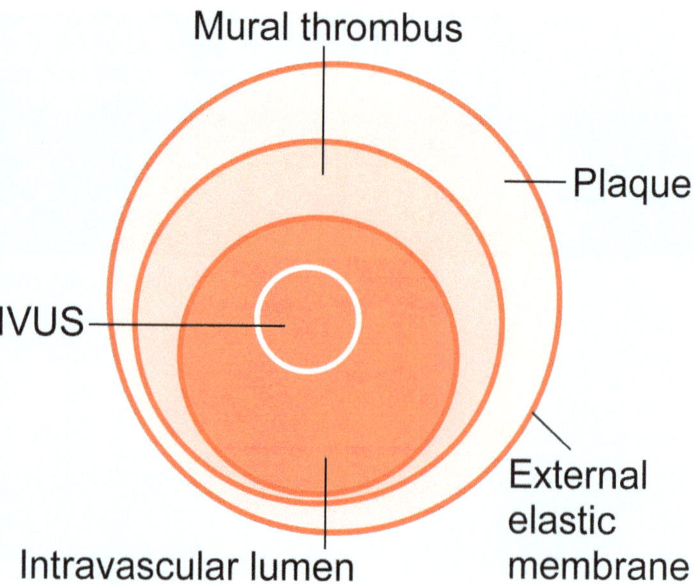

Fig. 3: Mural thrombus. (EEL: external elastic lamina; IVUS: intravascular ultrasound)

CHAPTER 14

Intravascular Ultrasound for Calcium Assessment

WHY DO WE NEED INTRAVASCULAR ULTRASOUND TO SEE CALCIUM?

Angiography is only moderately sensitive to detect calcium and it all depends upon the quadrants of calcium present **(Fig. 1)**.

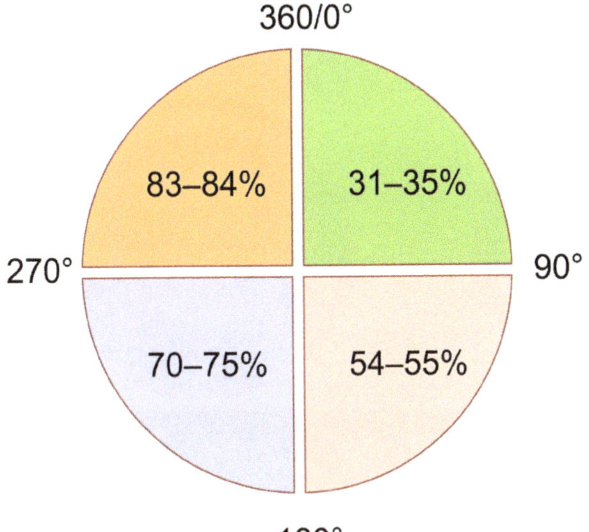

Fig. 1: Sensitivity of angiography in detecting calcium with reference to quadrants of calcium. (IVUS: intravascular ultrasound; OCT: optical coherence tomography)

HOW DOES CALCIUM LOOK ON INTRAVASCULAR ULTRASOUND?

Ultrasound waves reflect calcium strongly, so we get an echodense (bright white image). Also IVUS does not penetrate calcium, so we get acoustic shadowing (do not see anything beyond) **(Fig. 2)**.

Whenever we see calcium on IVUS, we have to assess basically things in two categories, i.e., calcium morphology and calcium severity.

Calcium morphology: It can be of three types: concentric, eccentric and nodular **(Fig. 3)**.

The plaque modifying device selection is based to some extent depending upon the morphology of the calcium. For example, if it is a concentric calcium, we may require OPN or intravascular lithotripsy (IVL) or ROTA [size of the burr should be more than the minimal luminal area (MLA) of the concentric calcium]. If it is an eccentric calcium, then a cutting balloon is preferred. In calcified nodule (CN), if there is a favorable wire bias, then ROTA, otherwise orbital atherectomy (OA) is a good choice.

Calcium severity is assessed under five headings:

1. **Arch of calcium:** If it is >270°, it is severe calcium **(Fig. 4)**.
2. **Length of calcium:** Length should be measured in L view **(Fig. 5)**. Any length >5 mm is severe calcium.
3. **Depth of calcium:** If it is located near the intima or lumen, it is superficial, but if it is located away from the lumen and toward adventitia, it is deep **(Fig. 6)**. It is the superficial calcium which causes hindrance in the passage of devices and stent expansion so should be taken seriously.
4. **Thickness of calcium:** Since IVUS does not penetrate the calcium, it is difficult to measure the thickness of calcium directly, but there are certain indirect parameters by which we can assess the thickness. Like if there are reverberations seen, it means it is thin and smooth calcium, if acoustic shadowing beyond the calcium is very deep, it is a thick calcium **(Fig. 7)**.
5. **Nodular protrusion:** CN can be of two types **(Fig. 8)**. If the fibrous cap is disrupted and the surface is irregular, it becomes an eruptive CN. If the fibrous cap is intact and the surface is smooth, it becomes noneruptive CN.

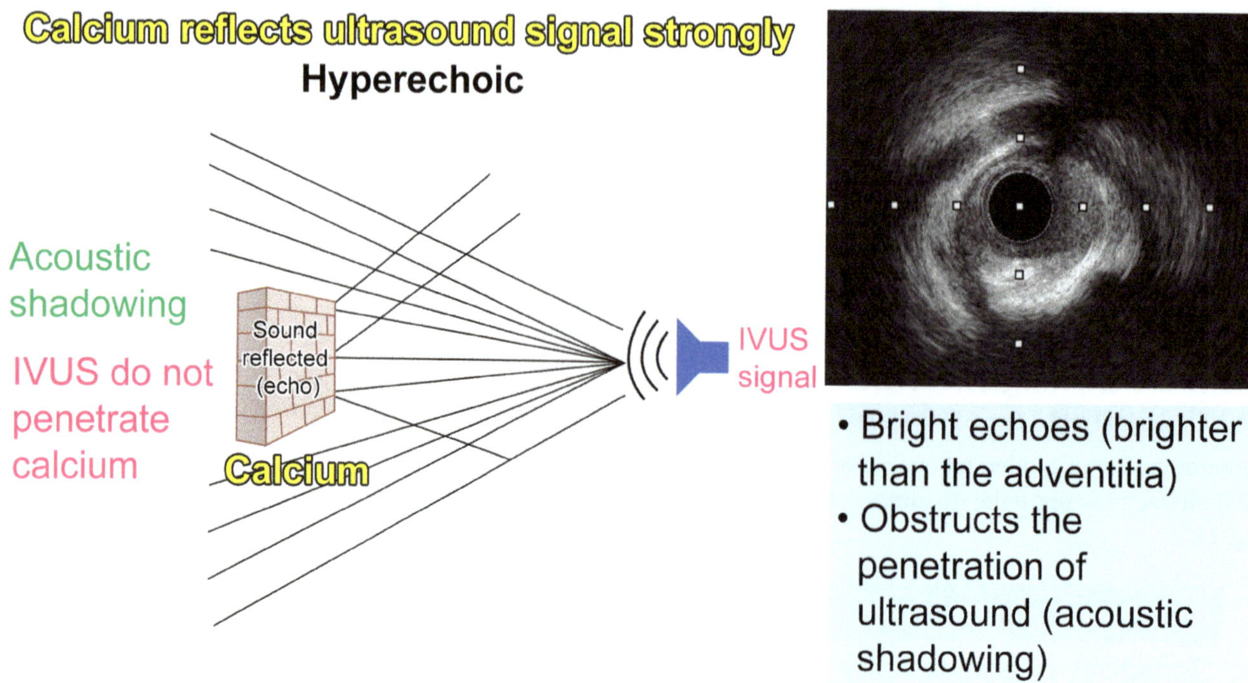

Fig. 2: How calcium looks on intravascular ultrasound (IVUS).

Calcium morphology

Concentric

Eccentric

Nodular

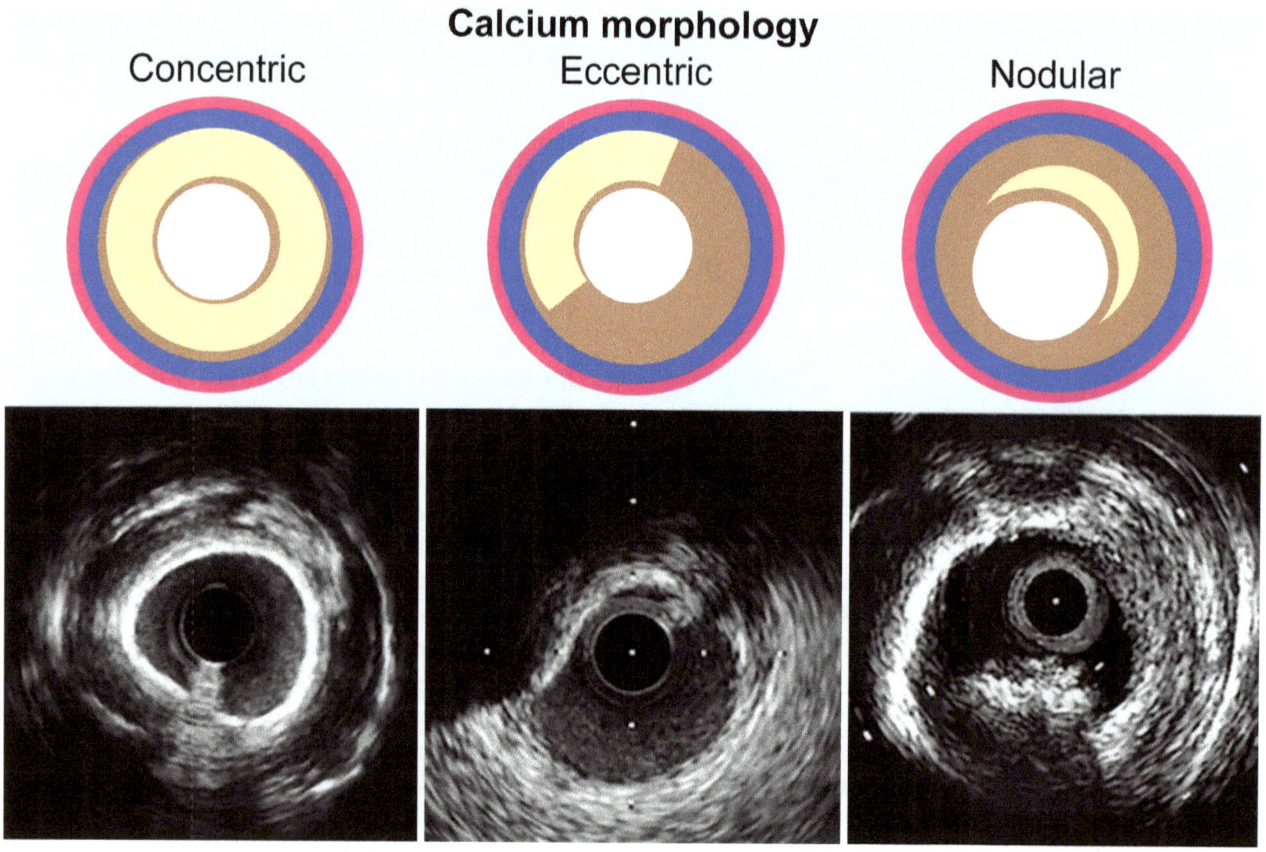

Fig. 3: Calcium morphology on intravascular ultrasound (IVUS).

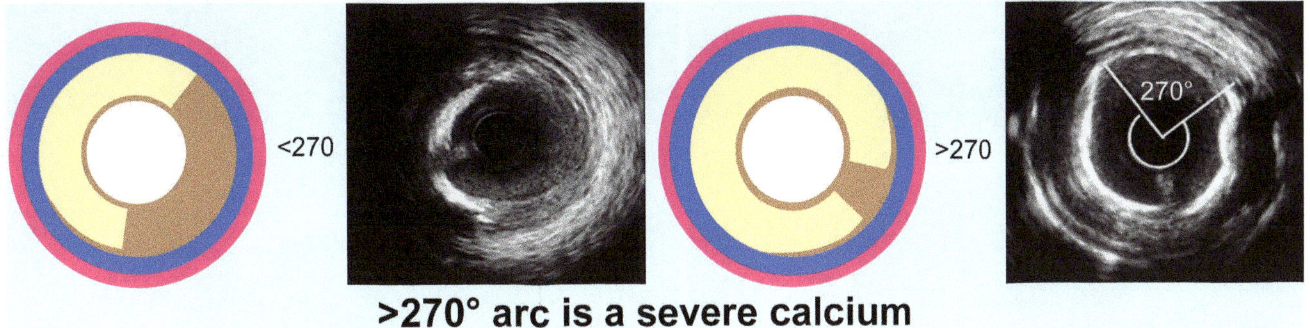

Fig. 4: Arch of calcium.

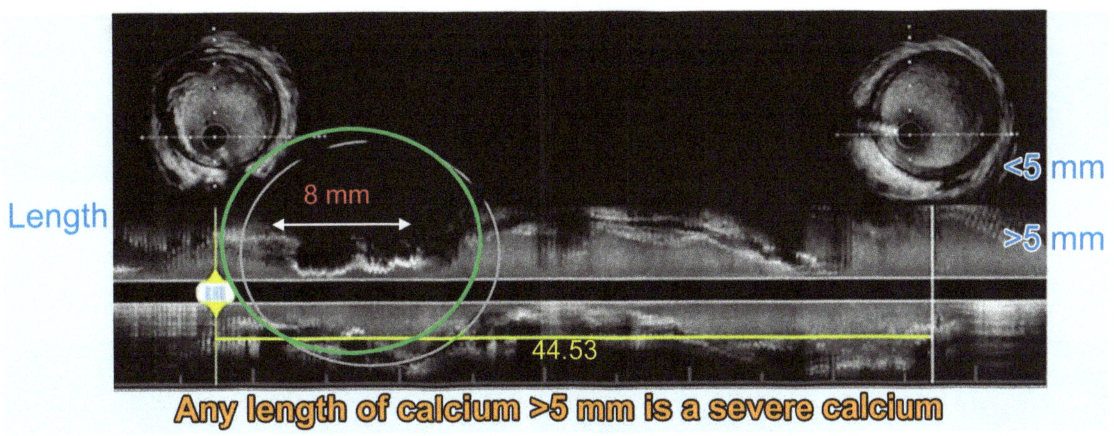

Fig. 5: Length of calcium.

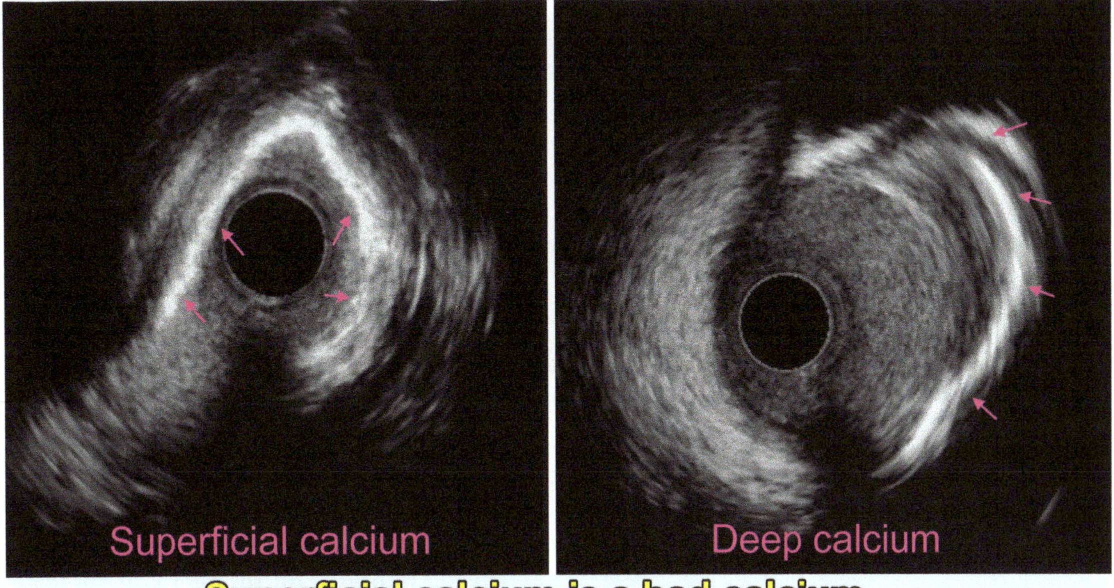

Fig. 6: Depth of calcium.

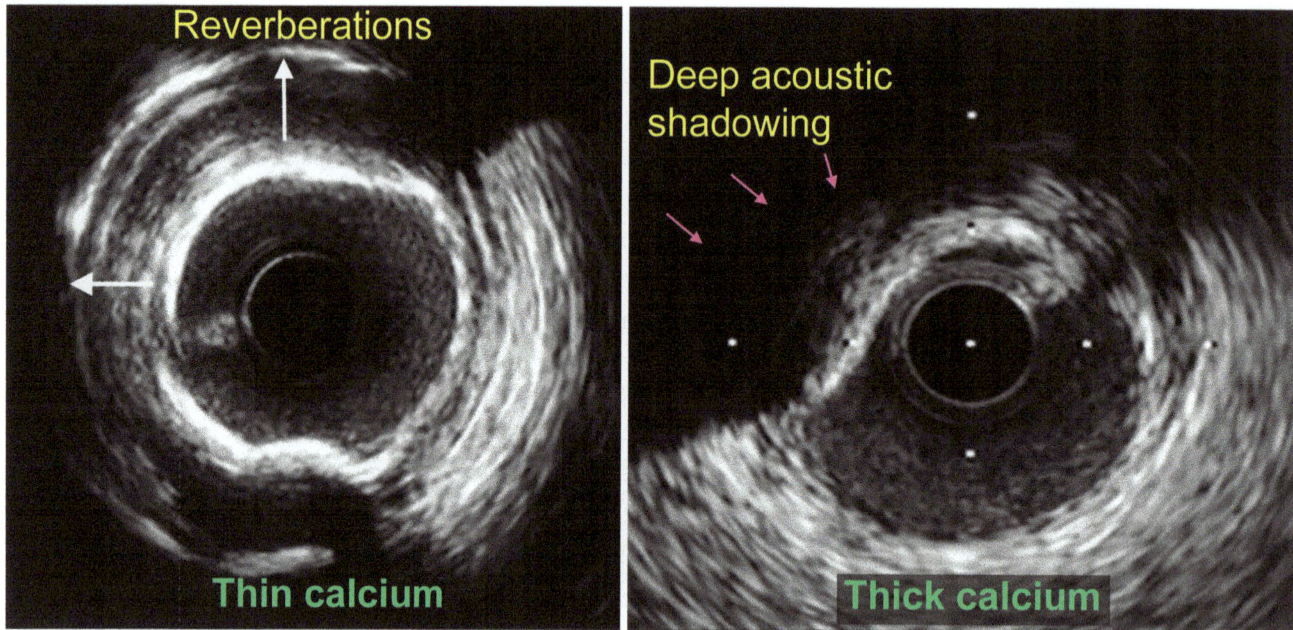

Fig. 7: Thickness of calcium.

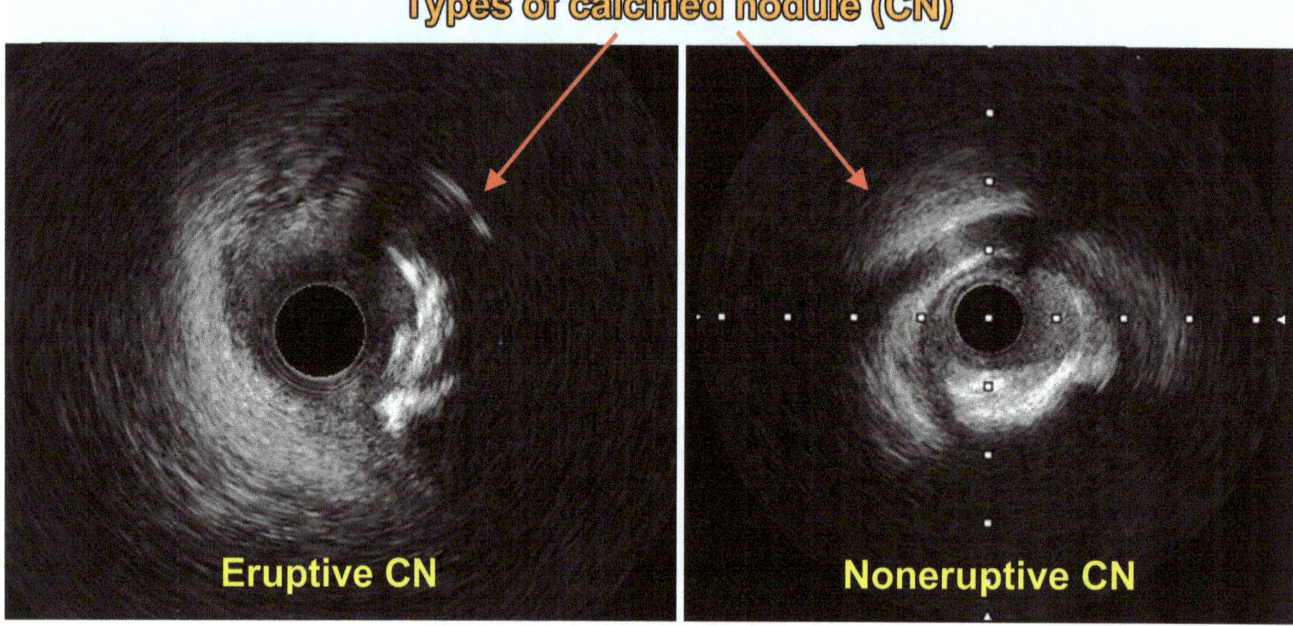

Fig. 8: Nodular protrusion.

CALCIUM SCORE

The IVUS-based calcium score has also been designed which will help you decide which patient requires atherectomy and which do not **(Fig. 9)**. If the score is 2 or more, the results are better with atherectomy.

The IVUS should be done at least three times in a calcified lesion:

1. Preintervention to assess the severity of calcium
2. During intervention to identify if sufficient plaque modification is done
3. Postintervention to confirm stent expansion

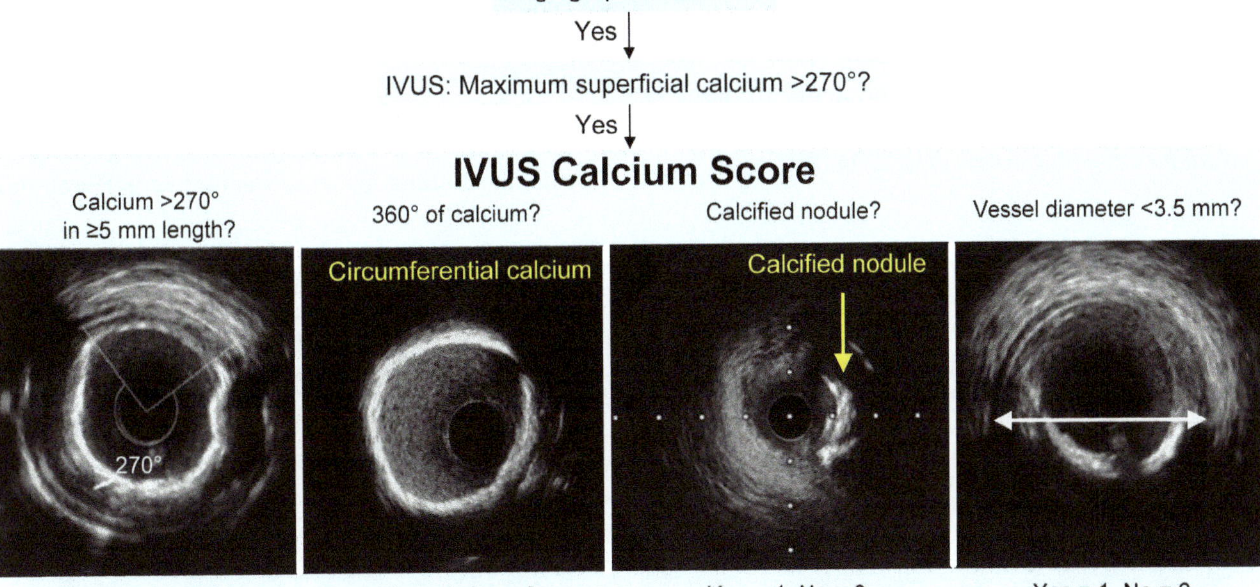

Fig. 9: Intravascular ultrasound (IVUS)-based calcium scoring.

HOW TO IDENTIFY IF SUFFICIENT PLAQUE MODIFICATION IS DONE OR NOT?

Four ways to do that:

1. *Look for calcium fractures:* Calcium hinders ultrasound waves penetration, and its fracture can be detected by observing ultrasound waves passing through it **(Fig. 10)**. Fracturing calcium entails observing at least two fractures 180° apart. These fractures indicate successful calcium modification.
2. *Reverberations:* When the surface of calcium is polished by ROTA or OA, it causes repeated reflection

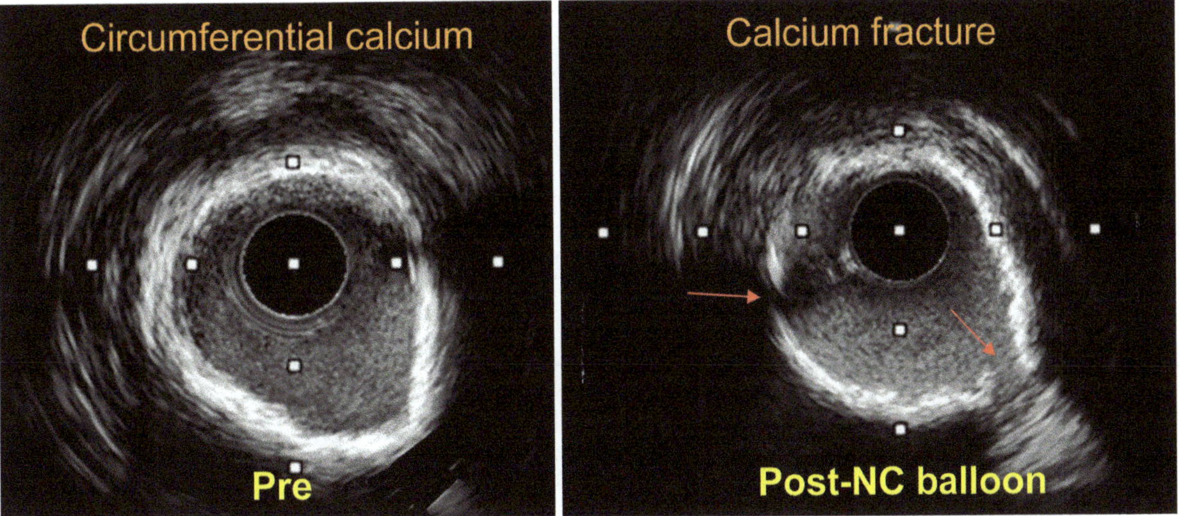

Fig. 10: Calcium fracture on IVUS. (IVUS: intravascular ultrasound; NC: noncompliant)

of these ultrasound waves, which causes these reverberations **(Fig. 11)**. Reverberations indicate that the thick calcium has been converted into thin calcium, making it easier to be broken down by a noncompliant (NC) balloon.

3. Look for *luminal gain* by comparing the MLA before and after debulking **(Fig. 12)**.
4. *Nodular debulking* in case of CN **(Fig. 13)**.

OPTIMIZING STENT EXPANSION IN CALCIFIED LESIONS

- Look for absolute minimum stent area (MSA) > 5.5 mm^2 as criteria for optimal stent expansion.
- Eccentric expansion is acceptable if absolute MSAs are good **(Fig. 14)**.
- Be cautious of mistaking post-stenting images in calcified lesions for stent fracture or perforation as

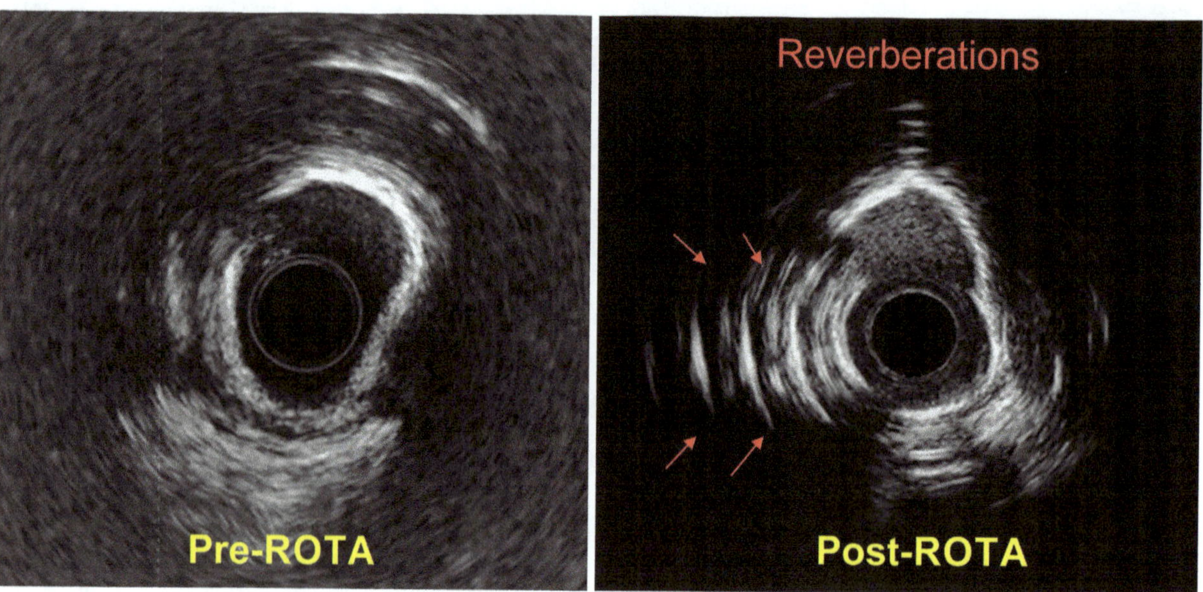

Fig. 11: Reverberation on intravascular ultrasound (IVUS) post-ROTA.

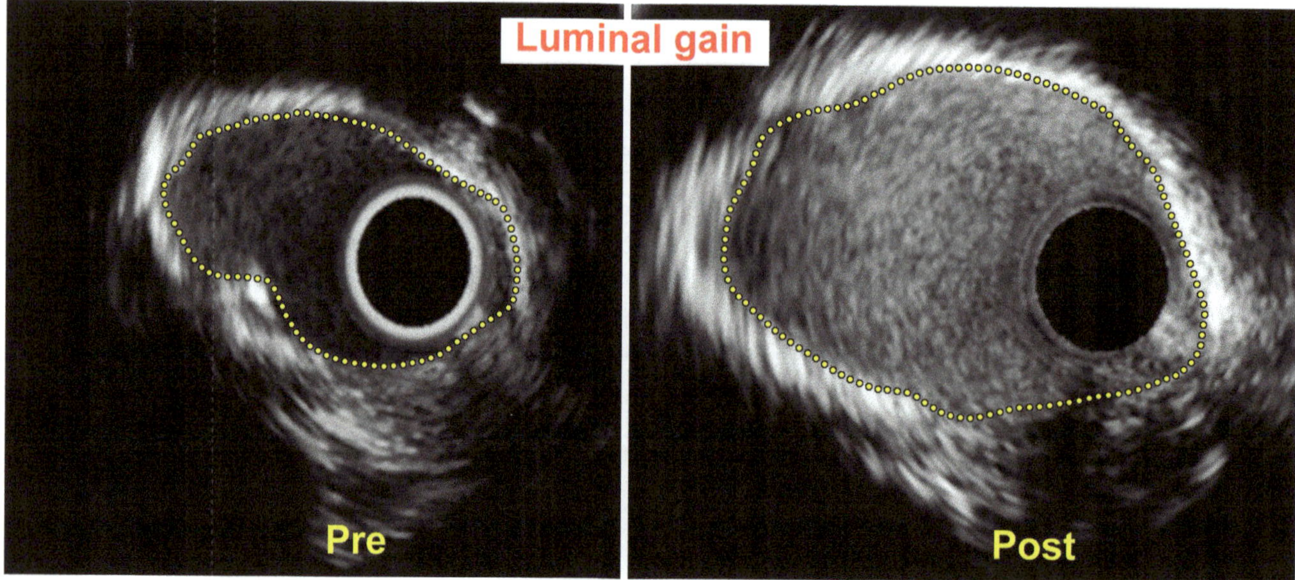

Fig. 12: Assessing luminal gain on intravascular ultrasound (IVUS).

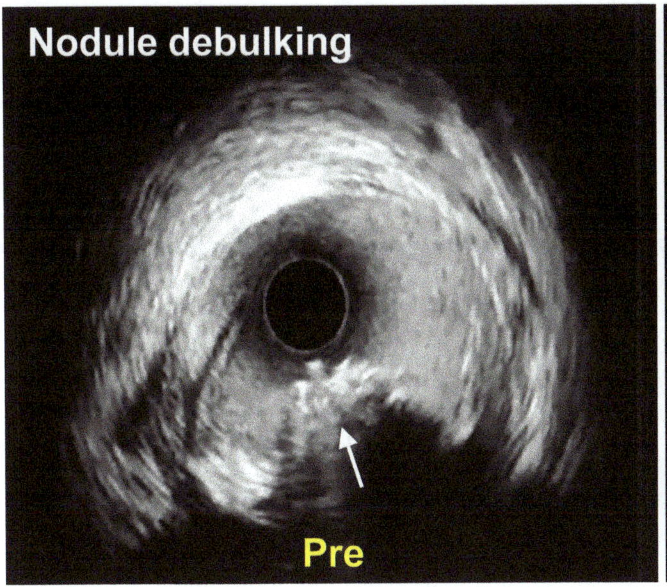

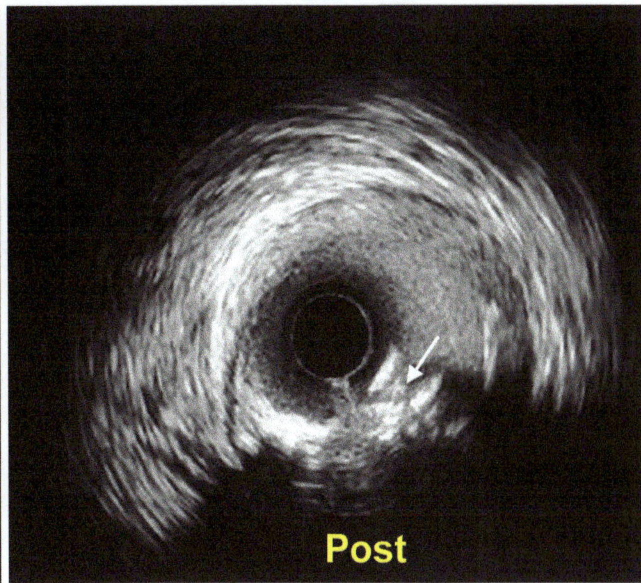

Fig. 13: Nodular debulking.

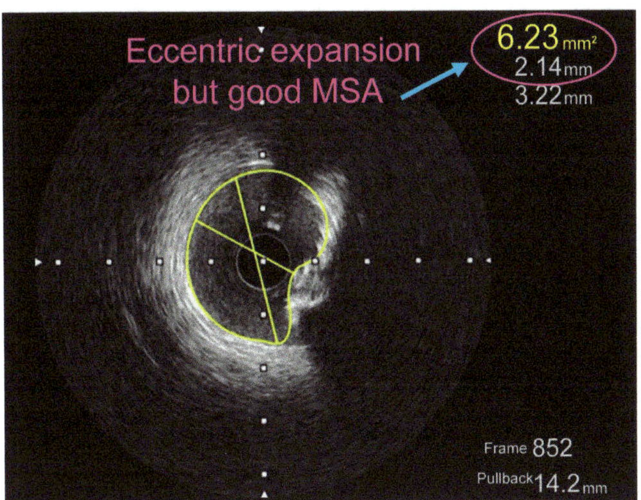

Fig. 14: Eccentric expansion but good minimum stent area (MSA).

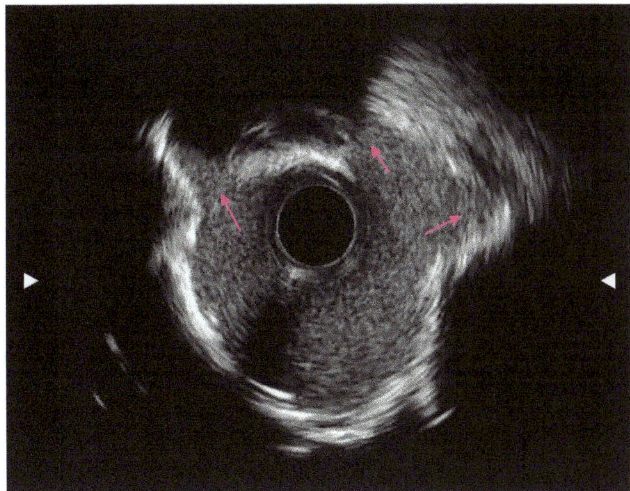

Fig. 15: Post-stenting image in a calcified lesion showing compressed calcium behind stent struts.

shown in **Figure 15**. Such images **(Fig. 15)** are due to adventitial stretching with compressed calcium behind the stent. In fact, if we see such images post-stenting in calcified lesion, it means calcium modification has been done adequately.

"By leveraging IVUS, clinicians gain a 360° perspective on calcified lesions, empowering them to make informed and confident decisions."

CHAPTER 15

Plaque Rupture on Intravascular Ultrasound

Rupture or superficial erosion of vulnerable plaque with subsequent thrombus formation represents the principal pathophysiology underlying most acute coronary syndromes (ACSs).

With high-definition intravascular ultrasound (HD IVUS), we can detect plaque rupture and differentiate it from plaque erosion.

Plaque rupture can be defined as a cavity in the vessel wall with disruption of the intima and flow observed within the plaque cavity **(Figs. 1 and 2)**.

Plaque erosion on IVUS is identified by superficial irregularities in the intima with an intact fibrous cap, often with thrombus formation on the eroded surface **(Fig. 3)**. Having said that it is difficult to appreciate plaque erosion on HD IVUS and it is usually the diagnosis of exclusion. Unlike plaque rupture, which involves a deep and complete breach of the fibrous cap and often leads to significant clinical events like myocardial infarction, plaque erosion tends to be more subtle and may not always lead to such severe outcomes immediately. Therefore, it is recommended that after ACS, if we see only plaque erosion on imaging, it can be managed conservatively, whereas plaque rupture usually requires stenting.

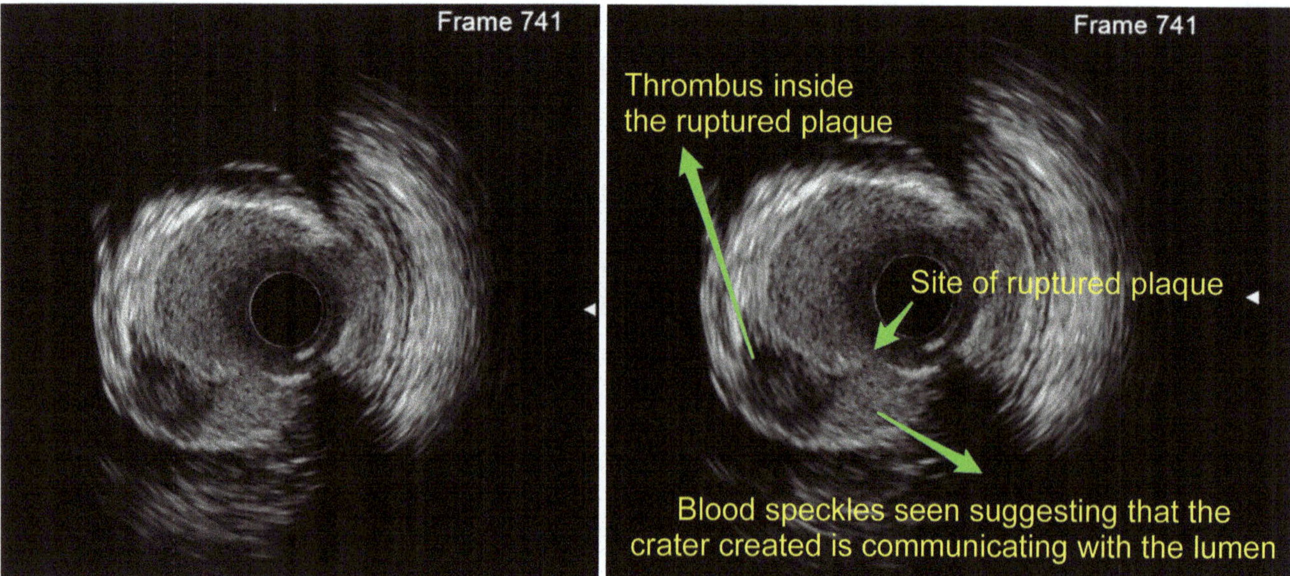

Fig. 1: Plaque rupture with thrombus seen inside the ruptured plaque.

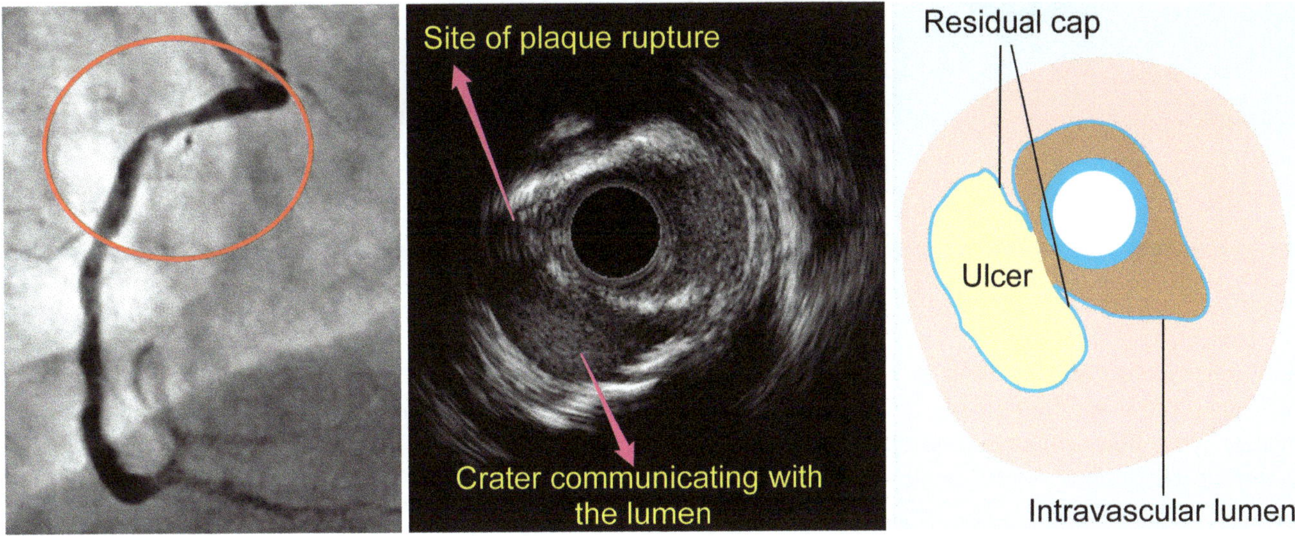

Fig. 2: Plaque rupture seen along with the crater communicating with lumen.

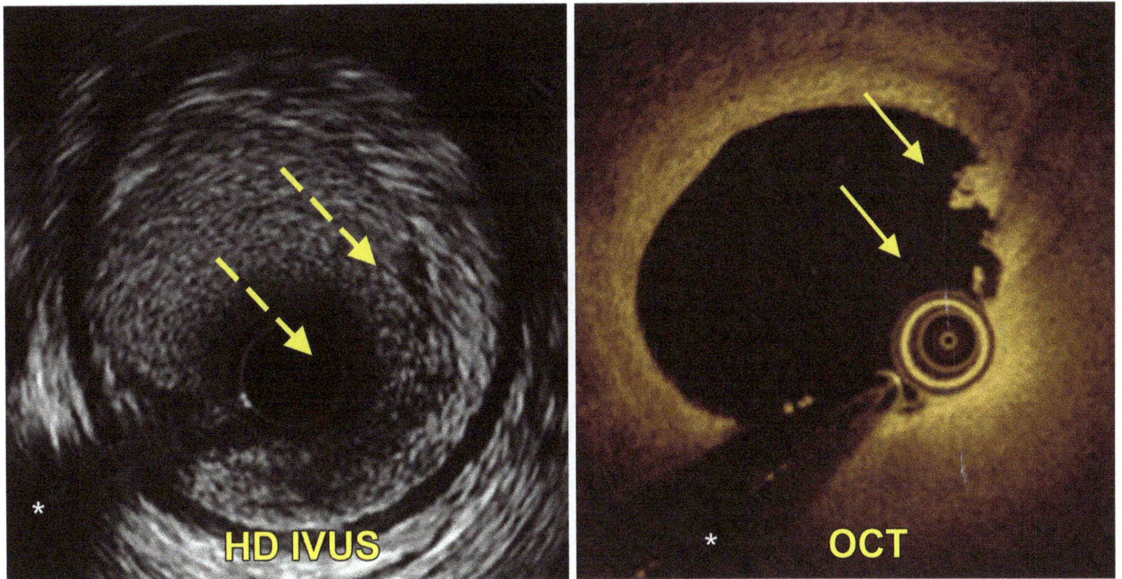

Fig. 3: Plaque erosion as suggested by superficial irregularities in the intima with intact fibrous cap along with thrombus. (HD IVUS: high-definition intravascular ultrasound; OCT: optical coherence tomography)

"IVUS is like a selfie for your blood vessels, but way more professional."

CHAPTER 16

Attenuated Plaque/Vulnerable Plaque

Attenuated plaque is defined as hypoechoic plaque with deep ultrasound attenuation without calcification or very dense fibrous plaque **(Fig. 1)**. Attenuated plaque is one of the predictors of slow flow and future major adverse cardiovascular event (MACE). Particularly those attenuated plaque with an angle of 180° or more and an attenuation distance of 5 mm or more in the longitudinal view.

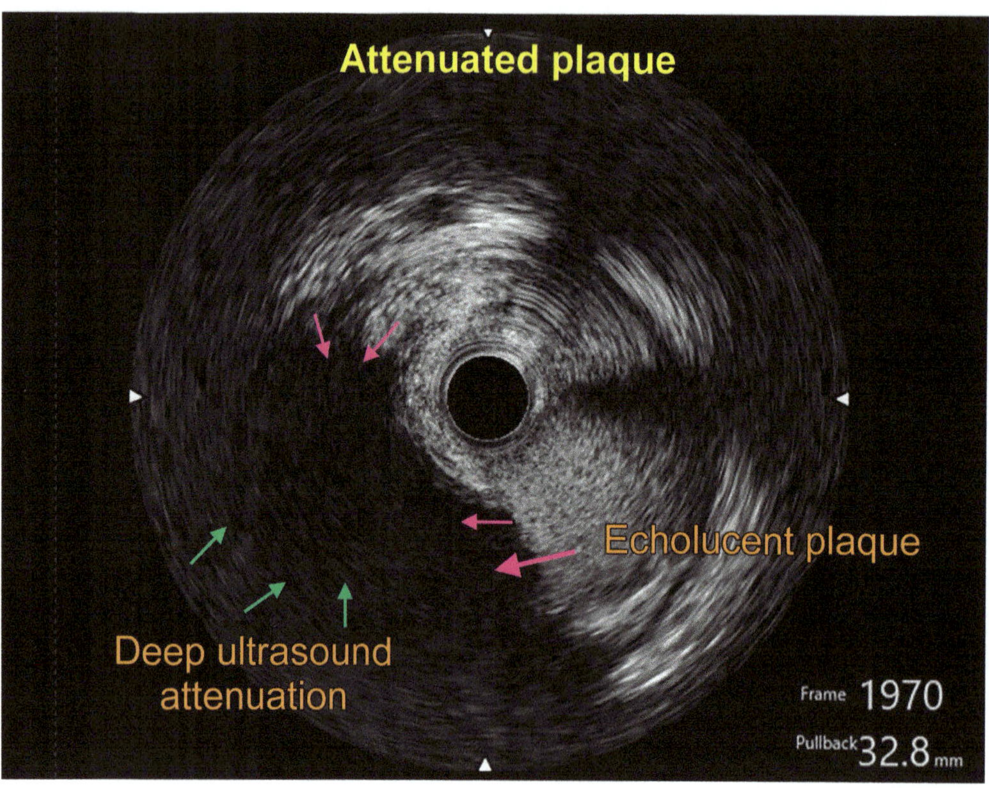

Fig. 1: Attenuated plaque on intravascular ultrasound (IVUS).

Vulnerable plaque: Identification of a thin fibrous cap (<65 μm) is not possible with intravascular ultrasound (IVUS) because of its resolution property. However, there are certain indirect parameters by which we can assess the vulnerability of the plaque **(Fig. 2)**.

- Plaque burden >50%
- Lipid pool occupying >40% of total lesion area
- 180 attenuation
- Remodeling index >1.05

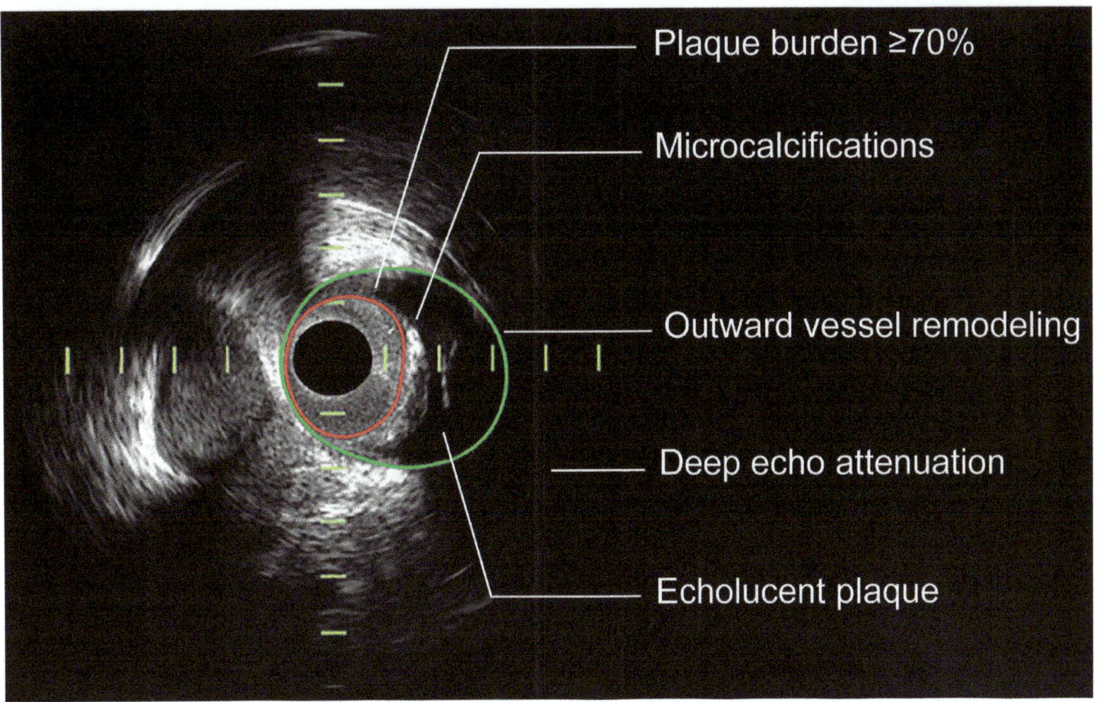

Fig. 2: Vulnerable plaque on intravascular ultrasound (IVUS).

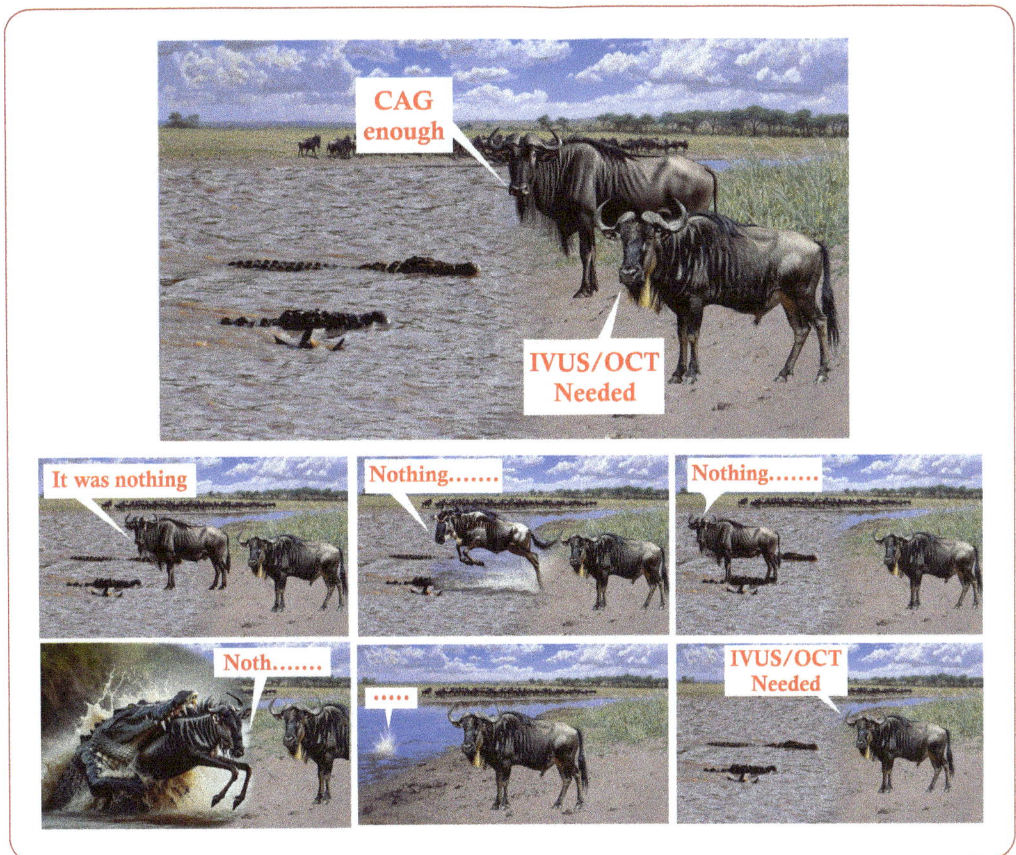

CHAPTER 17

Stent Sizing on Intravascular Ultrasound

Should stent sizing be based on distal reference lumen area or vessel area? The correct answer is it all depends upon the plaque burden (PB) at the distal landing zone.

- If the PB is >50%, then lumen area +0.25 mm
- If the PB is <50%, then vessel area -0.25 mm

For example, see in the **Figure 1**, the landing zone was completely plaque-free, so the stent chosen was according to the distal reference vessel area –0.25 mm, whereas the case shown in **Figure 2** has a PB >50% at the landing zone, so the stent chosen was according to the distal reference lumen area + 0.25 mm.

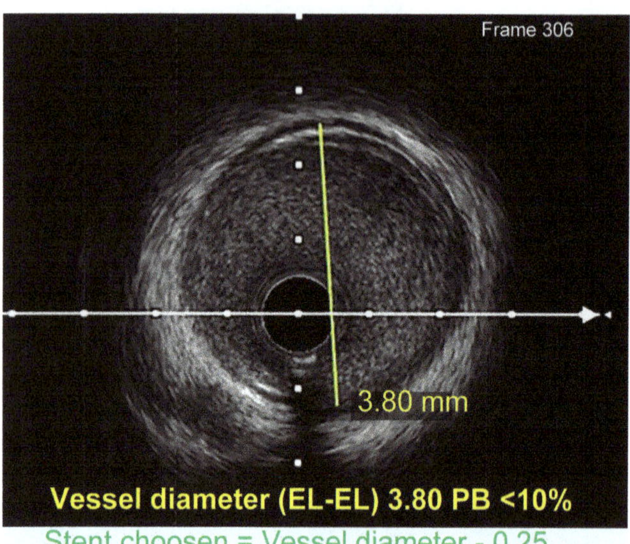

Fig. 1: Plaque burden (PB) at the landing site is less. Stent chosen according to the distal reference vessel area –0.25 mm.

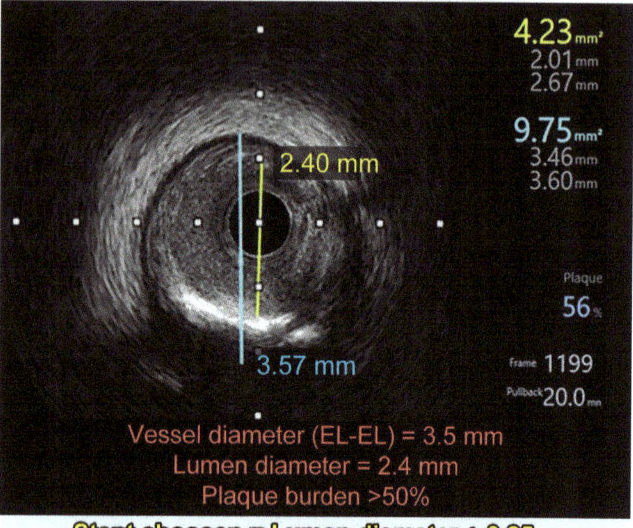

Fig. 2: Plaque burden (PB) at the landing site is >50%. Stent chosen according to the distal reference lumen area + 0.25 mm.

"DES implanted with image guidance can be called as a 5th generation DES"

CHAPTER 18

Stent Expansion

The main criteria's for stent expansion on intravascular ultrasound (IVUS) are:

- Stent expansion to its full ability [for example, if a 3.0 mm stent is fully expanded, it will achieve an area of 7 mm. But we know that the stent is expanded not in the air but against the plaque, so it may not be possible to get a 100% expansion always. Hence, we take 80% of the total expected minimal stent area (MSA) as a cut-off point for stent expansion. So, for example, any MSA of <5.7 mm in a 3.0 mm stent means it is <80% expansion, so it will be called an underexpanded stent] **(Table 1)**.
- MSA > 80–90% of distal reference lumen area **(Figs. 1 and 2)**
- Absolute MSA > 5.5 mm^2
- If you are not able to achieve any of the earlier mentioned three criteria then calculate the ratio of MSA/vessel area and if this ratio is exceeds 40%, indicating reasonable stent expansion **(Fig. 3)**. However, this is applicable to only to small MSA < 5 mm.

If we are not able to achieve any of the earlier mentioned criteria then it will be called as underexpanded stent **(Fig. 4)**. (If the stent is long, then divided into 2 and compare the MSA of the distal half of the stent with the distal reference lumen area and the proximal half of the stent with the proximal reference lumen area.)

Sometimes we can see eccentric expansion on IVUS, but as long as MSAs are good, eccentric expansion is acceptable **(Fig. 5)**. In some cases, even a good MSA may appear small compared to the vessel area. This occurs particularly in positively remodeled vessels. Instead of focusing on the vessel area, it is important to prioritize assessing stent expansion in relation to the distal reference lumen area or the absolute MSAs in these situations **(Fig. 6)**.

TABLE 1: Expected minimal stent area (MSA) depending upon stent diameter.

Stent diameter	*Ideal MSA (100%)*	*Optimal MSA (80–90%)*	*Underexpanded (<80%)*
2.5 mm	5.6 mm^2	4.5–4.9	<4.5
3.0 mm	7.1 mm^2	5.8–6.2	<5.7
3.5 mm	9.6 mm^2	7.7–8.6	<7.6
4.0 mm	12.4 mm^2	10.1–10.9	<10

"Numerical precision is the very soul of science"

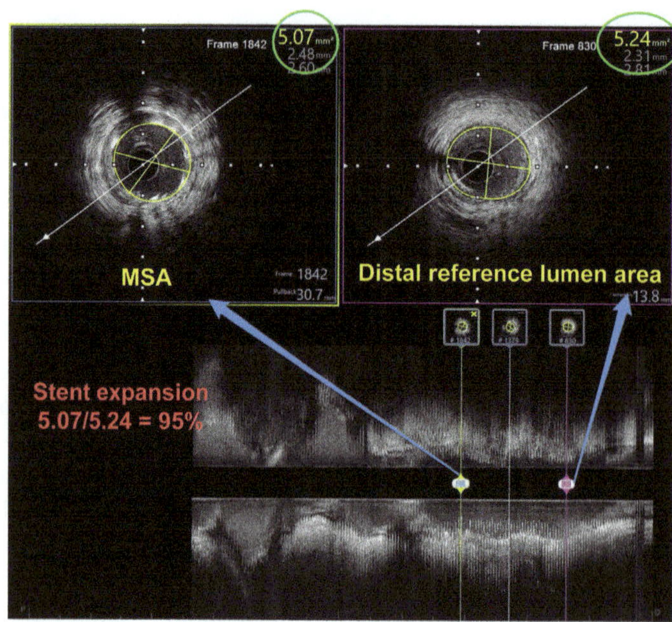

Fig. 1: Here the absolute minimal stent area (MSA) is 5.02 mm, but as compared to the distal reference, it is >95%, indicating good stent expansion.

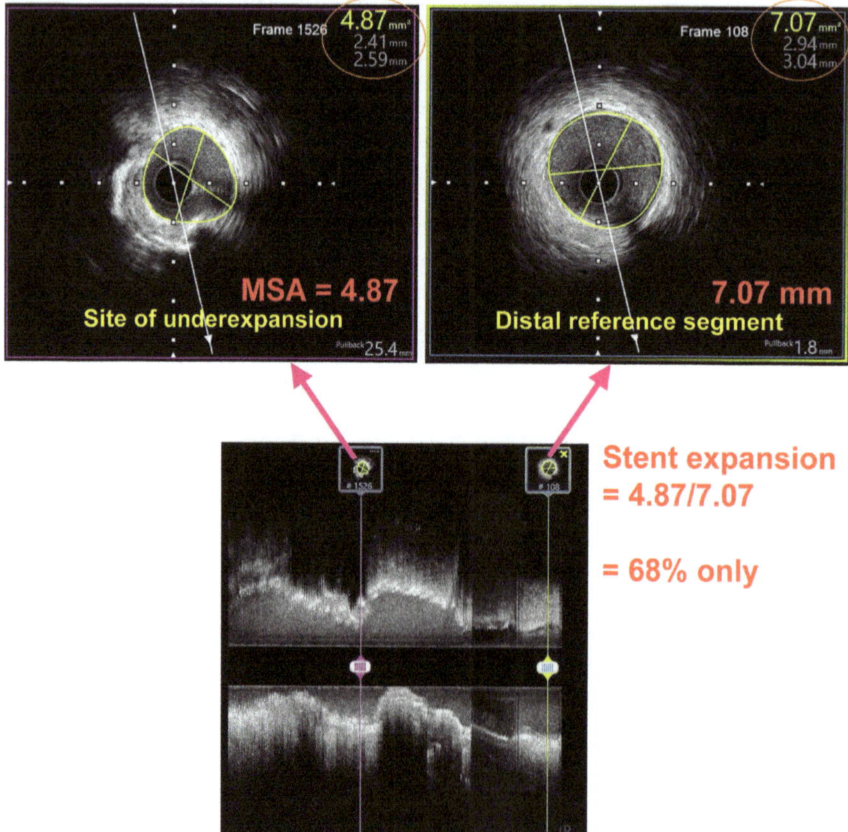

Fig. 2: Showing underexpanded stent since neither the absolute minimal stent areas (MSAs) are good nor the relative expansion with reference to the distal reference is satisfactory.

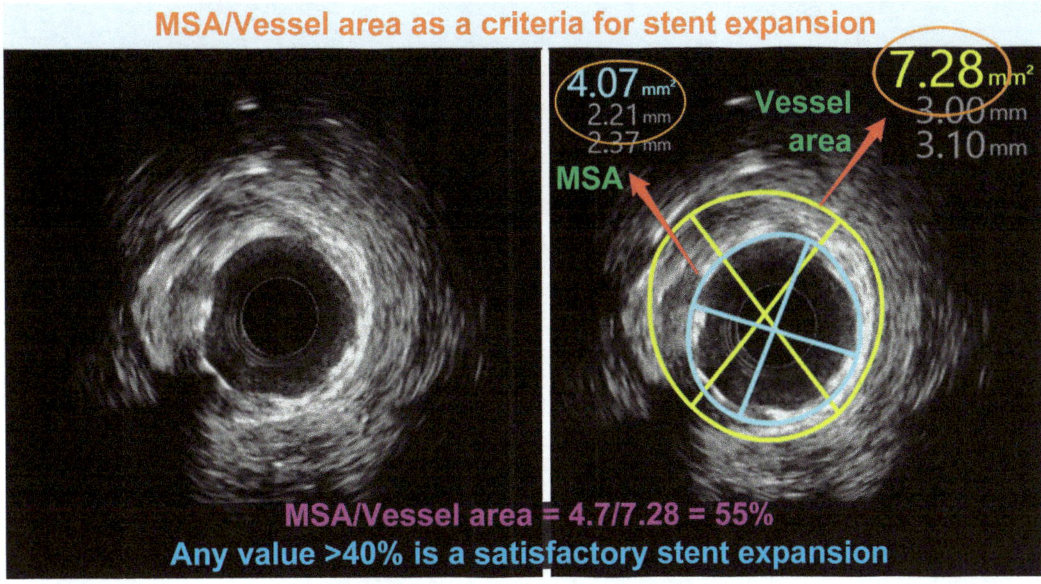

Fig. 3: The absolute minimum stent area is <5 mm, but the stent area to vessel area ratio exceeds 40%, indicating reasonable stent expansion.

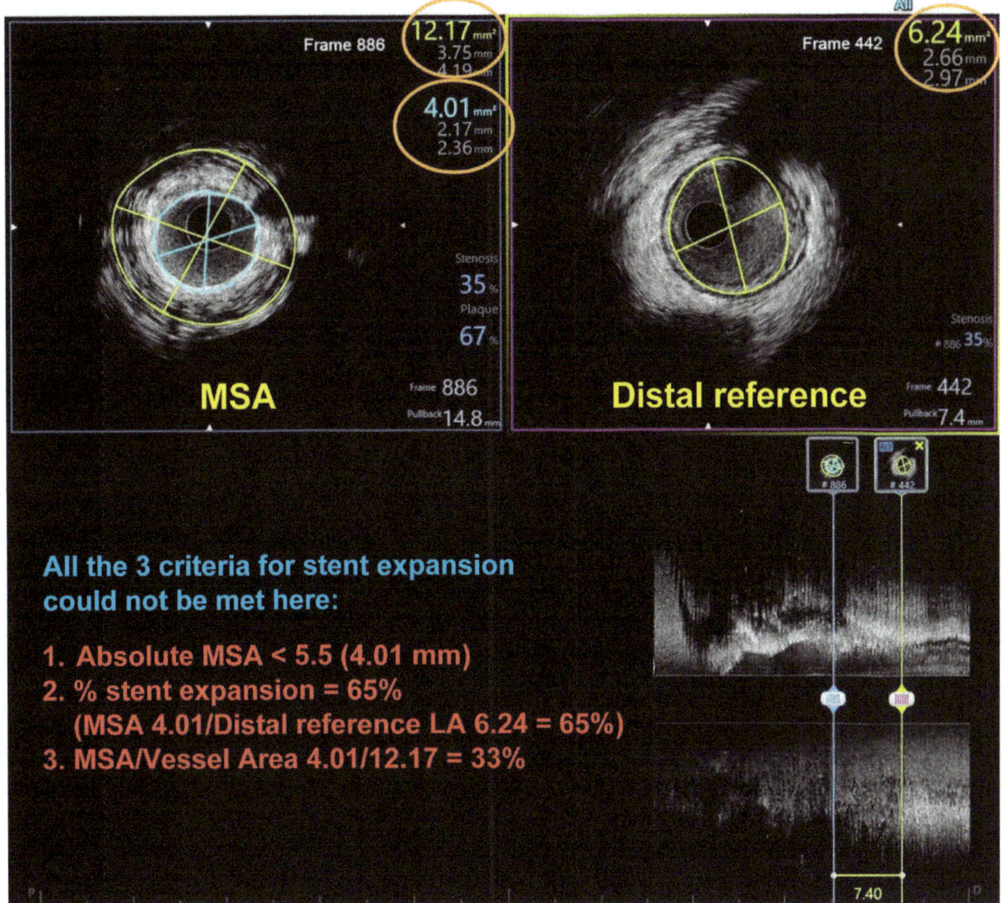

Fig. 4: Underexpanded stent failing to meet none of the criteria for stent expansion.

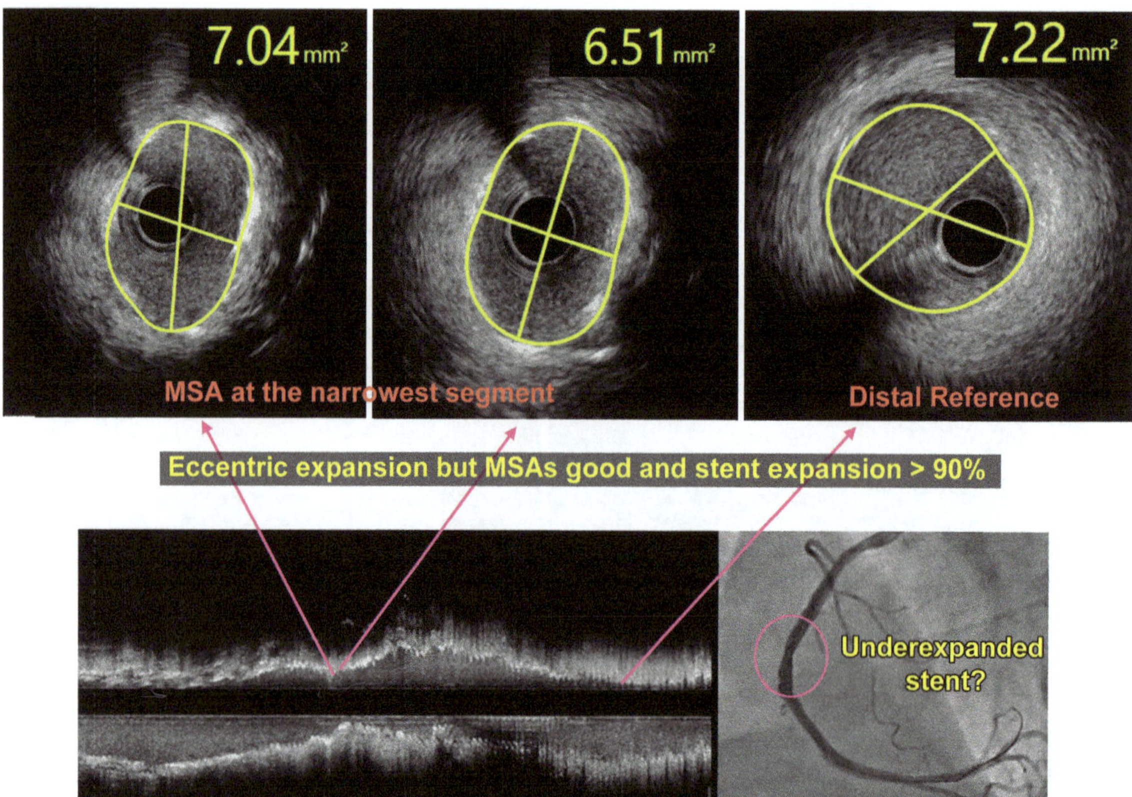

Fig. 5: Eccentric expansion on intravascular ultrasound (IVUS), but minimal stent areas (MSAs) are good, so it is acceptable.

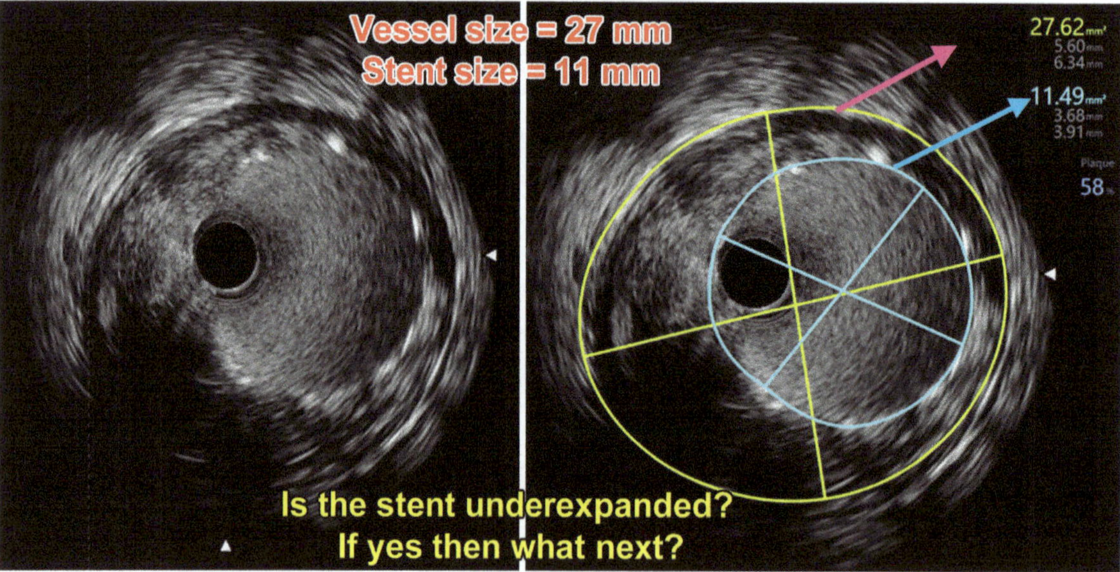

Fig. 6: In this cases, even a good MSA (11 mm) may appear small compared to the vessel area (27 mm). This is due to positive remodeling. Instead of focusing on the vessel area, it is important to prioritize assessing stent expansion in relation to the distal reference lumen area or the absolute MSAs in these situations.

CHAPTER 19

Malapposition

Malapposition means that there is some gap between the stent struts and vessel wall **(Figs. 1 and 2)**. It can be identified by seeing the blood speckles between the stent and vessel wall. Usually, malapposition does not lead to adverse long-term outcomes, but there are certain malappositions which need to be treated, such as:

- Malapposition >500 μm
- Malapposition associated with under expansion
- Proximal malapposition **(Fig. 3)** (if not treated the wire can go abluminal if rewiring is required during this index procedure or future intervention)

One more clue to diagnose malapposition is when we see the triangular shadow of stent struts **(Fig. 4)**.

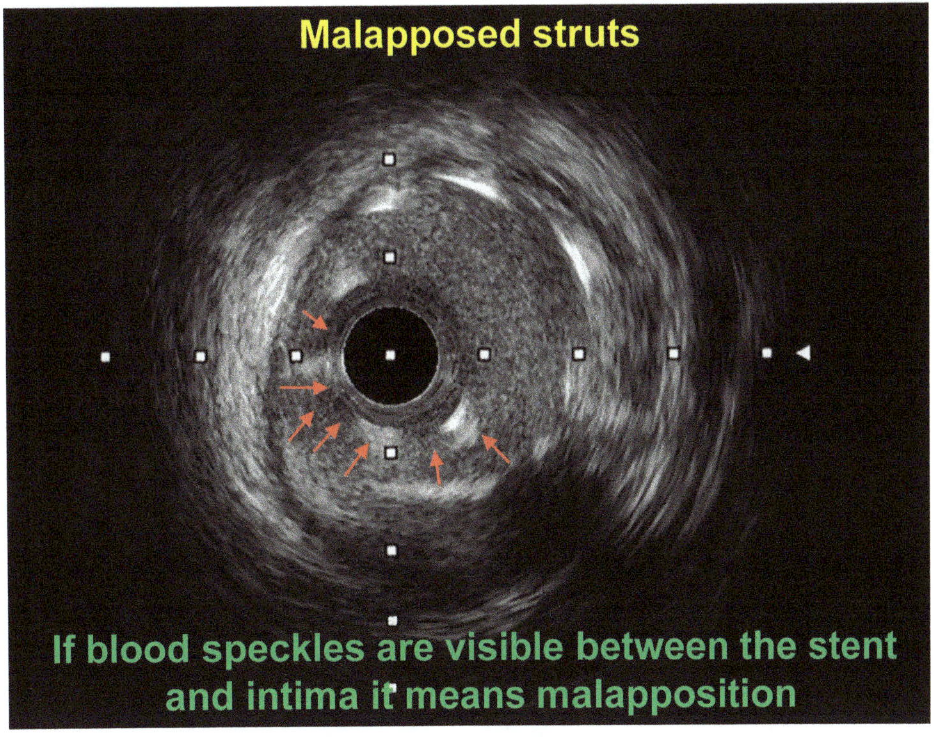

Fig. 1: Malapposed stent struts.

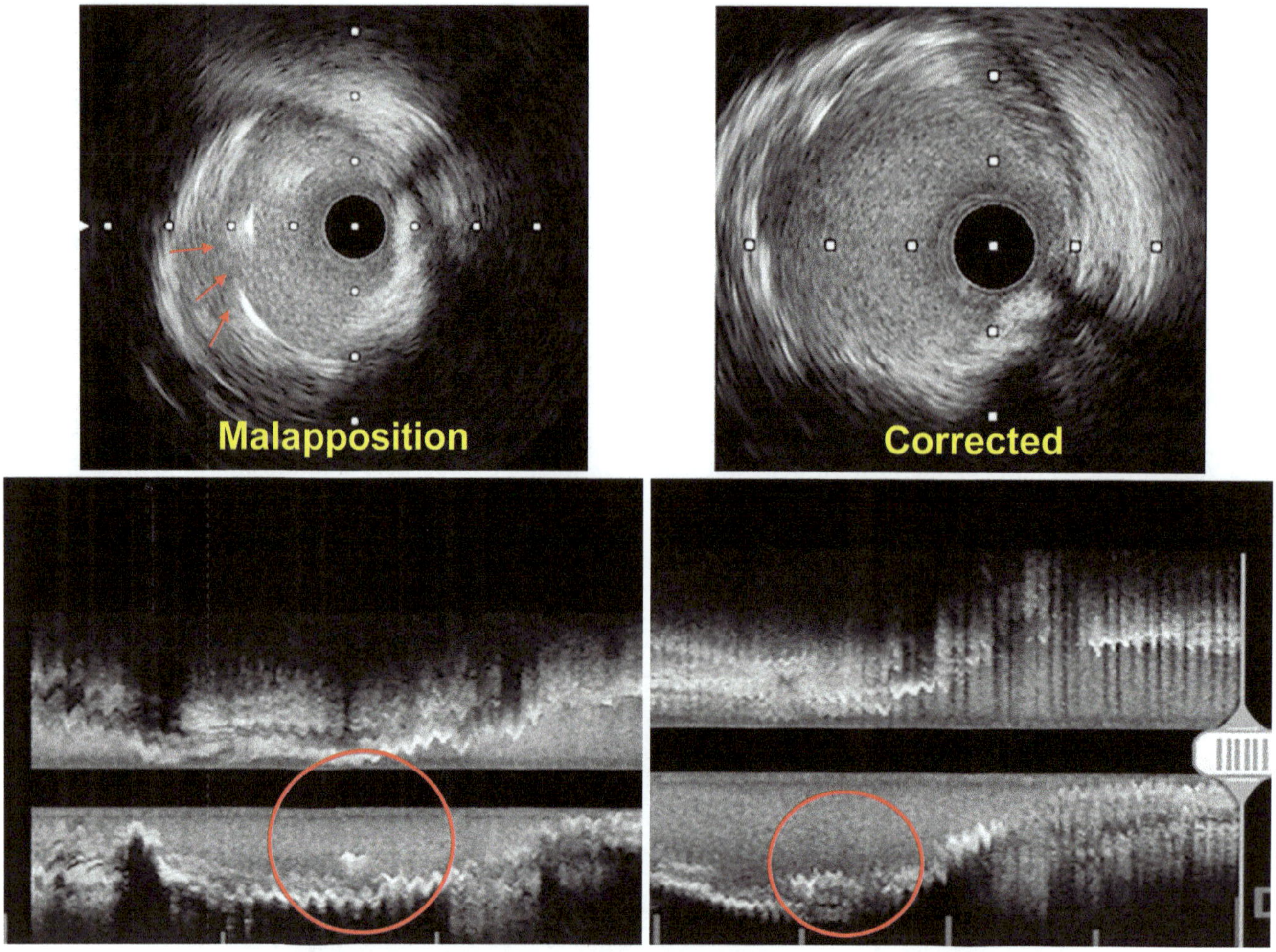

Malapposition

Corrected

Fig. 2: Malapposition seen in both short axis and L view and corrected.

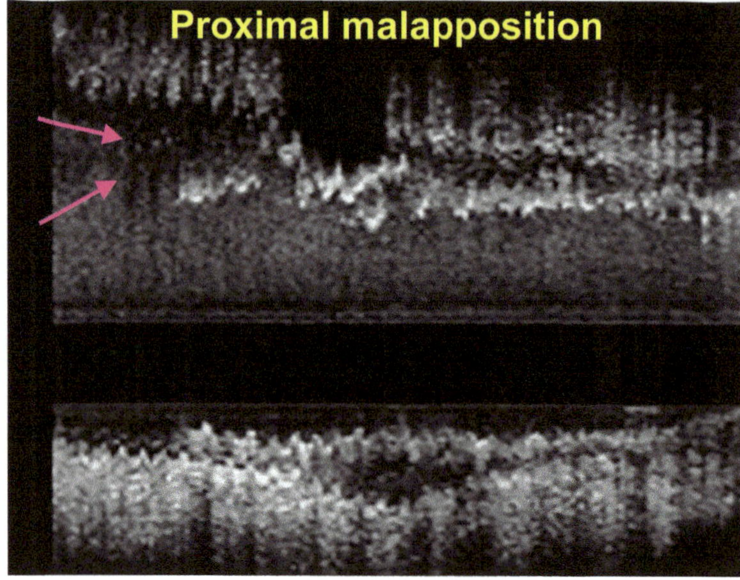

Fig. 3: Proximal malapposition seen in L view.

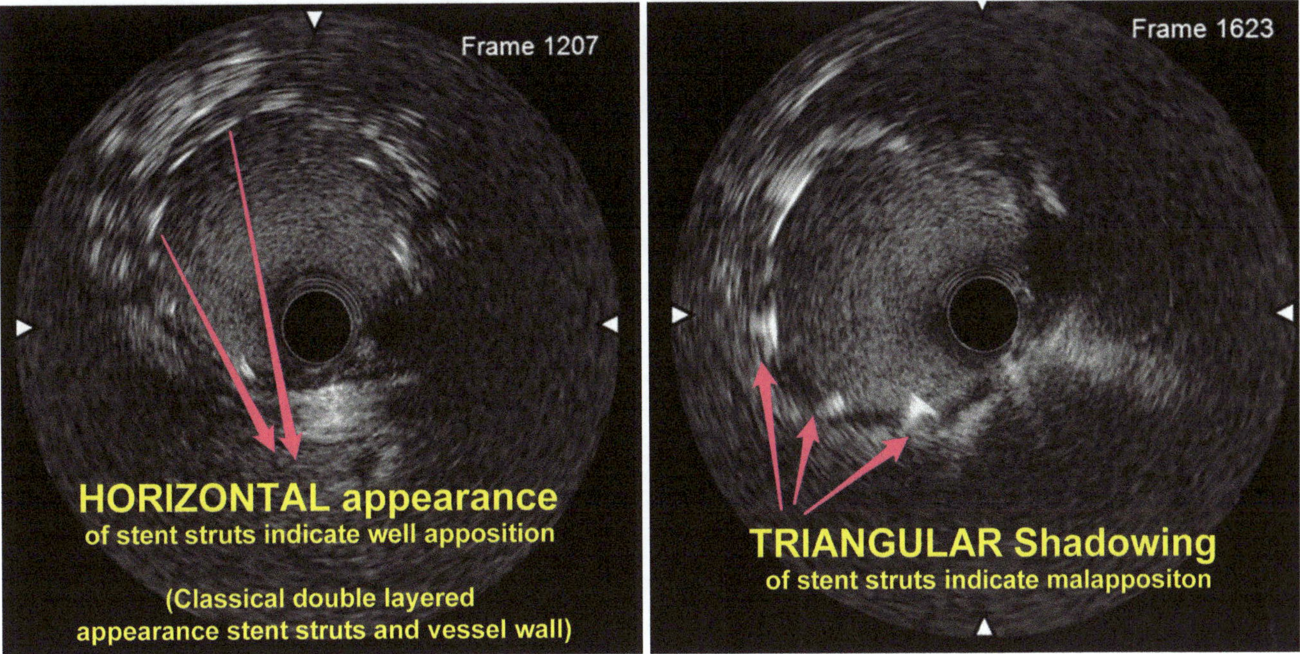

Fig. 4: Triangular shadow of stent struts indicating malapposition.

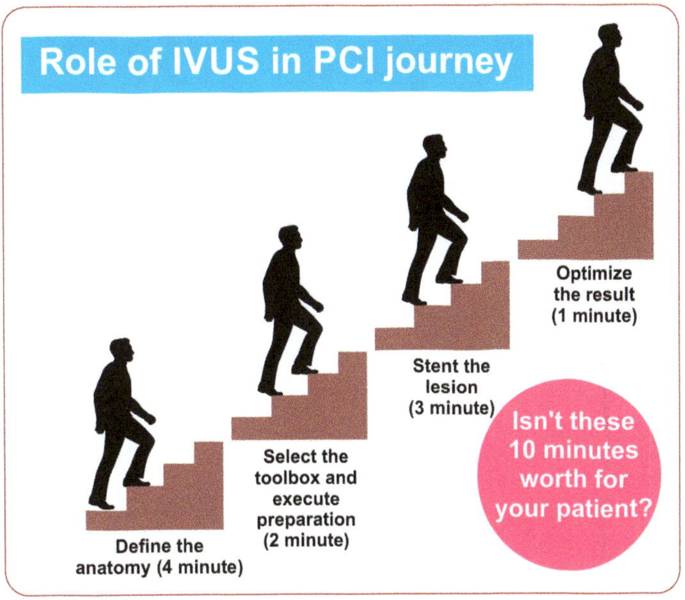

CHAPTER 20

Dissection Assessment on Intravascular Ultrasound

Dissection is a tear in the plaque parallel to the vessel wall with visualization of blood flow in the false lumen **(Fig. 1)**.

Whenever you see a dissection on intravascular ultrasound (IVUS), you have to tell these seven things **(Figs. 2 and 3)**:

1. **Axial extension:** It means intimal or medial or adventitial (any medial extension is significant)
2. **Circumferential:** It means the degree angle of arc (angle >60 is significant). (*See* **Fig. 4** to see how to measure dissection angle)
3. **Length** measure on longitudinal axis (length >5 mm significant)
4. **Intramural hematoma (IMH)** present or not
5. **Minimum lumen area (MLA)** at the dissection site (any MLA <4 mm significant)
6. **Pericardial or myocardial side** (pericardial is more dangerous than myocardial since surrounding muscle may constrain propagation in myocardial side)
7. Retrograde dissections are more forgiving than antegrade dissections **(Fig. 5)**

Any dissection occurring <5 mm to a stent edge is termed as stent edge dissection **(Fig. 6)**.

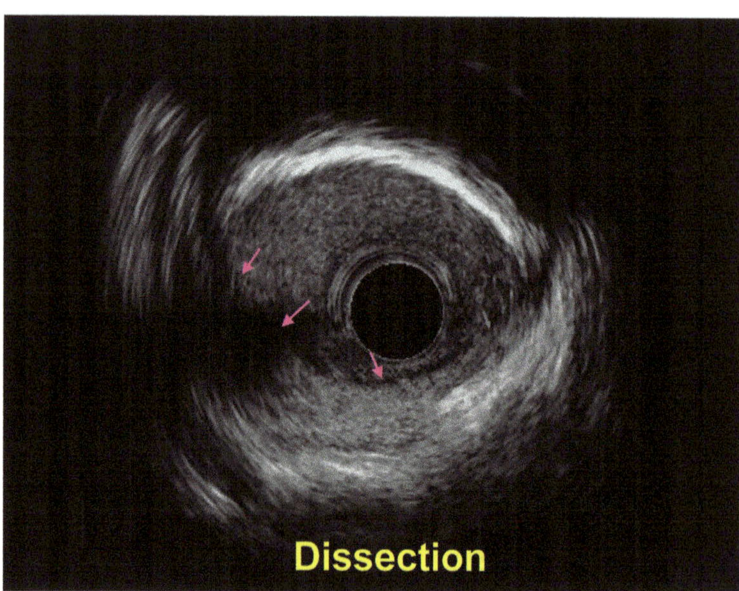

Fig. 1: Dissection on intravascular ultrasound (IVUS).

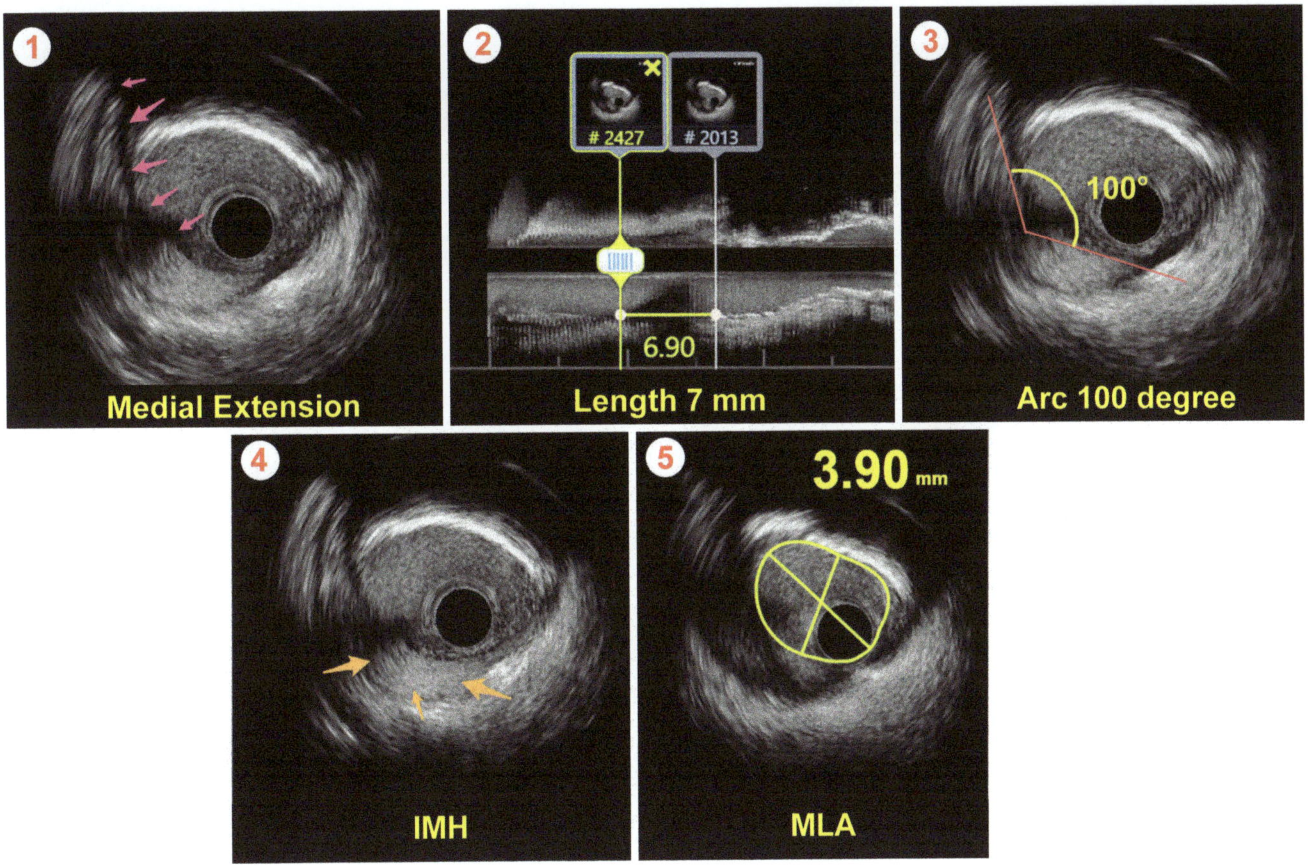

1
Medial Extension
2
2427
2013
6.90
Length 7 mm
3
100°
Arc 100 degree
4
IMH
5
3.90 mm
MLA

Fig. 2: Things to be looked for in a dissection.

Frame 37
2: IMH
1: Medial dissection
3: Arc >90°
5: MLA 5.1 mm
8 mm
4: Length of dissection >8 mm

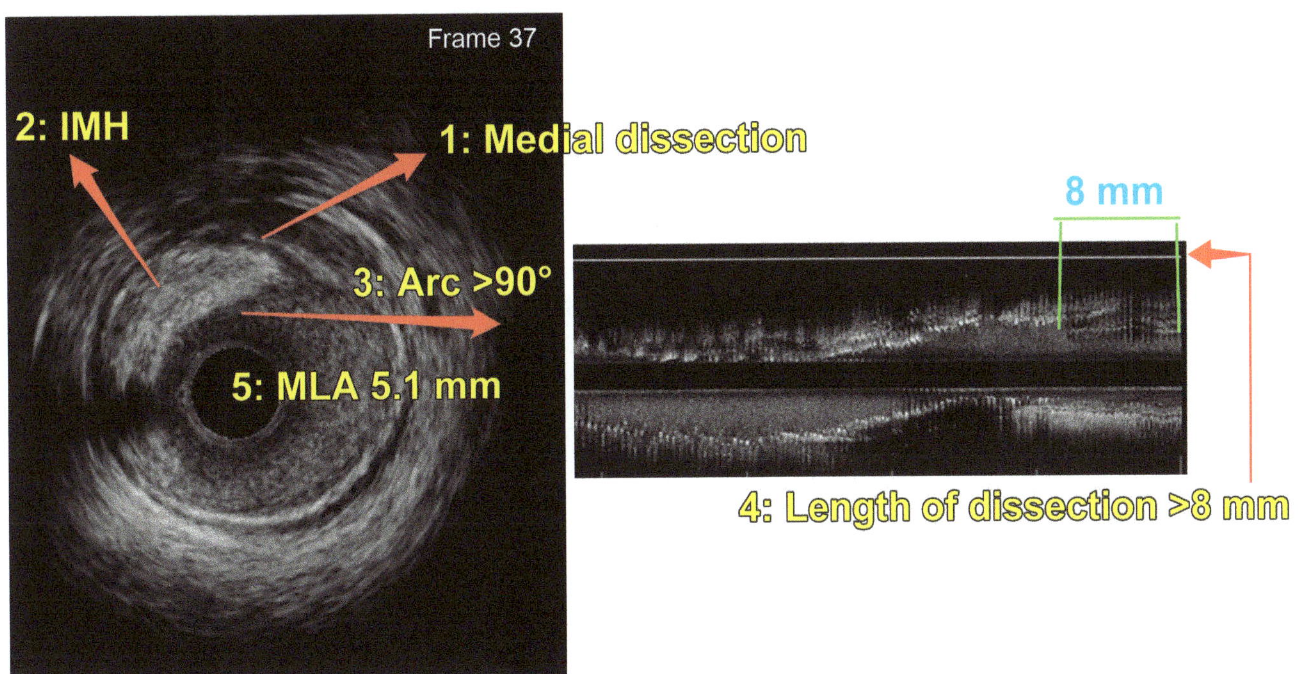

Fig. 3: Things to be looked for in this dissection. (IMH: intramural hematoma)

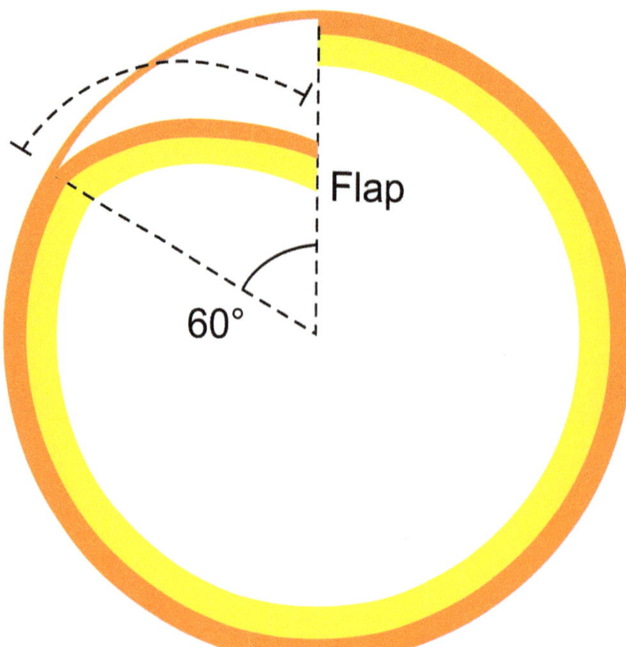

Fig. 4: How to measure dissection angle.

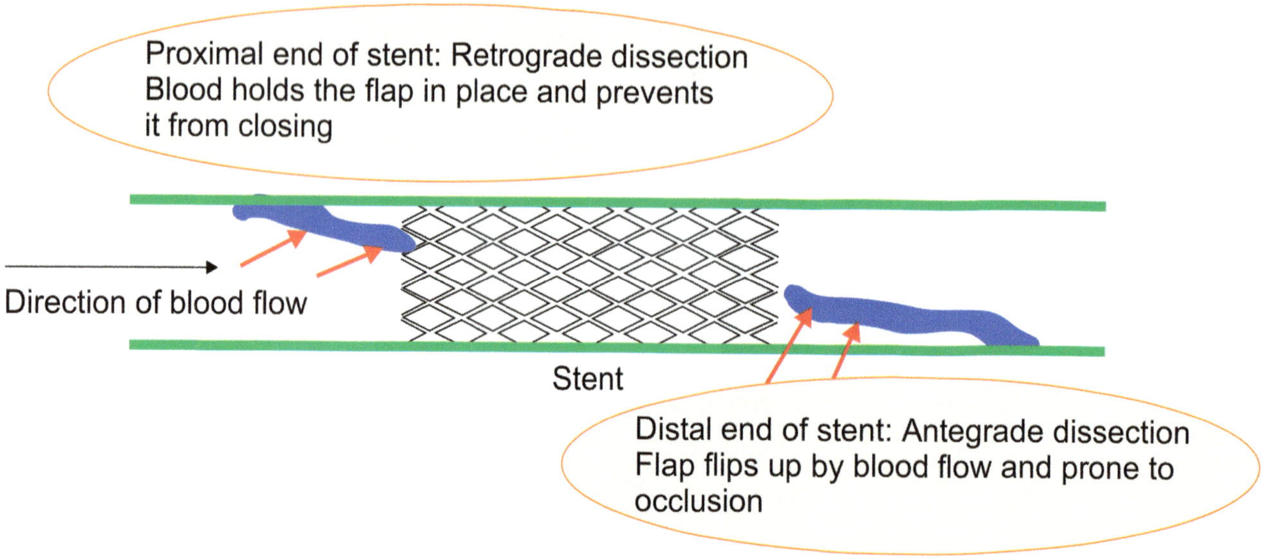

Proximal end of stent: Retrograde dissection
Blood holds the flap in place and prevents
it from closing

Direction of blood flow

Stent

Distal end of stent: Antegrade dissection
Flap flips up by blood flow and prone to
occlusion

Fig. 5: In retrograde dissections, the direction of blood hold the flap in place and prevent it from closing where as in antegrade dissection the flap fills up by blood flow and can cause occlusion.

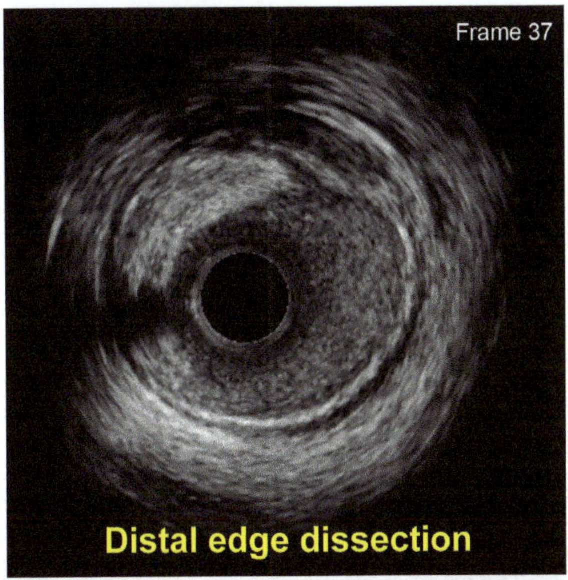

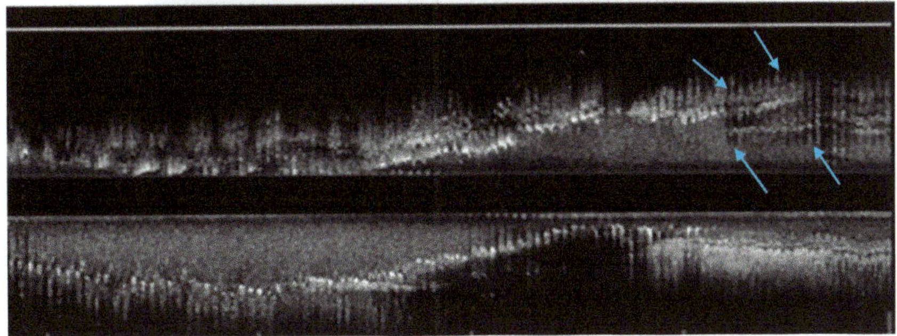

Fig. 6: Stent edge dissection.

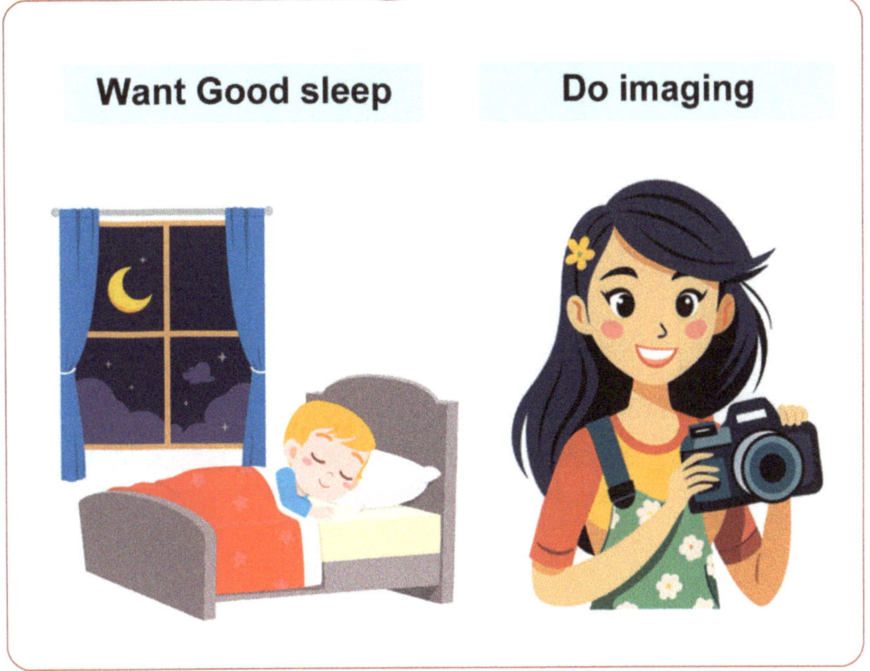

CHAPTER 21

Intramural and Extramural Hematoma

Intramural hematoma (IMH) can be defined as collection of blood within the medial space. If reentry is not created in a dissection that extends to the media, the distal end where the dissection occurs becomes a blind end, causing blood accumulation in the dissection cavity and formation of a hematoma. It occurs more often in the eccentric and less plaque areas. The external elastic membrane (EEM) is pushed backward while intima is pushed inward to cause lumen compromise.

On high-definition intravascular ultrasound (HD IVUS) it appears as hyperechoic crescent (helmet) shape homogenous opacity within the medial space **(Figs. 1 and 2)**. Whenever we see IMH try to define the entry and exit point **(Fig. 3)**.

Five types of IMH are worse:

1. Entry site not covered
2. Antegrade hematoma
3. Hematoma entering in normal segment (meaning no calcium, no side branch, etc.)
4. Extramural hematoma
5. Vessel size small

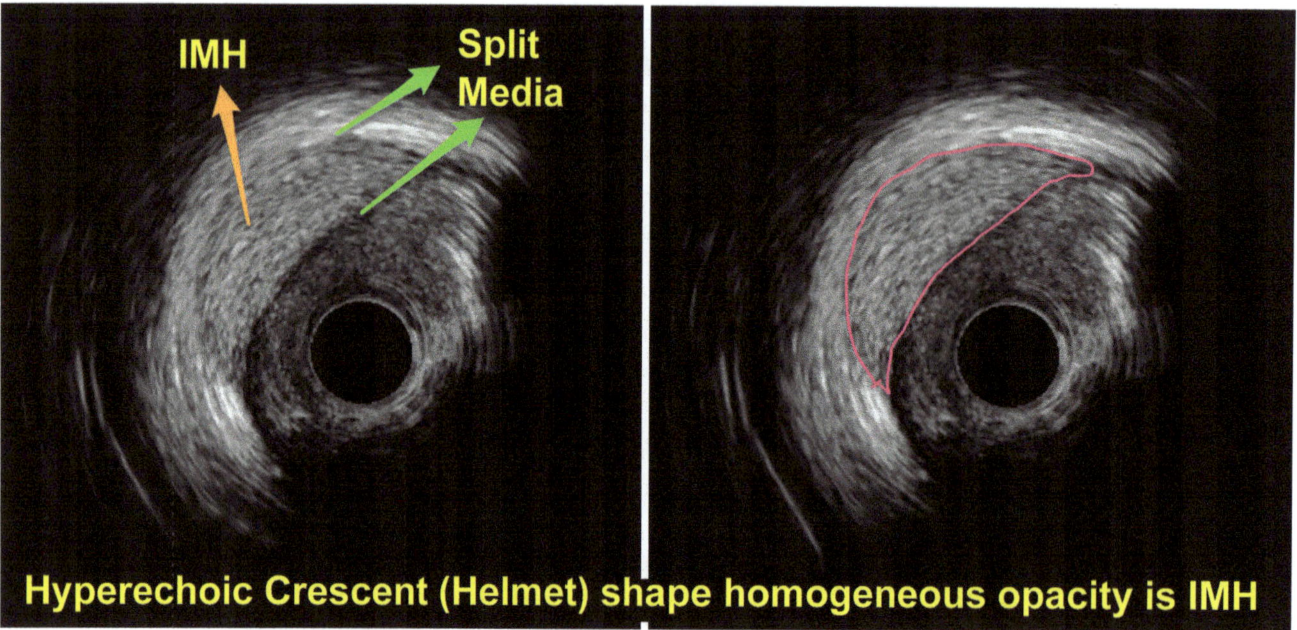

Fig. 1: Intramural hematoma (IMH).

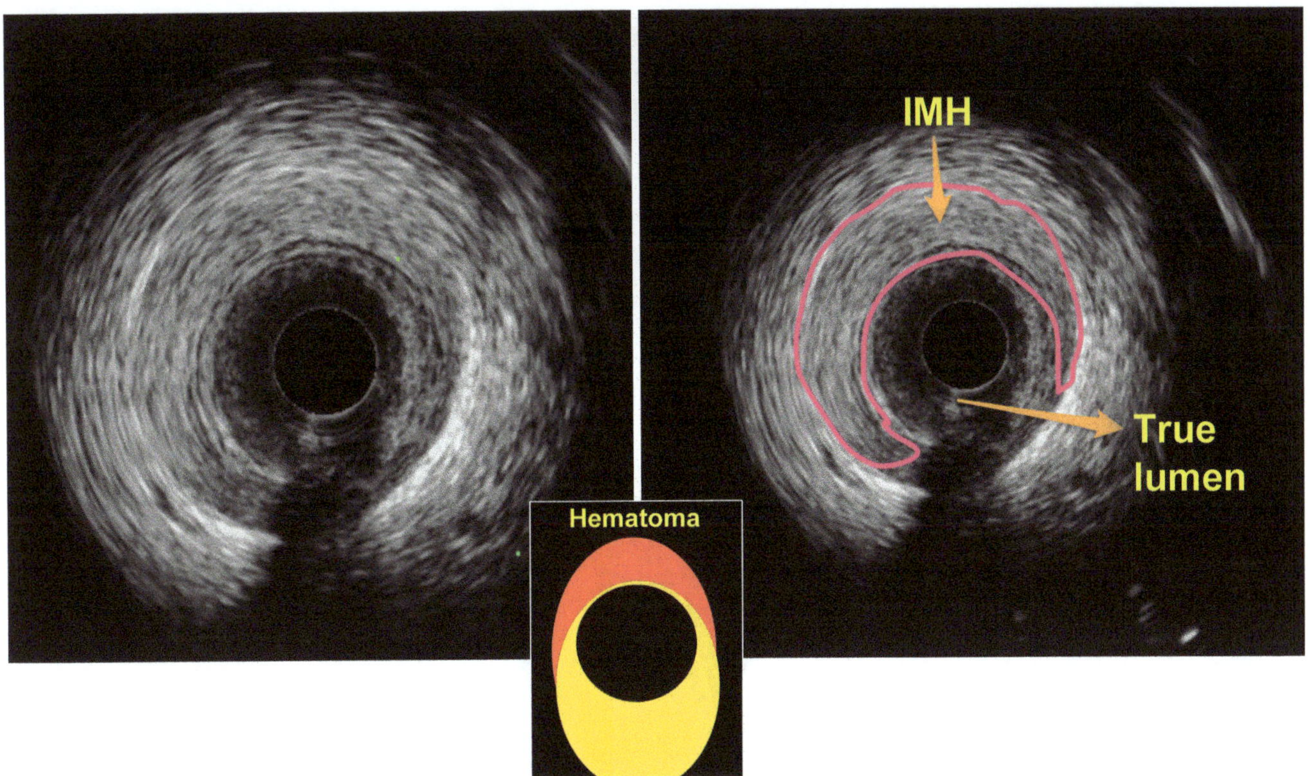

Fig. 2: Intramural hematoma compressing the true lumen.

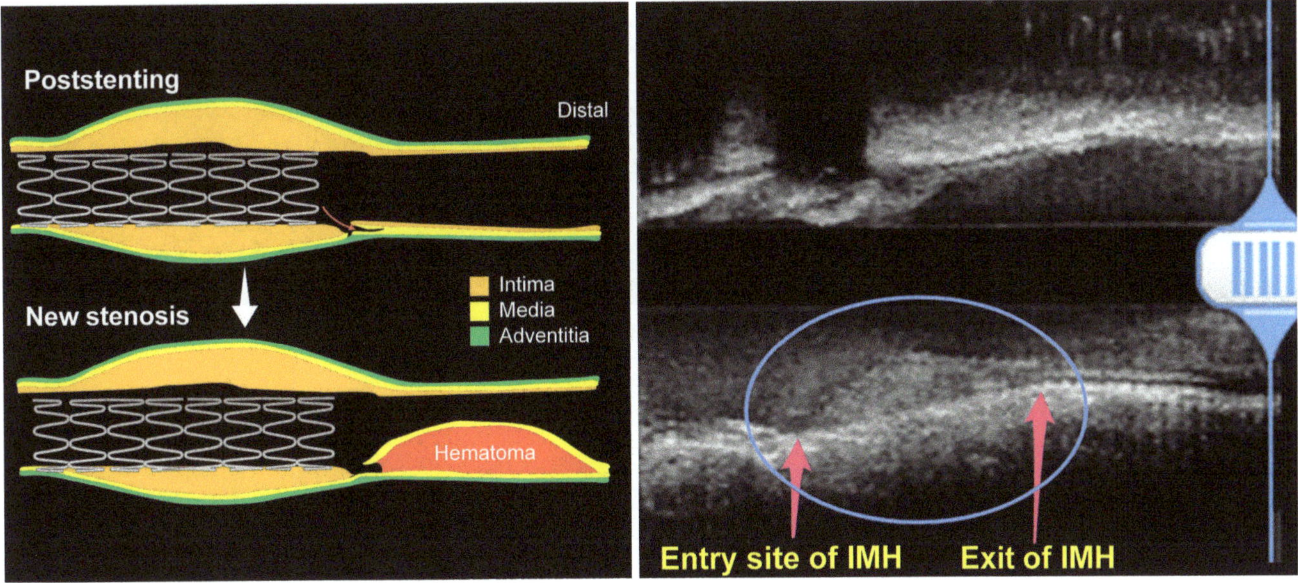

Fig. 3: The mechanism of intramural hematoma (IMH) with entry and exit point.

Utility of IVUS in IMH:

- Identifying the exact location of IMH
- Marking its exact entry and exit point
- Asssessing its impact on side branches.
- Development of treatment strategies without the use of contrast media, such as determining vessel diameter at the hematoma site to guide the selection of a cutting balloon for decompression the hematoma.

WHAT IS EXTRAMURAL HEMATOMA?

It is extravasation of blood or contrast, which may appear as echodense structure outside the vessel wall which happens due to adventitial dissection. This indicates that either this is already a contained perforation or an impending perforation **(Fig. 4)**.

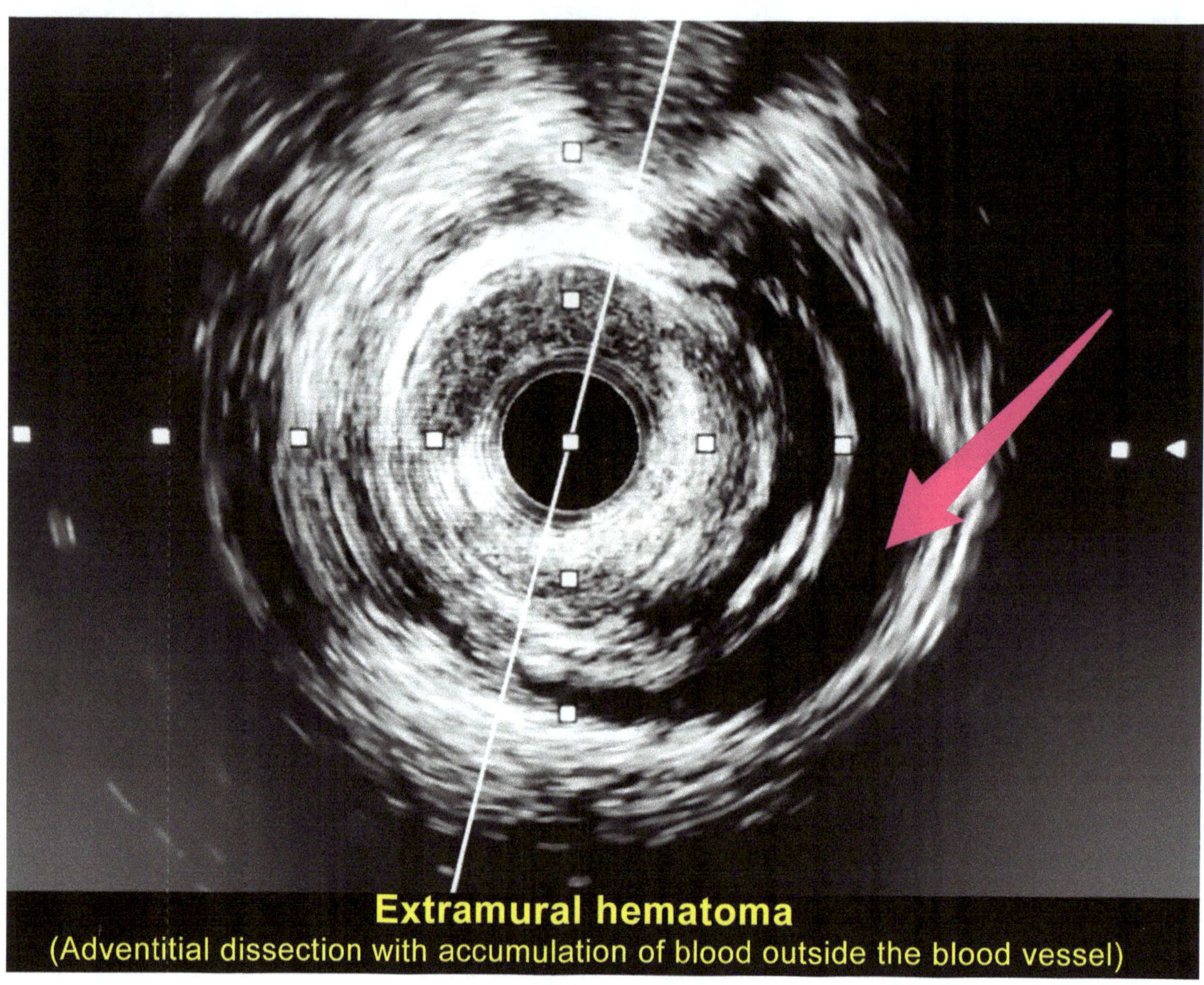

Fig. 4: Extramural hematoma.

"IVUS – because sometimes, the road to a healthy heart needs a GPS!"

CHAPTER 22

Geographical Miss on Intravascular Ultrasound

The term "geographical miss" is used when a stent misses the proper landing zone. The ideal landing zone should have a plaque burden of <50% with no lipidic plaque or calcium within 5 mm of the stent edge on both sides. Geographical miss is considered one of the predictors of stent failure **(Fig. 1)**.

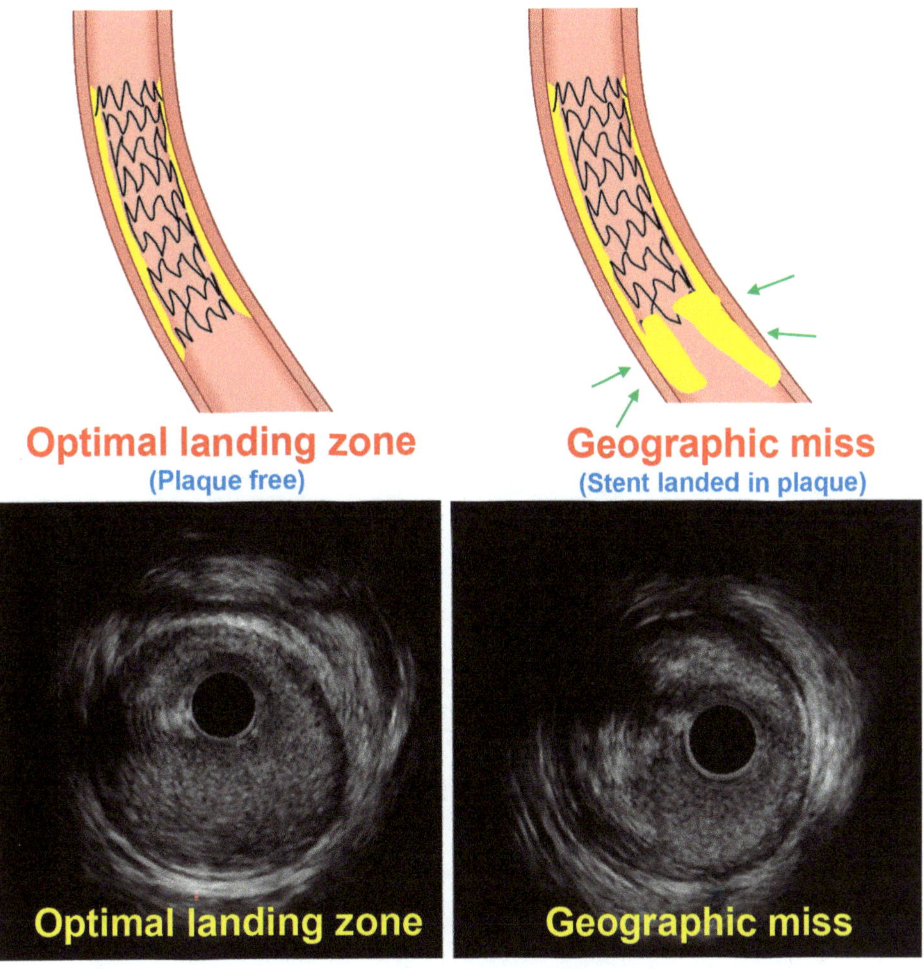

Fig. 2: Optimal landing zone and geographic miss.

"Trying to solve coronary mysteries? IVUS is your X-ray vision without the cape."

CHAPTER 23

Tissue/Plaque Prolapse

Tissue prolapse (TP) is defined as tissue extrusion through the stent struts assessed postintervention. The accurate discrimination of atherosclerotic plaque and thrombus within stent is very difficult because of limited resolution of intravascular ultrasound (IVUS). Thus, TP includes plaque and/or thrombus extrusion within stent. A few examples of TP are given in **Figures 1A and B**.

The volume of TP can be calculated by taking a ratio of total protrusion area to total minimal stent area (MSA). In this case **(Fig. 2)**, the protrusion area is around 1.98 mm

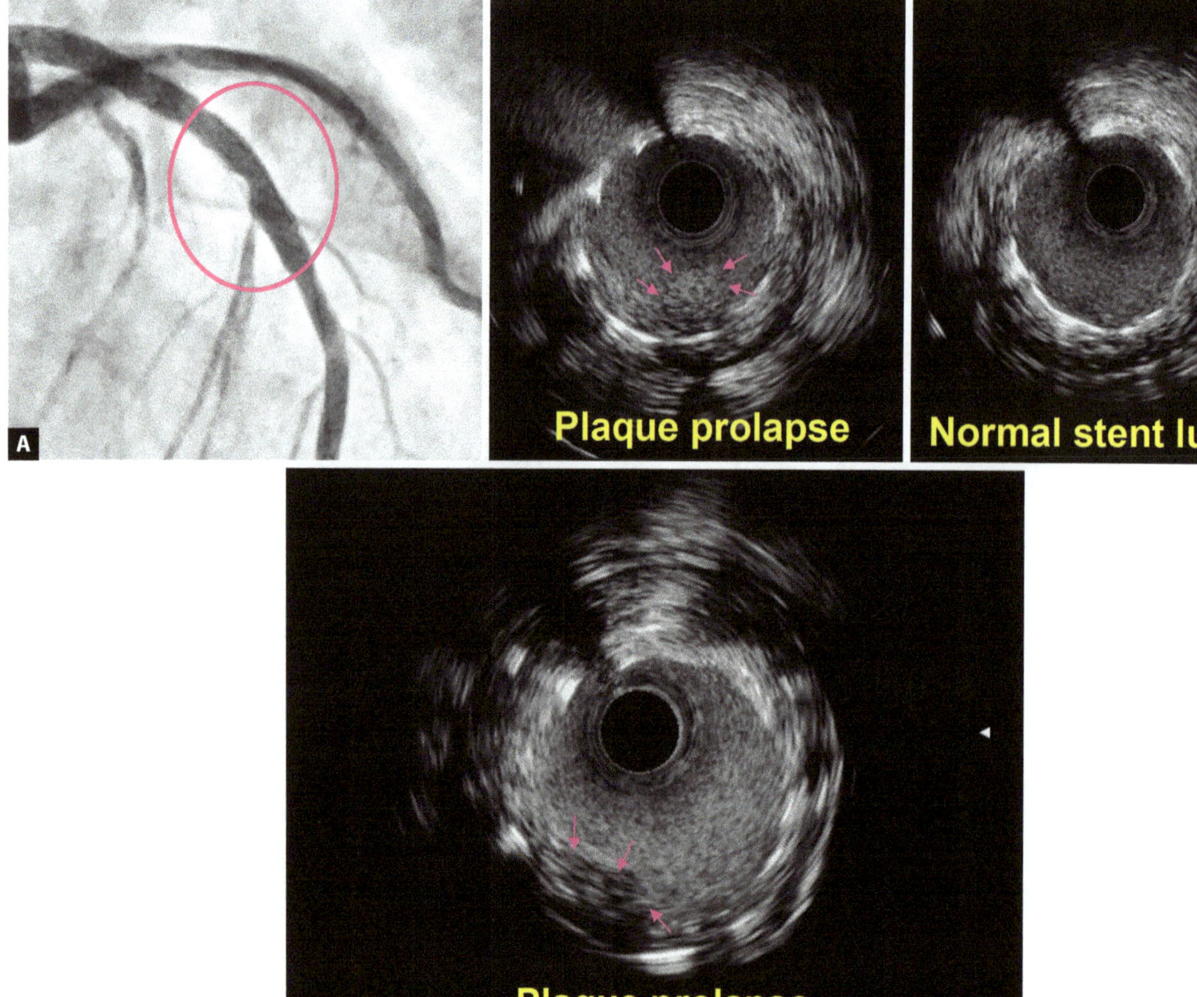

Figs. 1A and B: Tissue/plaque prolapse seen on intravascular ultrasound (IVUS).

and MSA is 10.05 mm. Therefore, the total protrusion volume % will be 1.98/10.05 = 20%. Any protrusion volume >10% requires treatment. Calculating the ratio of protrusion area to MSA helps determine the necessity of treatment for protrusion volumes.

Tissue prolapse usually disappears with time and is not associated with stent failure. But there are a few that require treatment such as:

- Protrusion area or volume >10%
- MSA <4.5
- Irregular TP >500 μm

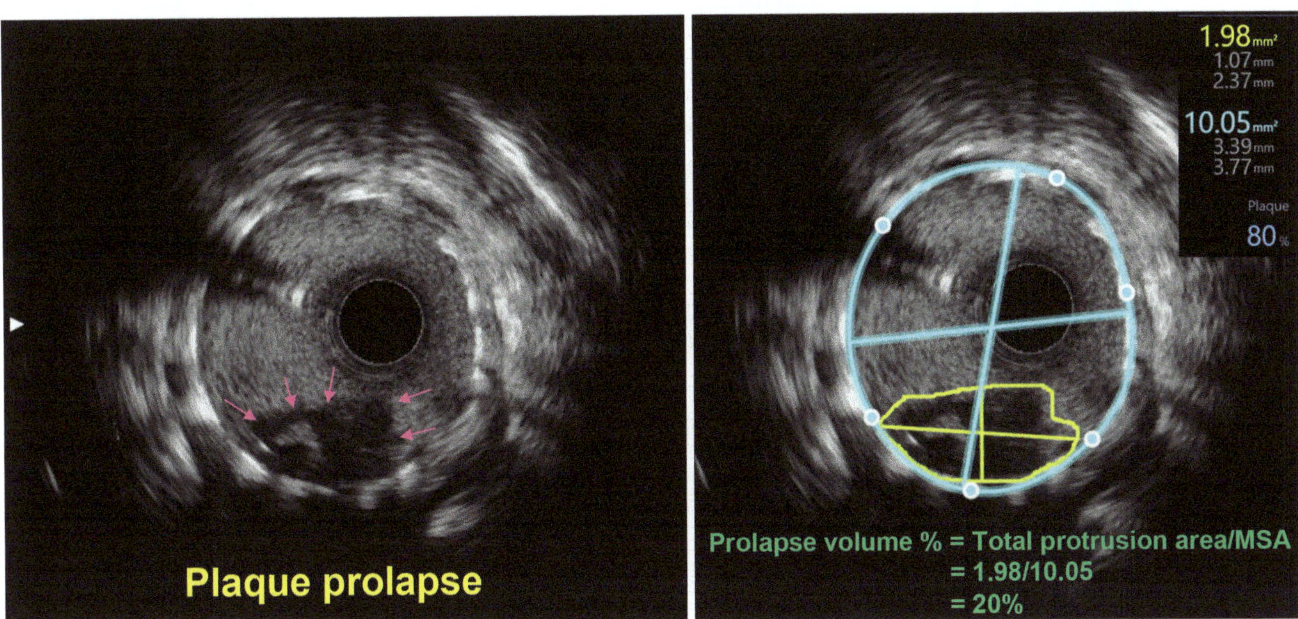

Fig. 2: Total protrusion volume % calculation. (MSA: minimal stent area)

CHAPTER 24

Intravascular Ultrasound in In-stent Restenosis

Intravascular imaging is a must in all cases of in-stent restenosis (ISR) since it helps us in identifying the cause of restenosis so that the treatment can be planned accordingly. It can be basically because of four reasons:

1. Stent fracture
2. Under expansion **(Fig. 1)**
3. Neointimal hyperplasia **(Fig. 2)**
4. Neoatherosclerosis **(Fig. 3)**

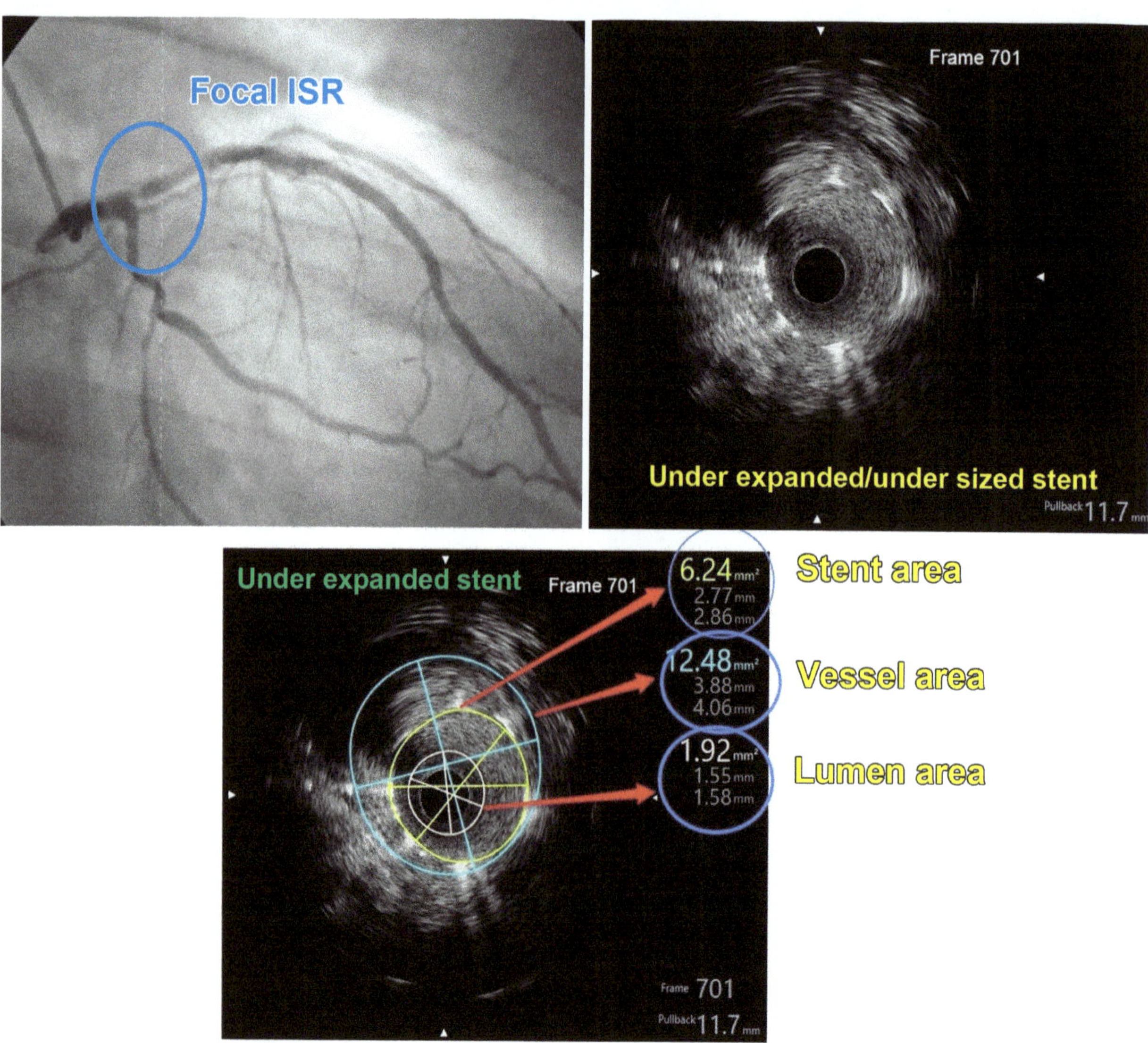

Fig. 1: Underexpansion as the mechanism of in-stent restenosis (ISR).

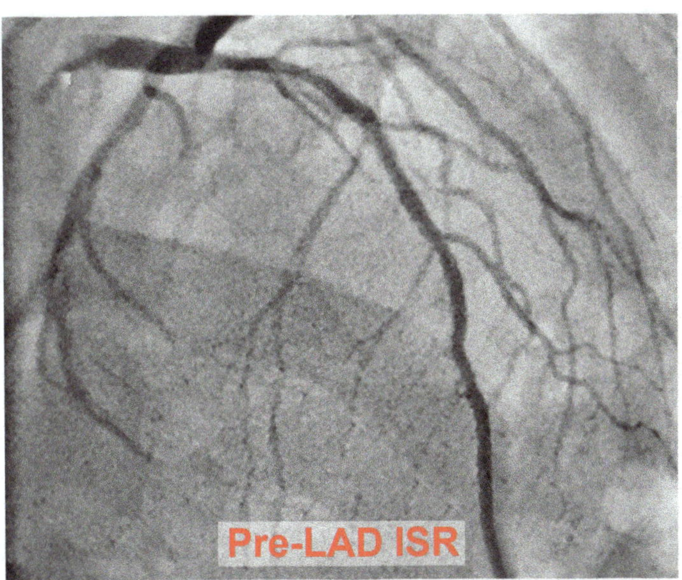

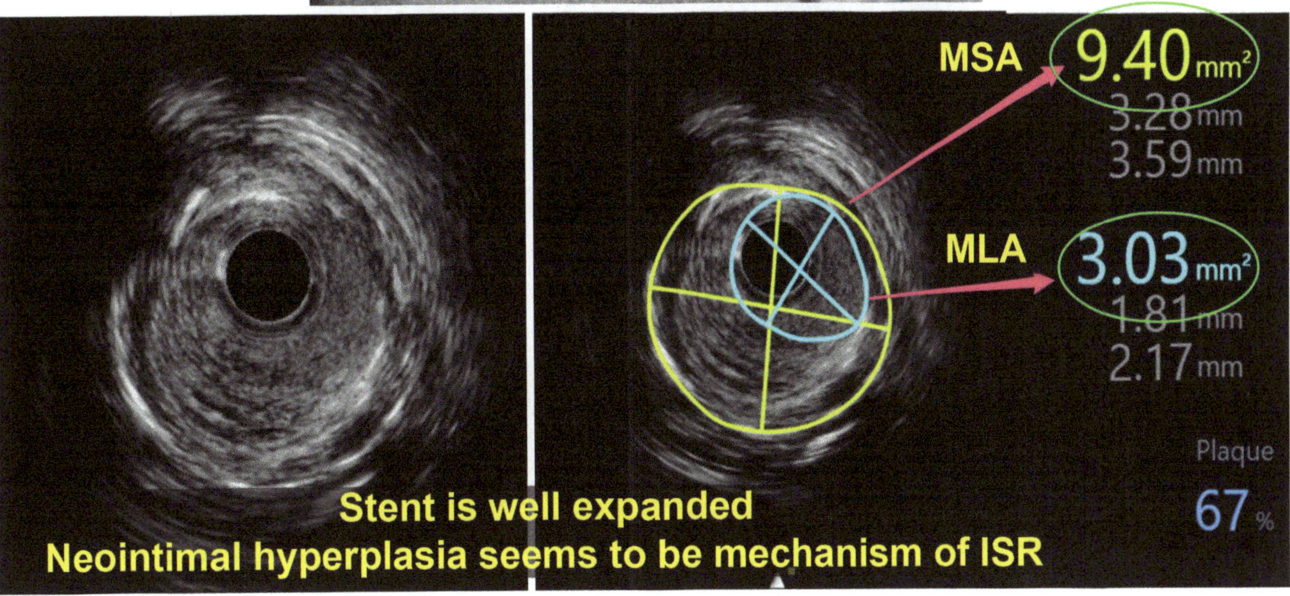

Fig. 2: Under NIH as the mechanism of ISR. (ISR: in-stent restenosis; LAD: left anterior descending; MLA: minimal lumen area; MSA: minimal stent area; NIH: neointimal hyperplasia)

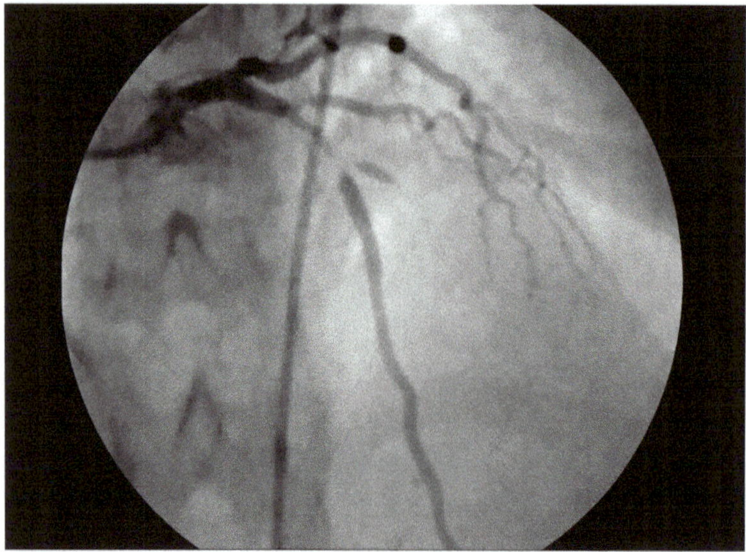

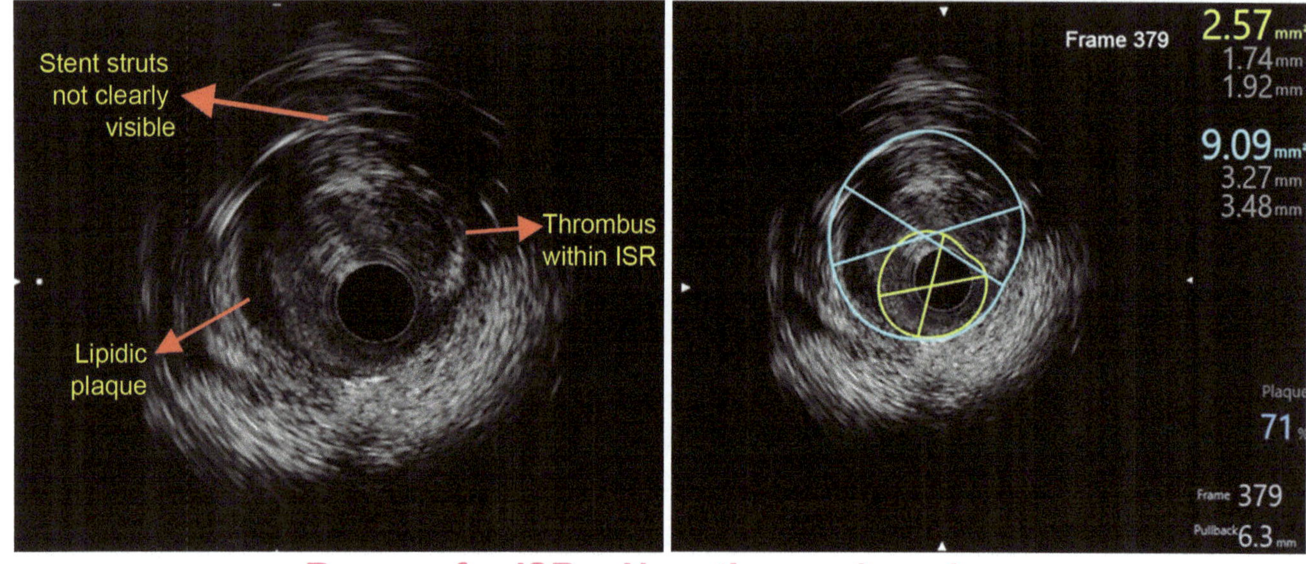

Fig. 3: Neoatherosclerosis as the mechanism of ISR. (ISR: in-stent restenosis; MSA: minimal stent area)

Differentiating neoatherosclerosis from neointimal hyperplasia is difficult on intravascular ultrasound (IVUS), but there are certain indicators on high-definition (HD) IVUS which can suggest that it is neoatherosclerosis:

- Presence of calcium within the ISR segment **(Fig. 4)**
- Thrombus visible
- Intrastent dissection defined as a disruption of the vessel luminal surface within the stent segment **(Fig. 5)**
- Plaque rupture in ISR **(Fig. 6)**
- Heterogeneous appearance (weak sign)
- Presence of lipid in ISR
- Stent struts not visible **(Fig. 4)**

(All these features suggest neoatherosclerosis is the possible mechanism of ISR)

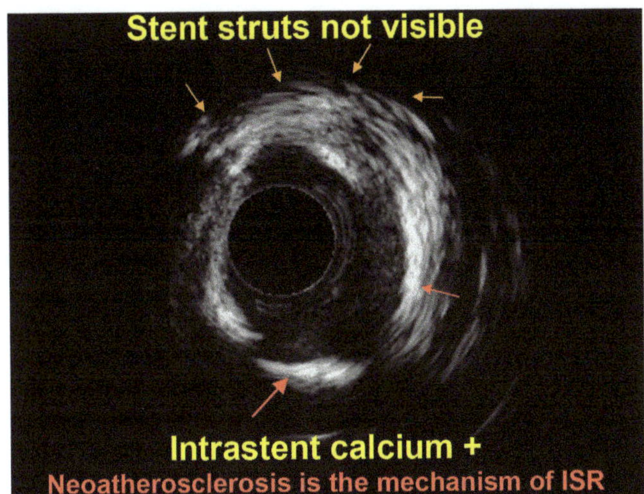

Fig. 4: Intrastent calcium seen plus lack of visibility of stent struts seen suggesting neoatherosclerosis as the mechanism of in-stent restenosis (ISR).

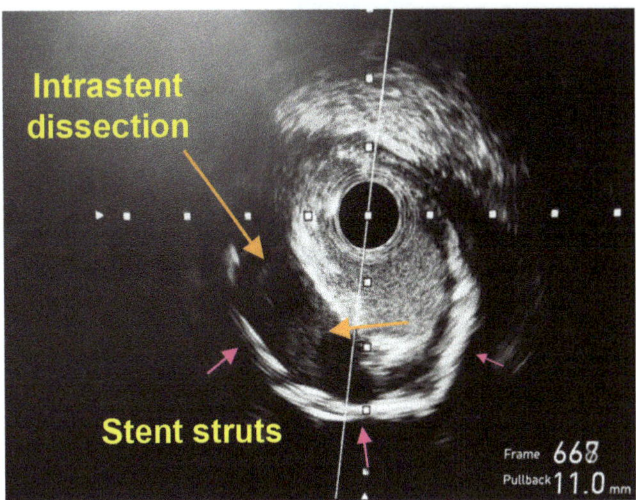

Fig. 5: Intrastent dissection.

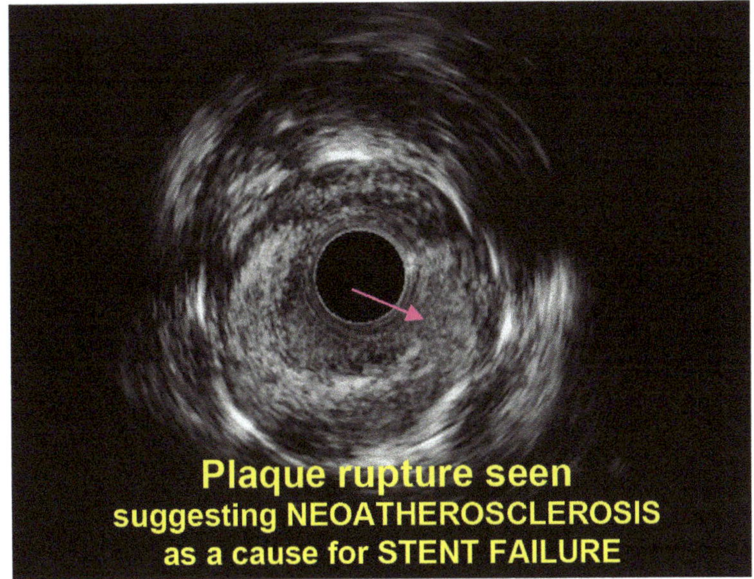

Fig. 6: Plaque rupture seen suggesting neoatherosclerosis as the mechanism of in-stent restenosis (ISR).

CHAPTER 25

Goals for Left Main Stenting: In Pursuit for the Magic Numbers

The main goal of left main (LM) stenting is to achieve a good minimum stent area (MSA) after LM bifurcation angioplasty for a positive long-term prognosis. In the past, we used to follow the Kang's criteria of 5-6-7-8 and then the EXCEL criteria of 6-7-10 but now in the current era, the MSAs to aim for are 6, 8, and 10 for left circumflex (LCX), left anterior descending (LAD), and left main coronary artery (LMCA), respectively **(Fig. 1)**. Additionally, if possible achieving a score of 7, 9, and 12 for the respective arteries may be more beneficial. Attaining these MSA targets is crucial for successful LM stenting and positive patient outcomes. The pursuit for these "magic numbers" is essential for the effectiveness of the procedure.

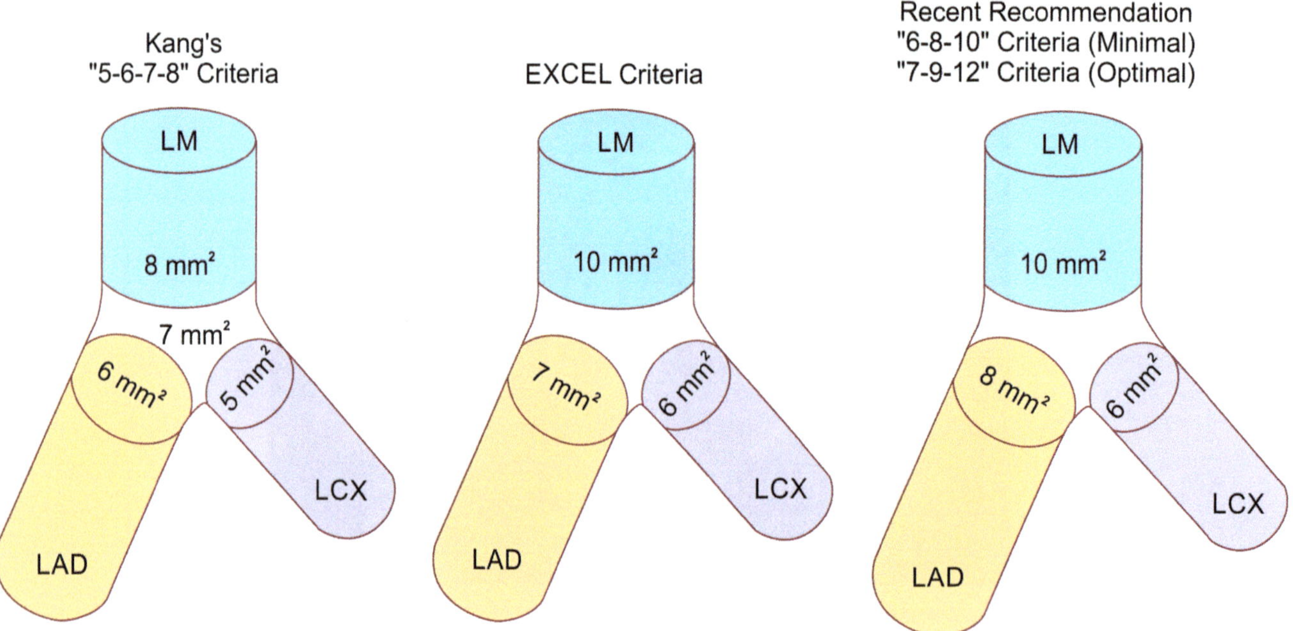

Fig. 1: Target MSAs for LMCA stenting. (LAD: left anterior descending; LCX: left circumflex; LM: left main; LMCA: left main coronary artery; MSAs: minimum stent areas)

"Be precise, lack of precision is dangerous when the margin of error is small"

CHAPTER 26

Intravascular Ultrasound in Ambiguous Left Main

Assessment of left main (LM) disease by angiography represents a particularly difficult clinical problem. Aortic cusp opacification or "streaming" of contrast may obscure the ostium. The short length of the vessel may leave no normal segment for comparison, and the distal LM artery may be concealed by the left anterior descending-left circumflex (LAD-LCX) bifurcation. In these situations, intravascular ultrasound (IVUS) can often provide additional information.

When we do IVUS to evaluate ambiguous left main coronary artery (LMCA), there are three possibilities **(Fig. 1)**:

1. Minimal lumen area (MLA) <4.5 mm (in that case, revascularize)
2. MLA >6.0 mm (defer revascularization)
3. MLA 4.5–6.0 mm [in that case, go for fractional flow reserve (FFR)]

If we see in **Figure 2**, angiographically it looked like a tight ostial LMCA, but on IVUS, it turned out to be noncritical with an MLA of around 6 mm. Even the FFR done, which was negative.

If we see in **Figure 3**, angiographically it does not look like a significant diseased LMCA, but on IVUS, it turned out to be critical with an MLA of around 4 mm **(Fig. 3)**.

Intravascular ultrasound can distinguish between true and pseudostenosis of LMCA caused by extrinsic compression, as illustrated by a case of LMCA compression by an enlarged pulmonary artery **(Fig. 4)**. **Key indicators of pseudostenosis due to extrinsic compression include:**

1. Dynamic compression
2. Absence of atherosclerosis
3. The whole vessel area is reduced, not the lumen area alone
4. Afolded appearance of the artery (circumferential blackout outside, visible media in the middle).

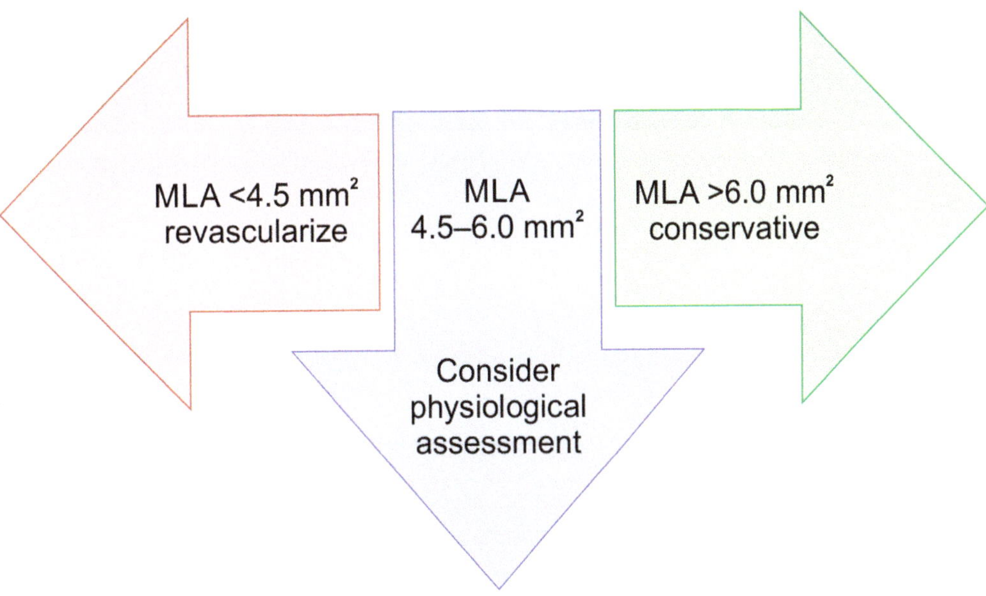

Fig. 1: Approach based on left main coronary artery (LMCA) minimal lumen area (MLA).

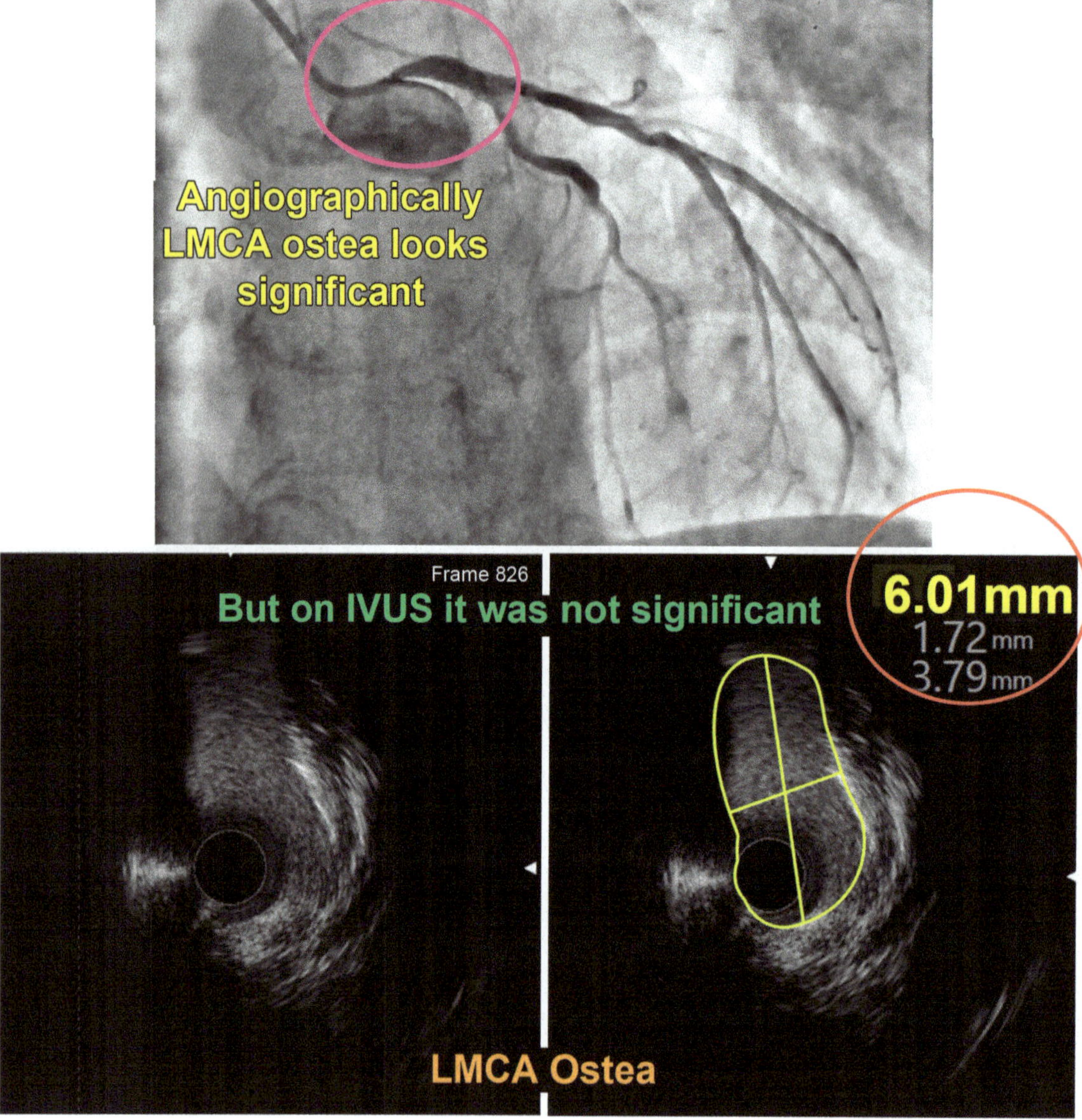

Fig. 2: Ambiguous left main coronary artery (LMCA) with intravascular ultrasound (IVUS) correlation.

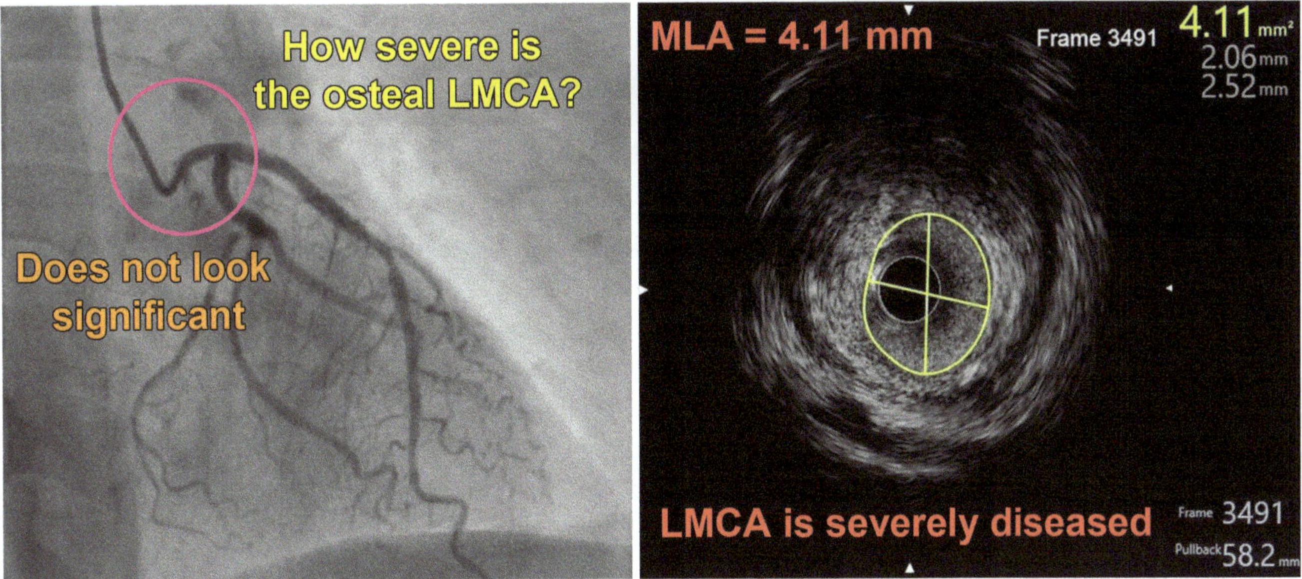

Fig. 3: Discrepancy in assessing the severity of LMCA between IVUS and angiography.

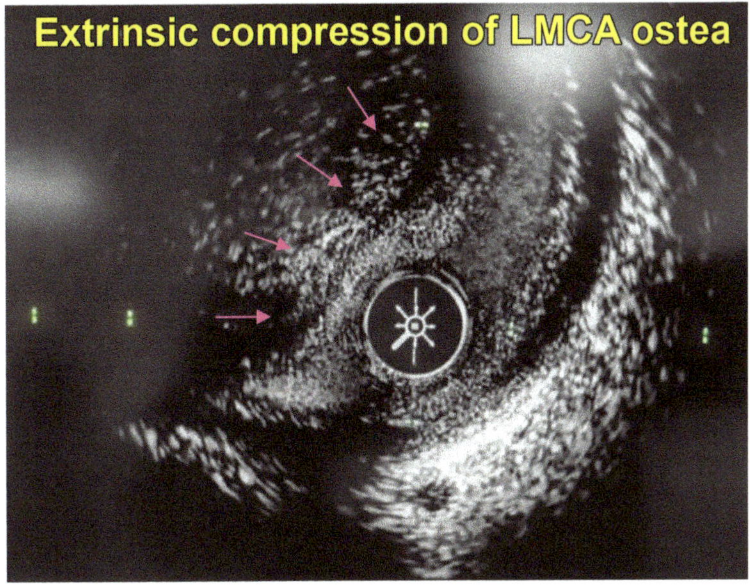

Fig. 4: Dilated pulmonary artery causing extrinsic compression of left main coronary artery (LMCA).

"Angiogram lies in the worst ways—it hides the things we need to know the most!"

CHAPTER 27

Intravascular Ultrasound in Deciding Two- versus One-stent in Left Main Coronary Artery Bifurcation

INTRAVASCULAR ULTRASOUND IN DECIDING UPFRONT TWO-STENT STRATEGY OR PROVISIONAL STENT STRATEGY IN A CASE OF LEFT MAIN CORONARY ARTERY BIFURCATION

In left main coronary artery (LMCA) lesions, intravascular ultrasound (IVUS) should be used initially to assess lesion characteristics and plaque distribution. Plaque in the left main coronary artery is typically found in the opposite portion of the carina. If there is plaque in the direction of the side branch or severe stenosis at the ostium, there is a high risk of side branch occlusion after stent placement **(Fig. 1)**.

In all cases of LMCA bifurcation, one should do a pullback from both the LAD and LCX. Studies have shown that if the preprocedural minimal lumen area (MLA) at the left circumflex (LCX) ostia is >3.7 mm and plaque burden (PB) <56% and length of lesion is <10 mm the need for a second stent after provisional approach is less.

For example, if we see **Figure 2**, both Cases 1 and 2 are LMCA bifurcation, and it is difficult to decide based on angiography alone. But when we do IVUS, it is clear in Case 1 that MLA at the LCX ostia is fine (9 mm). So, this is a good case for provisional stenting, whereas if we see the MLA of LCX in Case 2, it is around 2 mm and the length is >16 mm, suggesting that this is not a suitable case for provisional stenting, and one must go for upfront two-stent strategy.

Also, there are certain predictors of side branch (SB) pinching on IVUS such as eyebrow sign, BP-CT length <1.7 mm, calcium in the MB, opposite side branch, lipid-rich plaque at the ostia of SB, distal or circumferential plaque distribution of SB, etc. (*See* Chapter 28). If these signs are present, then one may think of opting for an upfront 2-stent strategy.

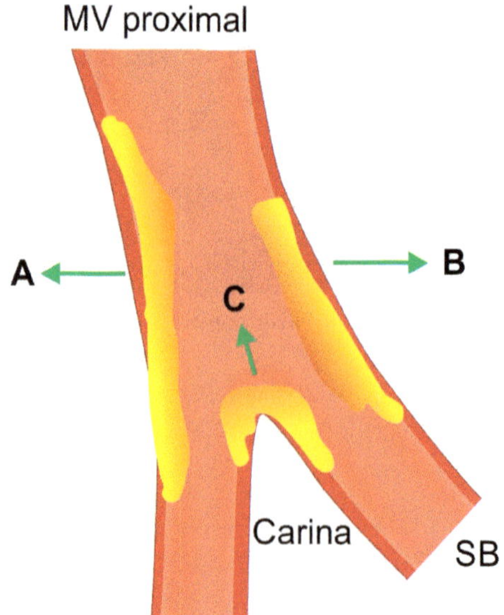

Fig. 1: Plaque distribution at bifurcation based on IVUS. (A) Plaque present on the opposite side of carina (MB). (B) Plaque is present in the direction of side branch (SB) and extends into the origin of SB. (C) Plaque is present on the carina side of SB. B and C will have high chance of SB occlusion after MB stenting.

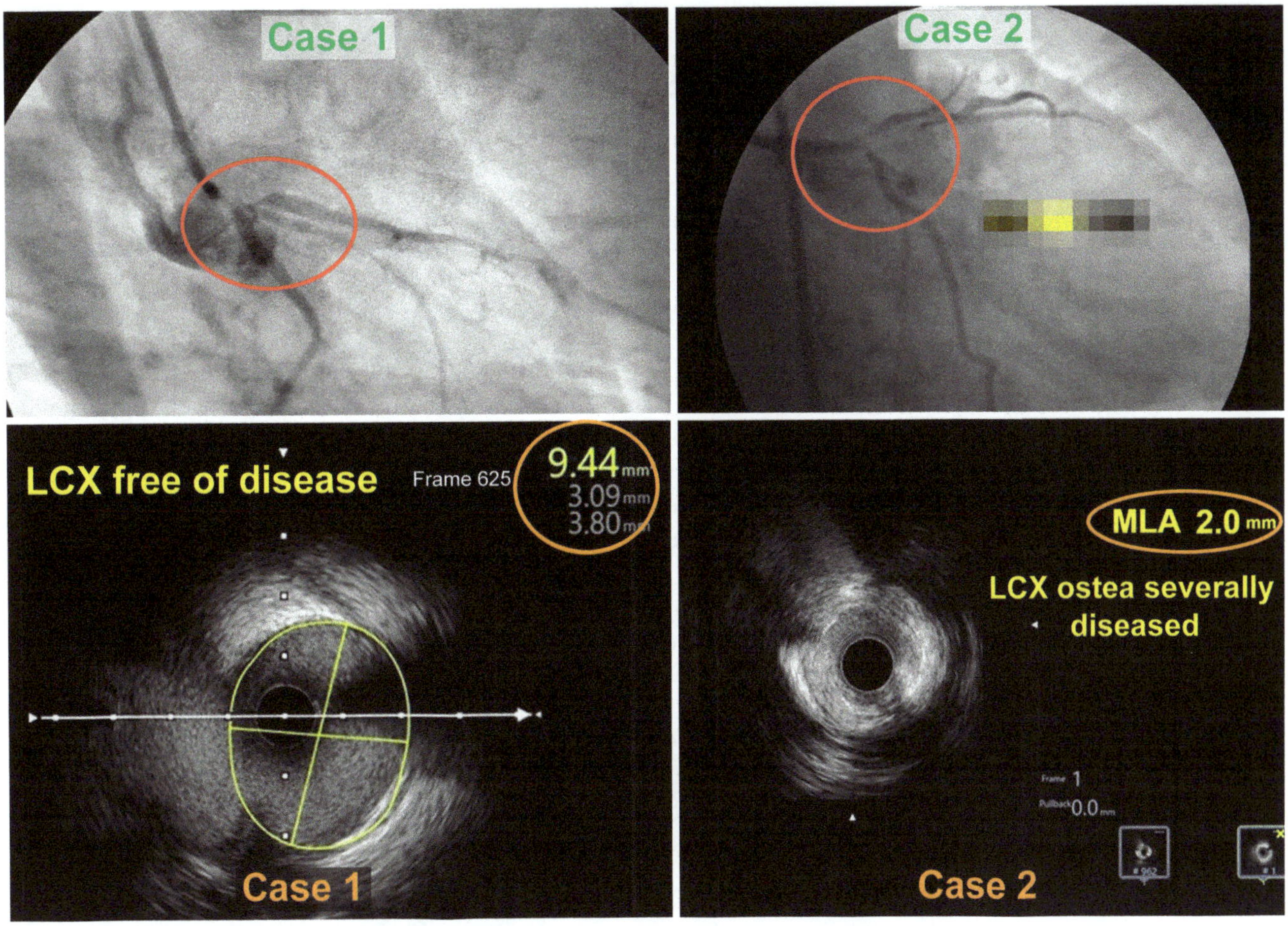

Fig. 2: Role of IVUS in deciding two- versus one-stent strategy in LMCA bifurcation. (IVUS: intravascular ultrasound; LCX: left circumflex; LMCA: left main coronary artery; MLA: minimal lumen area)

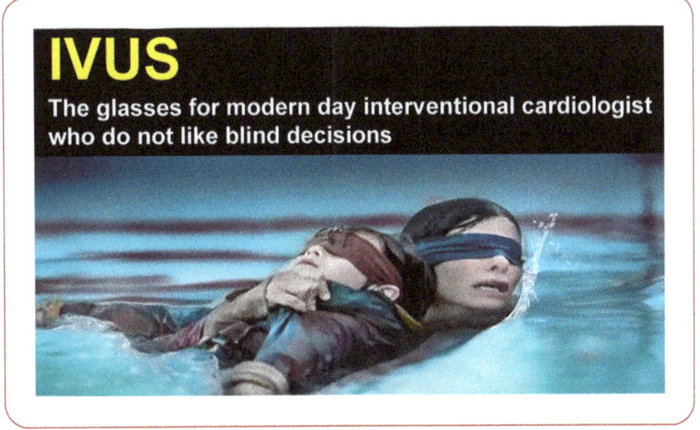

CHAPTER 28

Intravascular Ultrasound Predictors of Side Branch Pinching

Following are the intravascular ultrasound (IVUS) predictors of side branch (SB) pinching:

- **Hairy spiky carina (eyebrow sign)** ***(Figs. 1A to C):*** If the reconstructed carina, as seen on L view, appears pointed/elongated, then any crossover stenting can push the carina toward SB and can lead to occlusion of SB.
- **Branching point-carinal tip** *(BP-CT length <1.7 mm)* ***(Fig. 2):*** The shorter the BP-CT length, the more chances of carinal shift.
- **Calcium in the main branch (MB), opposite SB** ***(Figs. 3 and 4)*:** Any calcium on the MB opposite the carina will resist expansion of the stent on the calcium side and will, in turn, push the carina toward the SB (noncalcium side), leading to carinal shift.
- **Lipid-rich plaque at the ostia of SB** ***(Fig. 5):*** The lipid-rich plaque during crossover stenting can embolize distally, leading to SB compromise.
- **SB diameter ratio >1.5** ***(Fig. 6):*** It is the ratio of SB total diameter (EL-EL)/SB luminal diameter

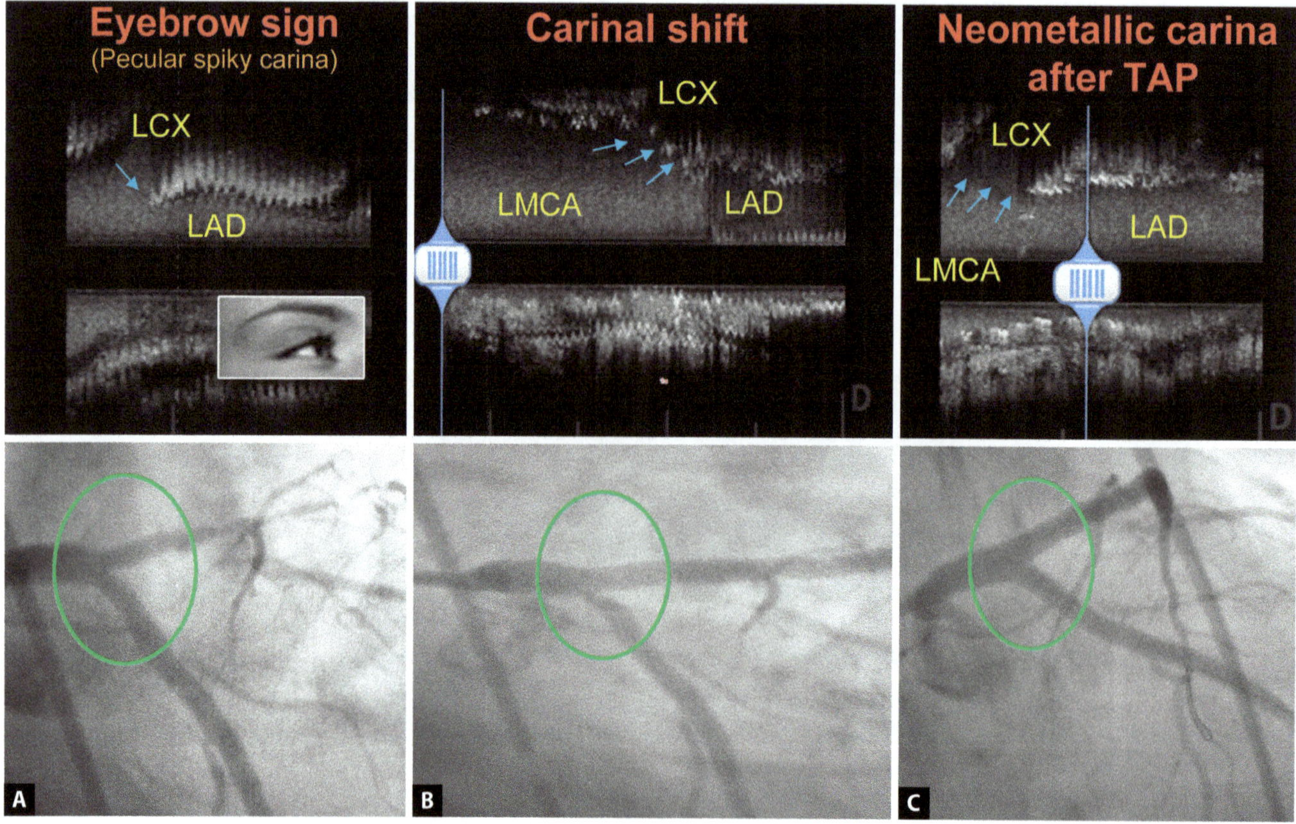

Figs. 1A to C: (A) Hairy spiky carina (eyebrow sign); (B) Carinal shift with pinching of left circumflex (LCX) after crossover stenting left main coronary artery (LMCA) to left anterior descending (LAD); (C) Carinal geometry restored after putting another stent by T and small protrusion (TAP) technique.

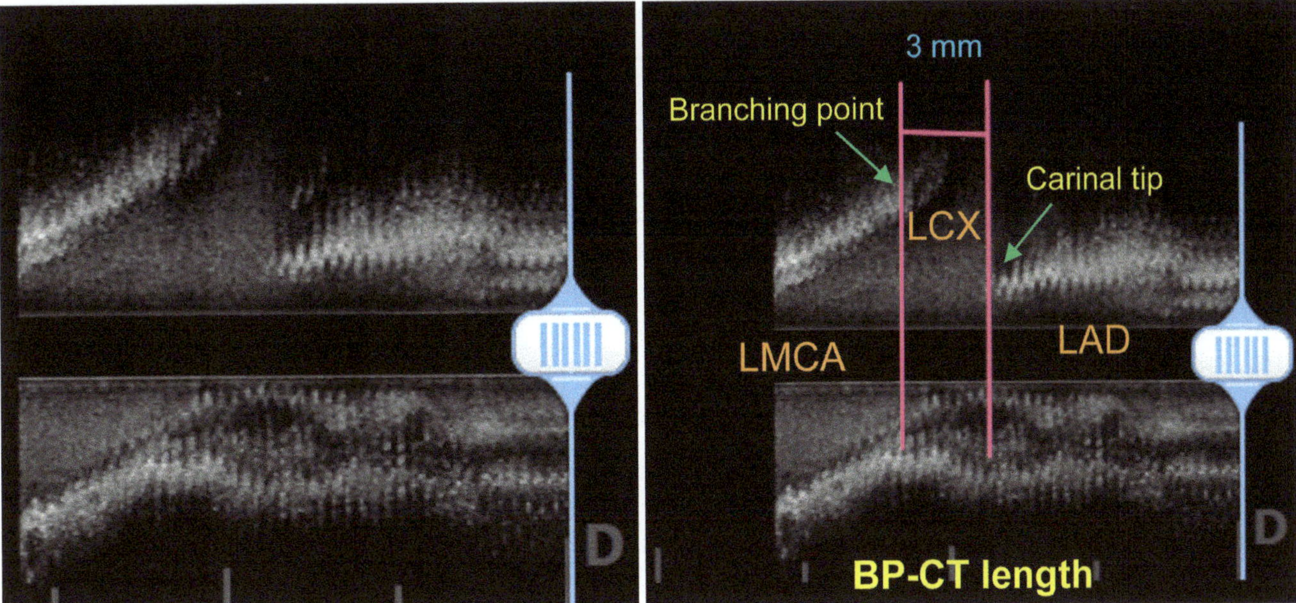

Fig. 2: BP-CT length on IVUS. (BP-CT: branching point-carinal tip; IVUS: intravascular ultrasound; LAD: left anterior descending; LCX: left circumflex; LMCA: left main coronary artery)

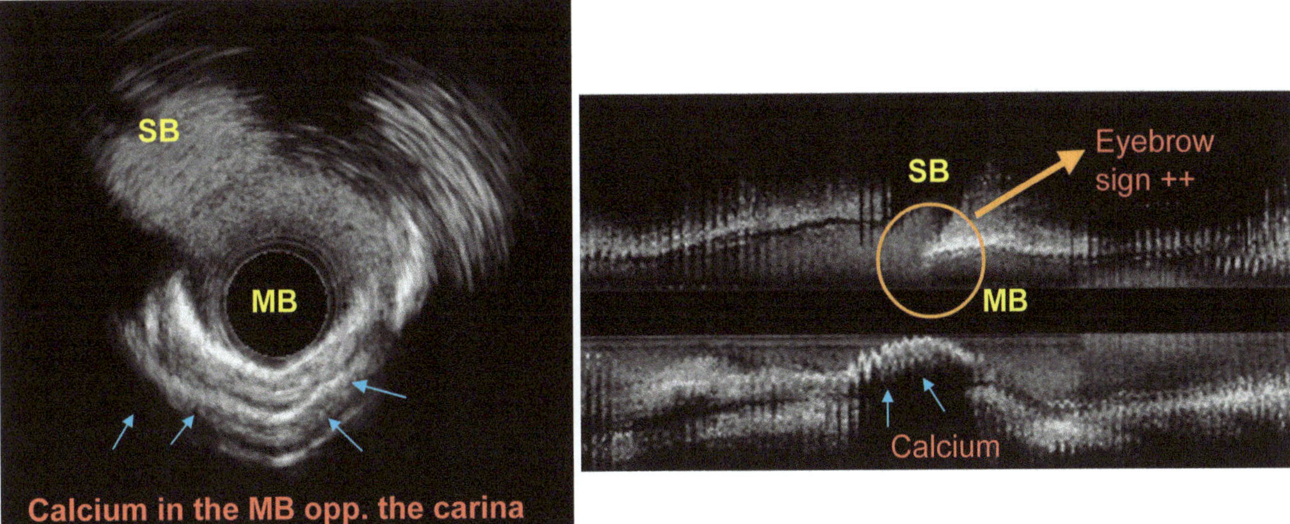

Fig. 3: Calcium in the main branch (MB), opposite side branch (SB).

(intima-intima). If the ratio is >1.5, it indicates significant plaque at the SB ostia and is a precursor of SB pinching.

- **Distal or circumfential plaque distribution of SB:** The side branch at the time of IVUS pullback from the main branch can predict side branch occlusion. There are 3 types of plaque distribution in the SB as assessed from the MB IVUS pullback **(Figs. 7A to C)**.

The first type is the No SB lesion group, where there may be visible stenosis in the ostia of SB on angio but no lesion found on IVUS (this has the least chance of SB occlusion). The second type is the SB lesion proximal type with the lesion only in the proximal part of SB. The third type is the SB lesion Distal or circumferential type with plaque in the distal part or entire circumferential of SB, having the maximum chance of SB occlusion.

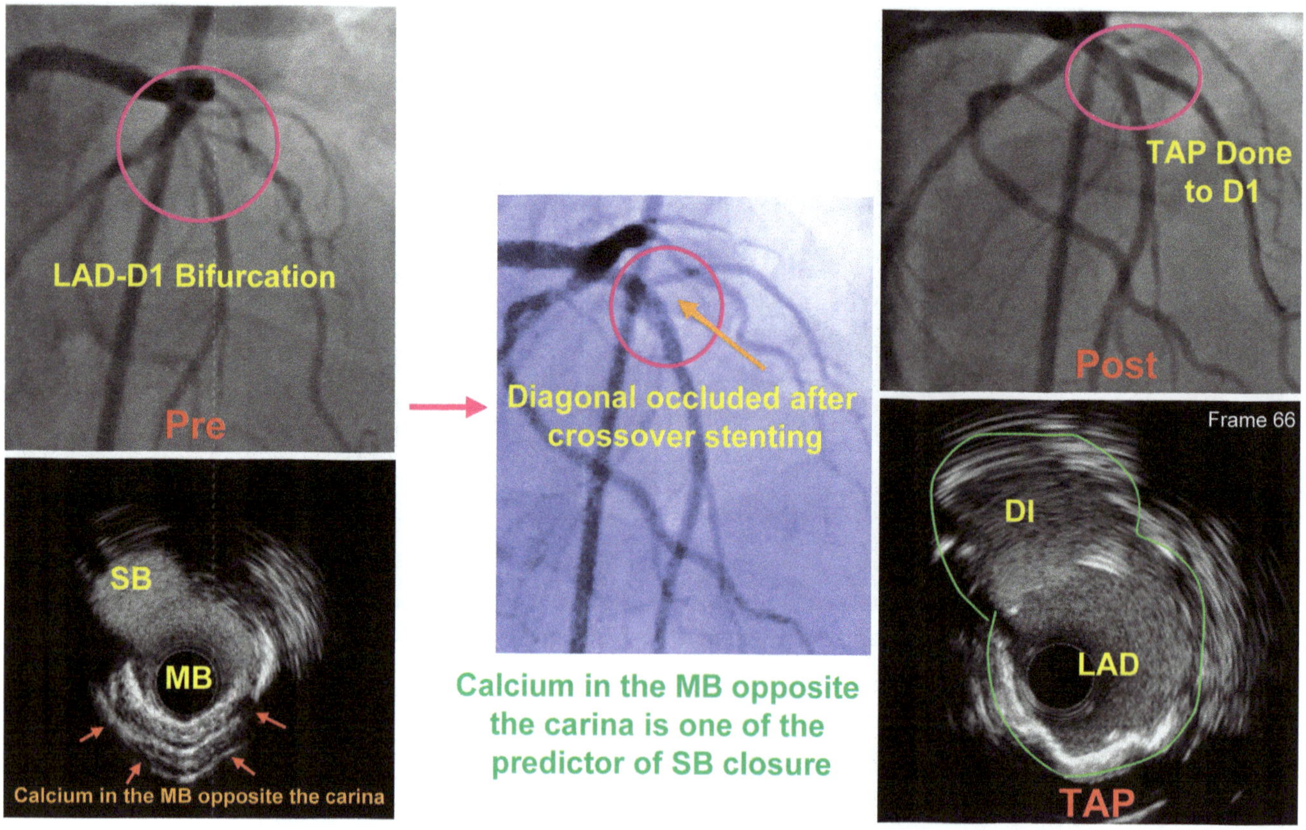

Fig. 4: There was a calcification in the MB (LAD) opposite the carina. During crossover stenting, the carina got shifted and led to occlusion of the SB (D1), which was, however, bailed out by doing a TAP stenting.

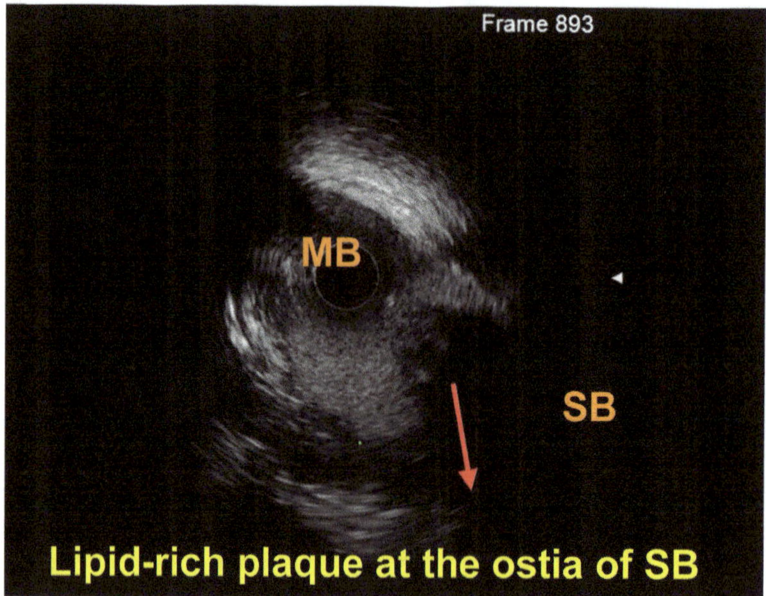

Fig. 5: Lipid-rich plaque at the ostia of SB is one of the predictor of SB occlusion.

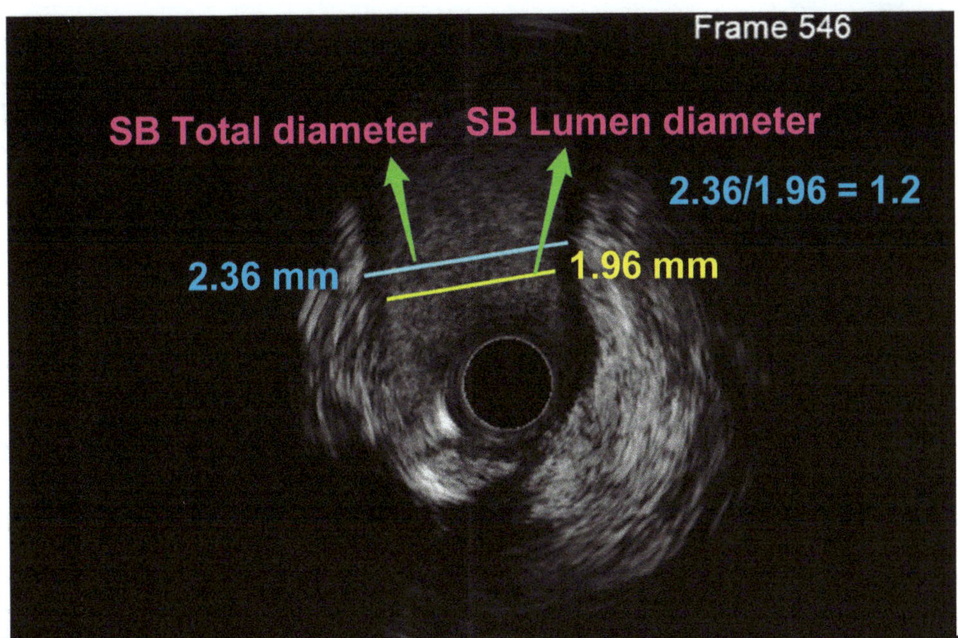

Fig. 6: SB diameter ratio estimation on IVUS. (IVUS: intravascular ultrasound; SB: side branch).

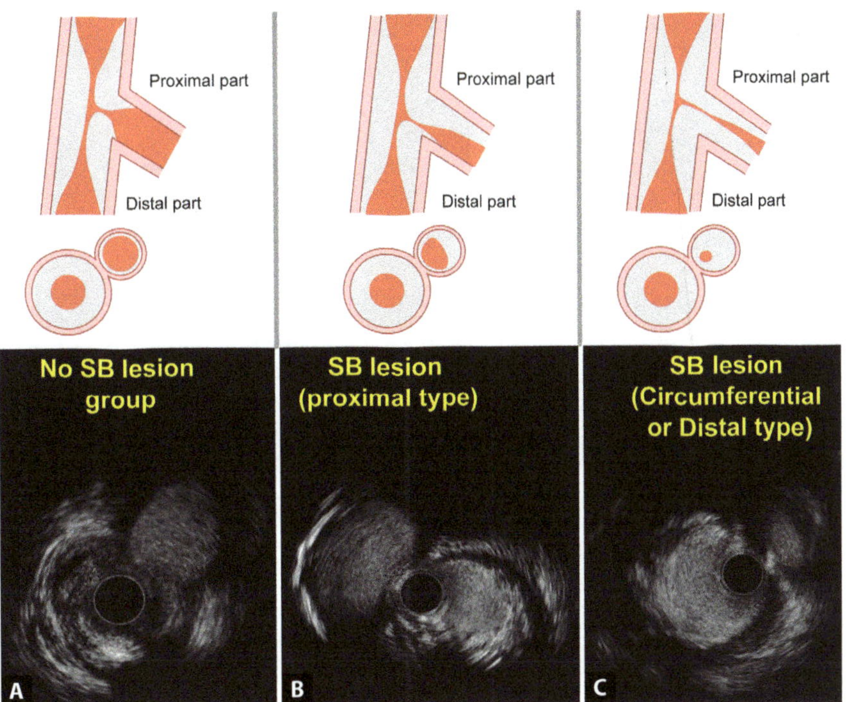

Figs. 7A to C: Classification according to the plaque distribution in the side branches assessed during IVUS pullback from the main branch.

CHAPTER 29

Identifying Good Final Kissing Balloon Inflation and Link-free Carina on Intravascular Ultrasound

A good final kissing balloon inflation (FKBI) will produce a symmetrical carina or what is called a figure of 8 sign or dumbbell sign.

If we see an asymmetrical carina, then repeat FKBI with appropriate size balloon **(Fig. 1)**.

After FKBI in a provisional stent strategy, one should aim for a link free carina. But if stent struts or links are seen in front of the side branch (SB) ostia even after FKBI, then there can be two possibilities **(Fig. 2)**:

1. Size of balloon was inadequate in SB during FKBI. In this case, repeat FKBI with a bigger size balloon.
2. Nondistal recross. Here, recross again with a distal strut.

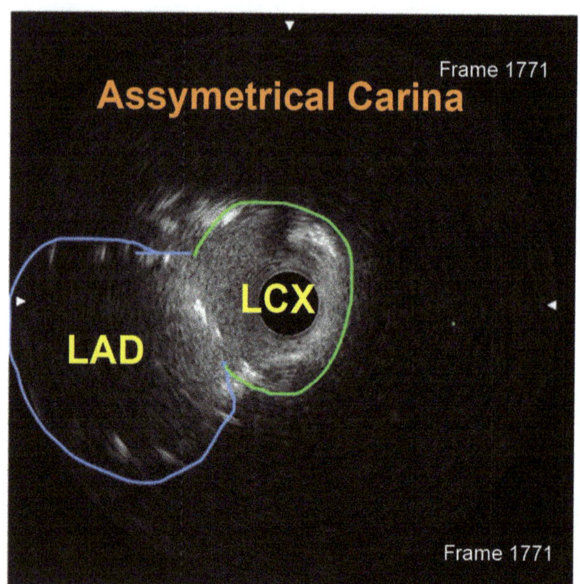

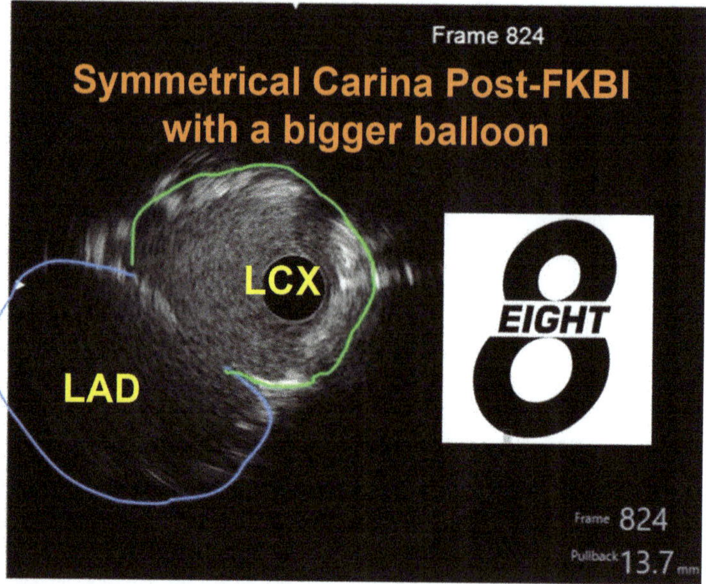

Identifying good FKBI on IVUS:
Look for symmetry of carina (figure of 8 sign)

Fig. 1: Symmetry of carina was restored after repeating FKBI with a bigger size balloon. (FKBI: final kissing balloon inflation; IVUS: intravascular ultrasound)

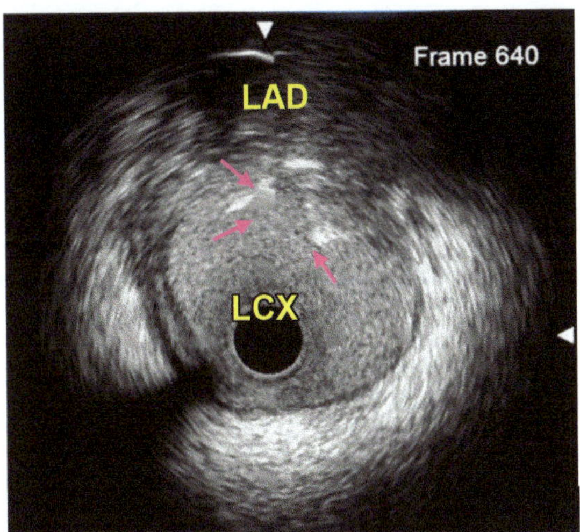

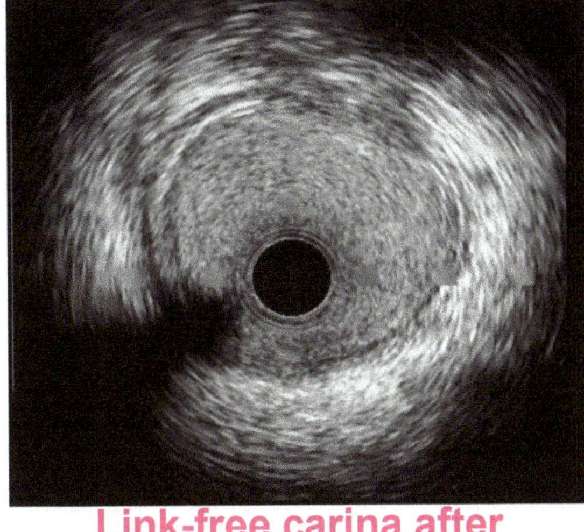

Struts in front of LCX ostea even after FKBI

Link-free carina after repeat FKBI from distal strut

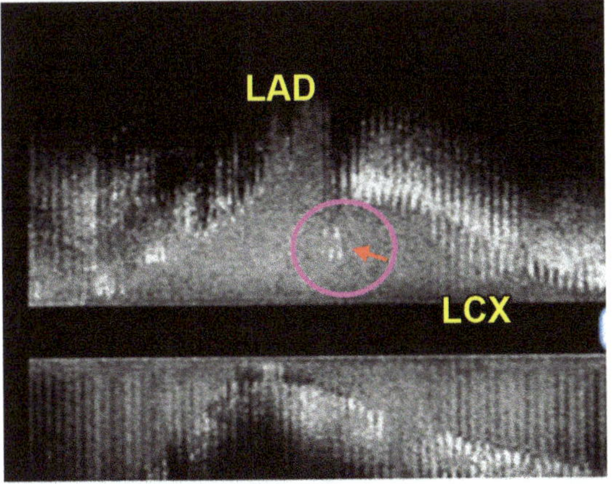

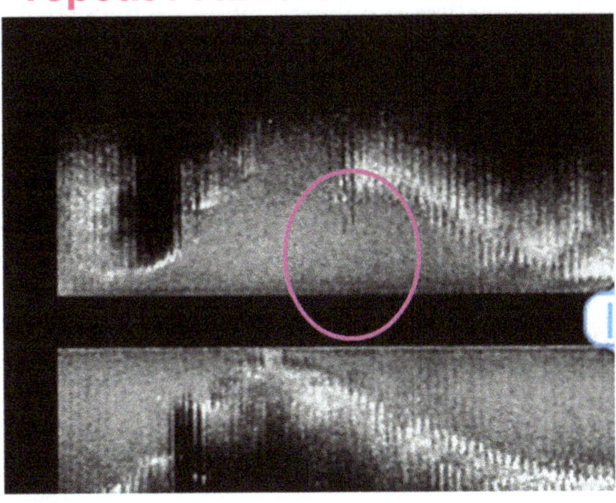

Fig. 2: Even after FKBI, several struts or links were seen. Repeating FKBI after recrossing with distal struts got them removed. (FKBI: final kissing balloon inflation; LAD: left anterior descending; LCX: left circumflex)

"IVUS: "Getting a clear view of your arteries is like cleaning your glasses—suddenly, everything makes sense."

CHAPTER 30

Differentiating Plaque Shift versus Carina Shift on Intravascular Ultrasound

Whenever a side branch gets compromised after a crossover stenting, it is very important to differentiate whether it is because of plaque shift or carina shift because if it is just a carina shift then usually it can be corrected by kissing balloon inflation at low pressure. But if it is a plaque shift then it usually requires high pressure kissing balloon dilation and there is always a high chance that it may require bailout stenting **(Table 1)**.

CLUE TO DIFFERENTIATING PLAQUE SHIFT VERSUS CARINA SHIFT ON INTRAVASCULAR ULTRASOUND (FIG. 1)

Plaque Shift

There is a decrease in the minimal lumen area (MLA), increase in the plaque burden with preserved vessel area (EL-EL).

Carina Shift

There is a decrease in both the MLA and the vessel area (EL-EL) without significant increase in the plaque area.

TABLE 1: Comparison of plaque shift and carina shift.

Points	*Plaque shift*	*Carina shift*
Vessel area (EL-EL)	Same	Reduced
Minimal lumen area (MLA)	Reduced	Reduced
Plaque burden	Increased	Same
Consequences	More injury, more dissection	Less injury, less dissection
Treatment	Large balloon, high pressure	Relatively small balloon, low pressure
Chances of side branch (SB) stenting	High	Low
Late loss	More	Less

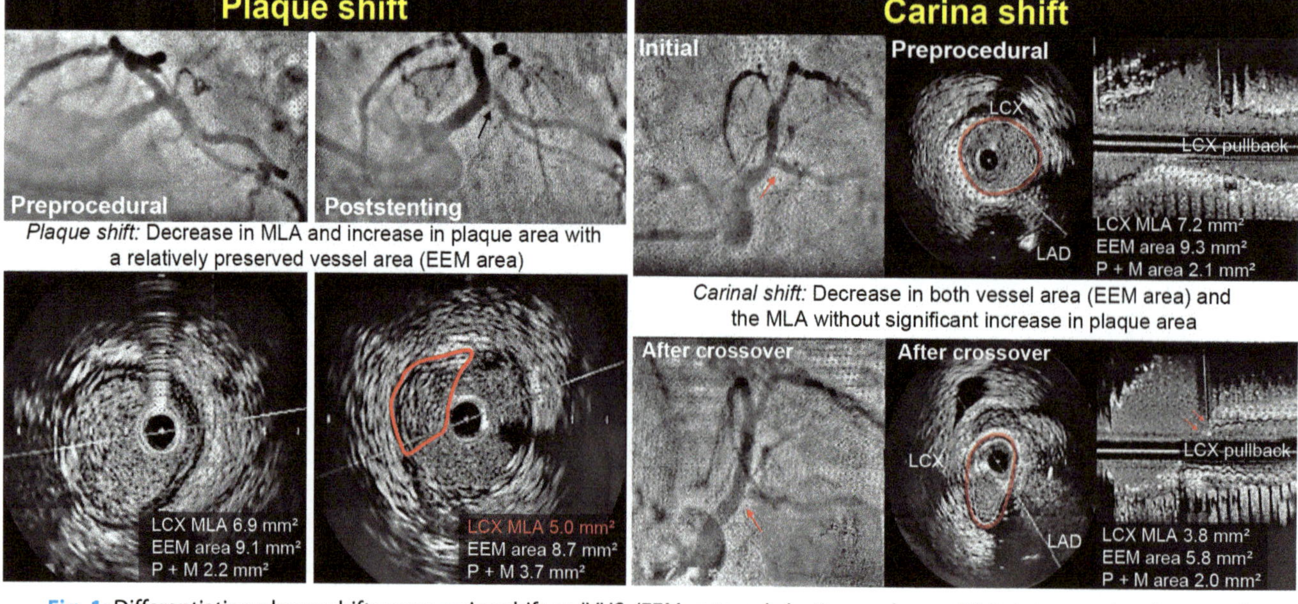

Fig. 1: Differentiating plaque shift versus carina shift on IVUS. (EEM: external elastic membrane; IVUS: intravascular ultrasound; LCX: left circumflex; MLA: minimal lumen area)

CHAPTER 31

Identifying Distal Wire Recrossing on Intravascular Ultrasound

Wire recrossing through distal struts is always desirable in a case of provisional intravascular ultrasound (LMCA) crossover stenting.

Though optical coherence tomography (OCT) is the best, but with high-definition (HD) IVUS also we can identify distal recrossing. Here are the steps to identify:

Step 1: The point where you start seeing the left circumflex (LCX) flow, bookmark that segment as A.

Step 2: The moment you start seeing the LCX wire, bookmark that segment as B.

Step 3: Measure the distance between A and B on L view.

If the distance is short, then it means it is a distal recross **(Fig. 1)**.

On the L view, we can actually see the wire recrossing the side branch **(Fig. 2)**.

If we do distal recrossing, it gives a good scaffolding of the side branch ostia with the main branch stent struts **(Fig. 3)**.

How to identify recrossing point by IVUS

1. When GW goes into the distal point

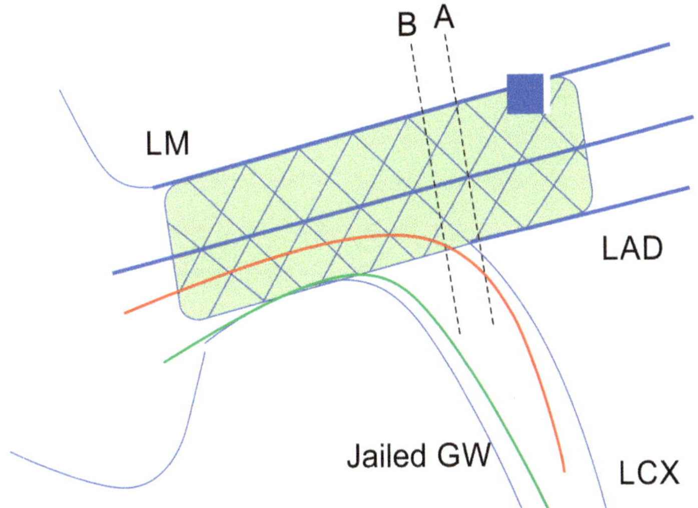

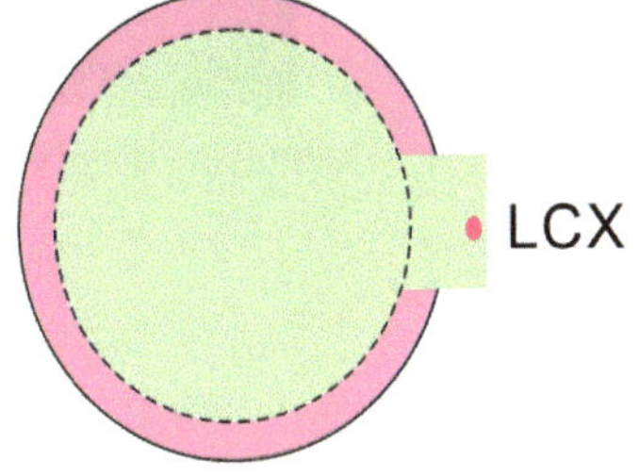

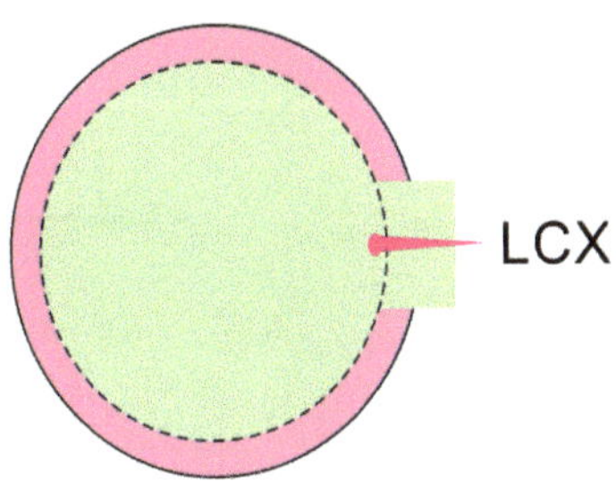

Contd...

Contd...

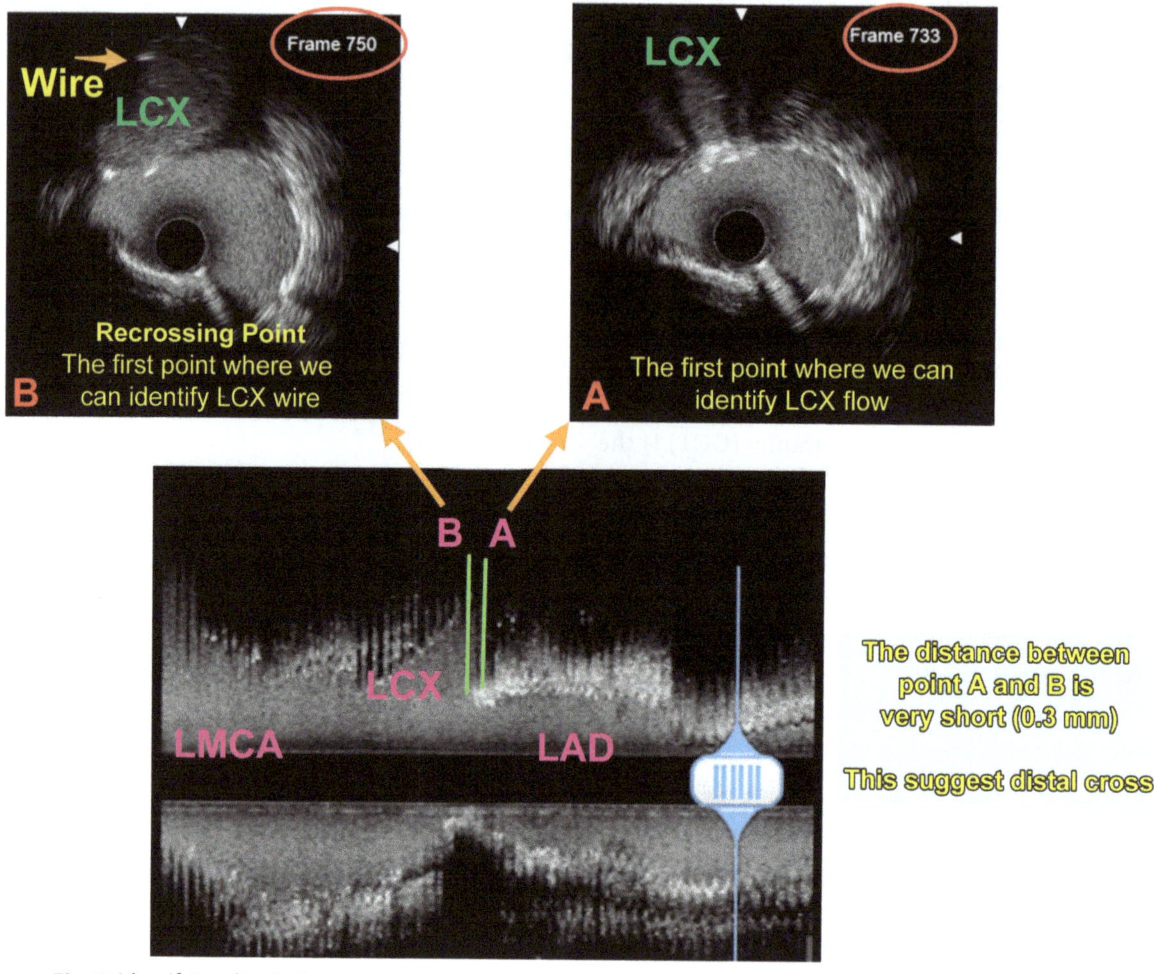

Fig. 1: Identifying distal wire recrossing on IVUS. (IVUS: intravascular ultrasound; LAD: left anterior descending; LCX: left circumflex; LMCA: left main coronary artery)

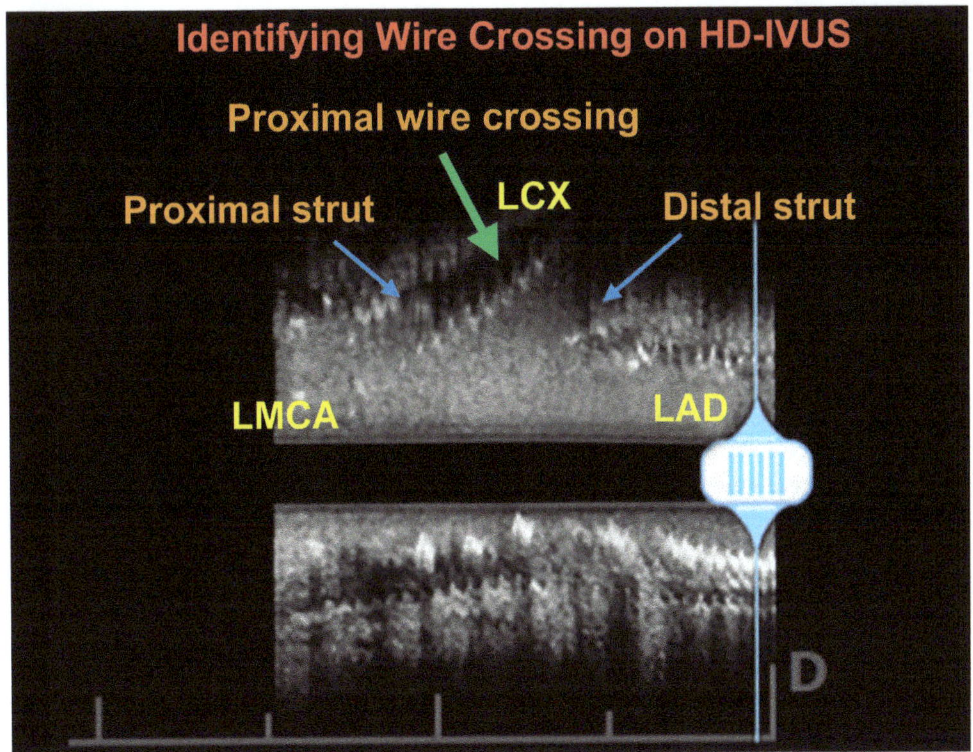

Fig. 2: Wire recrossing seen in the L view. (LAD: left anterior descending; LCX: left circumflex; LMCA: left main coronary artery)

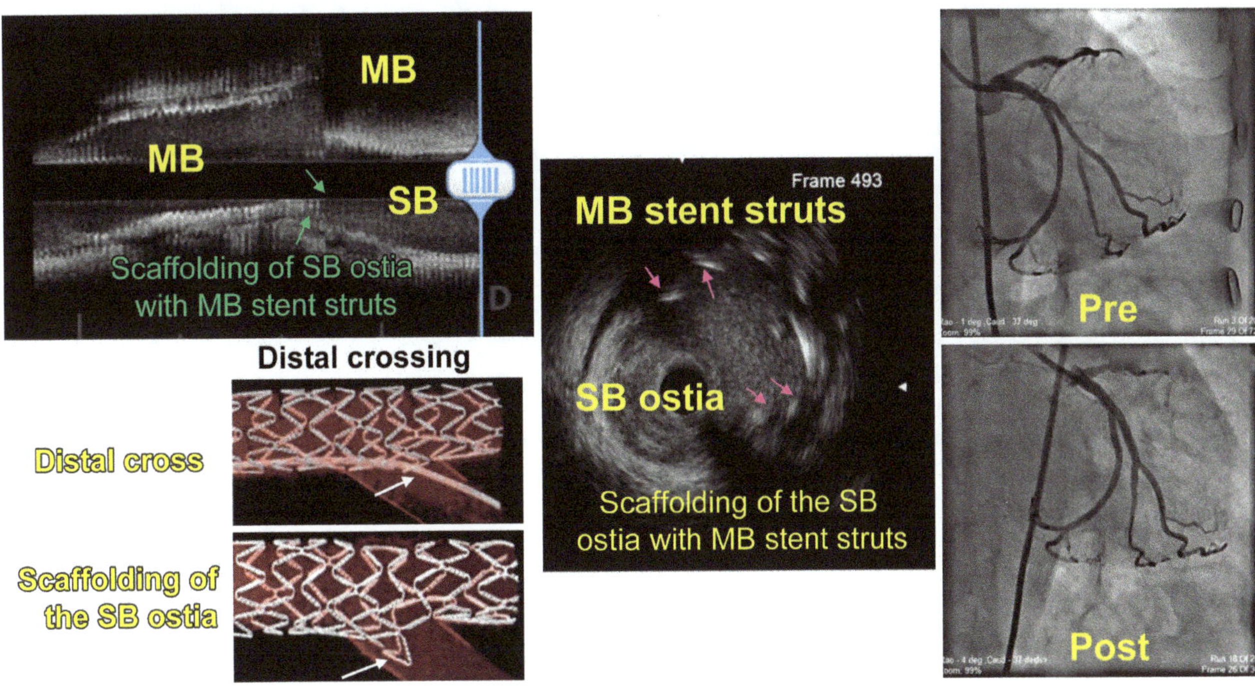

Fig. 3: Distal wire crossing causes a good SB scaffolding seen on IVUS. (IVUS: intravascular ultrasound; MB: main branch; SB: side branch)

"When you look at an artery with IVUS, it's like the artery is opening up and saying, 'Here's my story!"

CHAPTER 32

Identifying Abluminal Wiring on Intravascular Ultrasound

Intravascular ultrasound (IVUS) can easily identify abluminal wiring (wiring behind the stent struts). For example, you can see in **Figure 1** both the wire and the IVUS catheter are behind the stent struts.

In **Figure 2**, you can see the left anterior descending (LAD) wire is in the lumen, but the diagonal wire is seen behind the stent struts.

In **Figure 3**, you can see there is abluminal wiring of the left circumflex (LCX) wire behind the left main stent struts in the ostial proximal portion.

The LCX wire (yellow arrow) goes behind the stent struts (white arrow), causing distortion in the ostial proximal region.

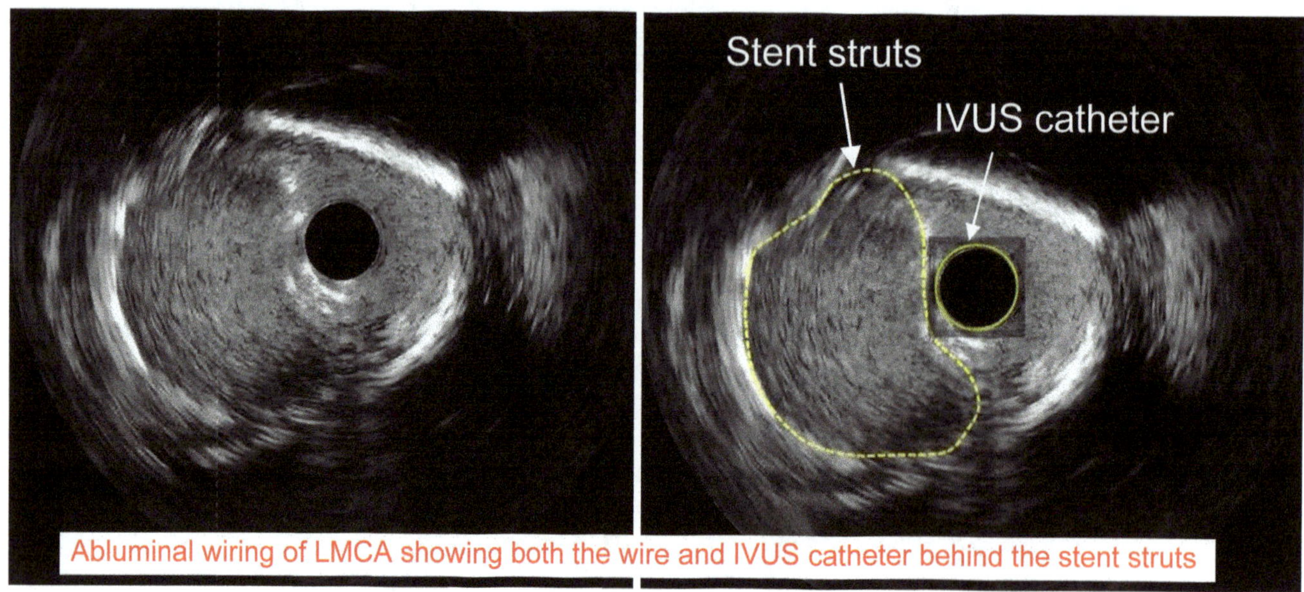

Fig. 1: Abluminal wiring of LMCA. (IVUS: intravascular ultrasound; LMCA: left main coronary artery)

"The experimenter who does not know what he is looking for will not understand what he finds"

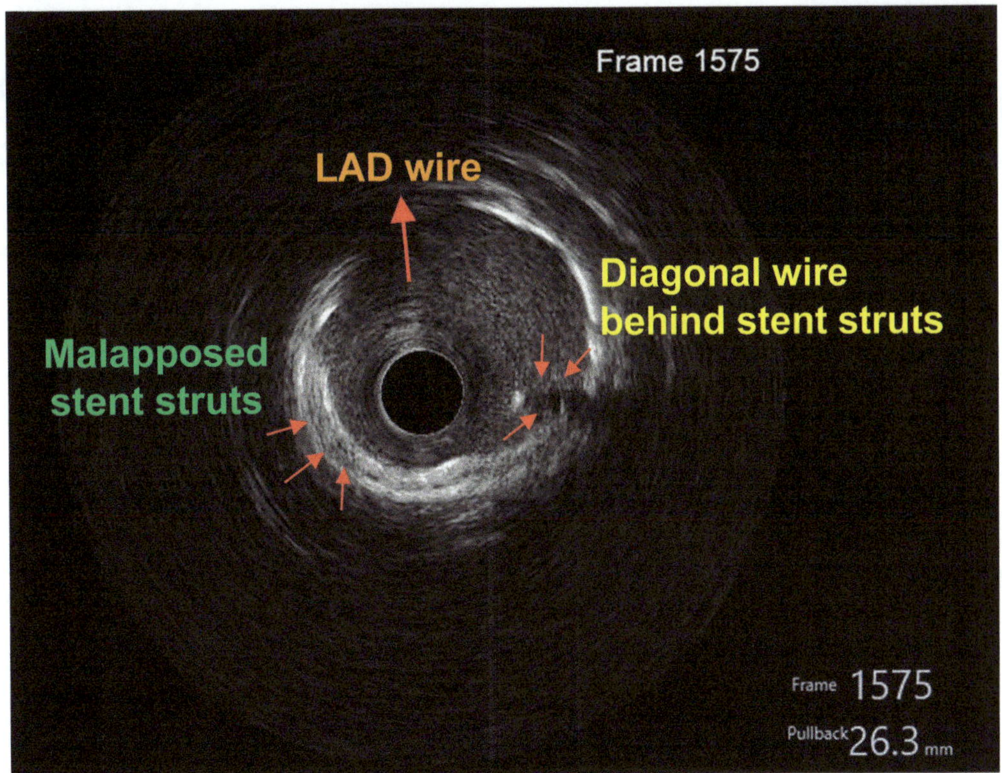

Fig. 2: Abluminal wiring of D1 during LAD-D bifurcation stenting. (LAD: left anterior diagonal; D: diagonal)

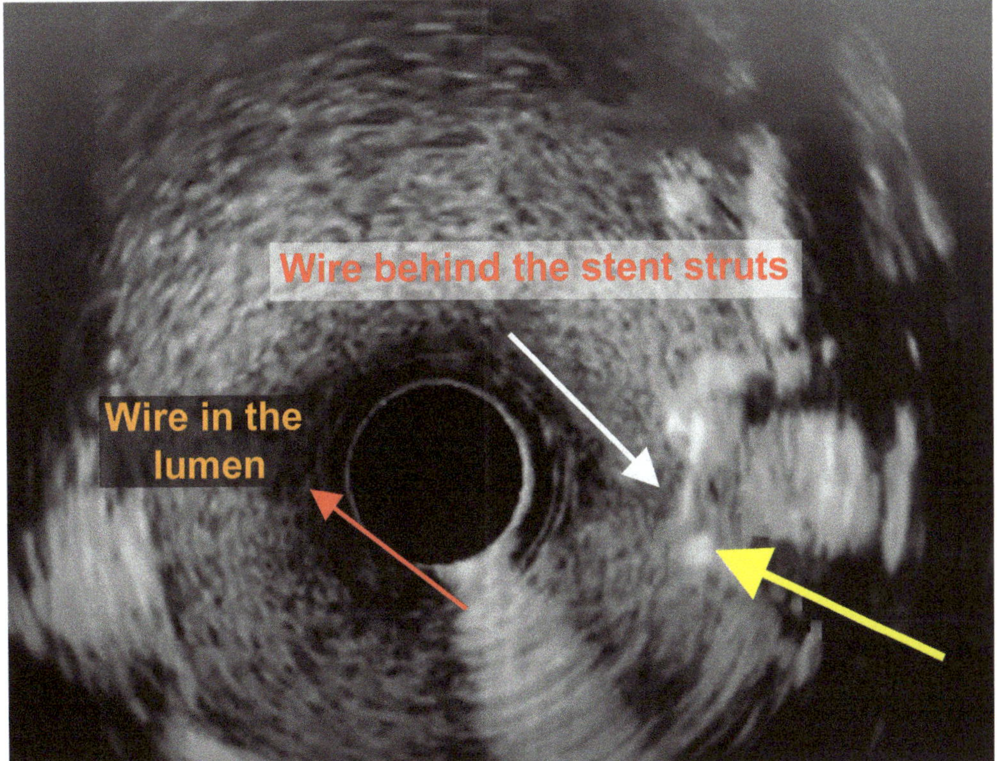

Fig. 3: Abluminal wiring of left circumflex (LCX) during left main coronary artery (LMCA) bifurcation stenting.

CHAPTER 33

Intravascular Ultrasound in Double Kissing Crush

The schematic diagram showing an overview of how double kissing (DK) crush looks on intravascular ultrasound (IVUS) is shown in **Figure 1**. Besides routine evaluation, one should look for the following things in IVUS in a case of DK crush:

- Adequate stent coverage of the side branch ostia (no stent gaps) **(Fig. 2)**
- *Identifying adequacy of crush* ***(Fig. 3)****:* An adequate crush means no stent struts hanging in the polygon of confluence (POC). Both main branch (MB) and side branch (SB) struts completely apposed to the MB vessel wall.
- *Minimal overlap:* It means a single layer of stent in the POC **(Fig. 4)**.
- *Identifying good final kissing balloon inflation on IVUS:* Look for symmetry of carina, what is called the figure of 8 sign or dumbbell sign **(Fig. 5)**.
- *Ensuring adequate stent expansion and knowing your final score:* The minimum MSAs to aim for are 6, 8, and 10 for LCX, LAD, and LMCA, respectively. Additionally, if possible achieving a score more than 7, 9, and 12 for the respective arteries may be more beneficial **(Fig. 6)**.

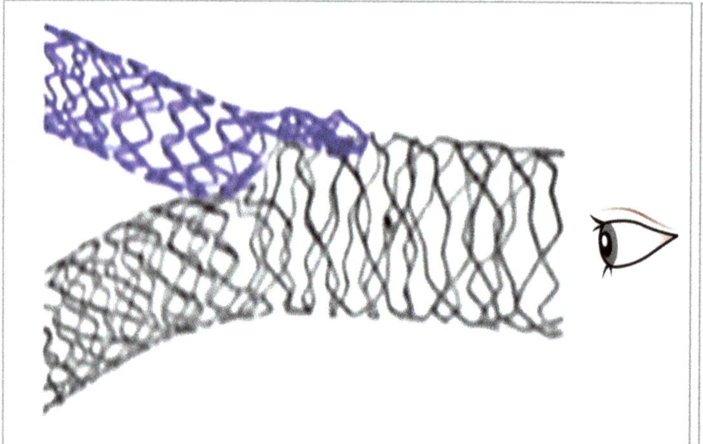

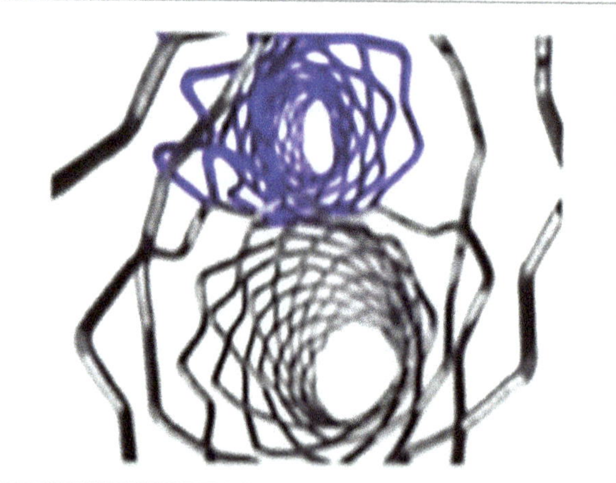

Fig. 1: Schematic diagram showing how double kissing (DK) crush looks on intravascular ultrasound (IVUS).

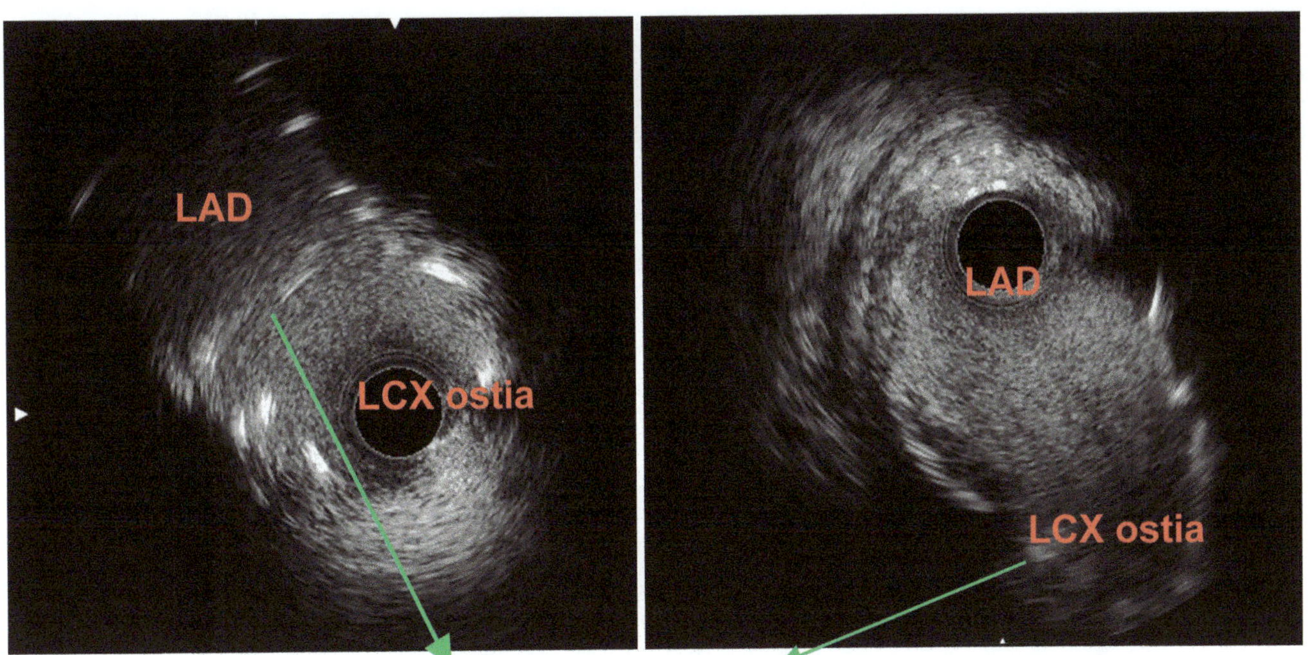

Fig. 2: Ensuring no stent gaps in SB ostium. (LAD: left anterior descending; LCX: left circumflex; SB: side branch)

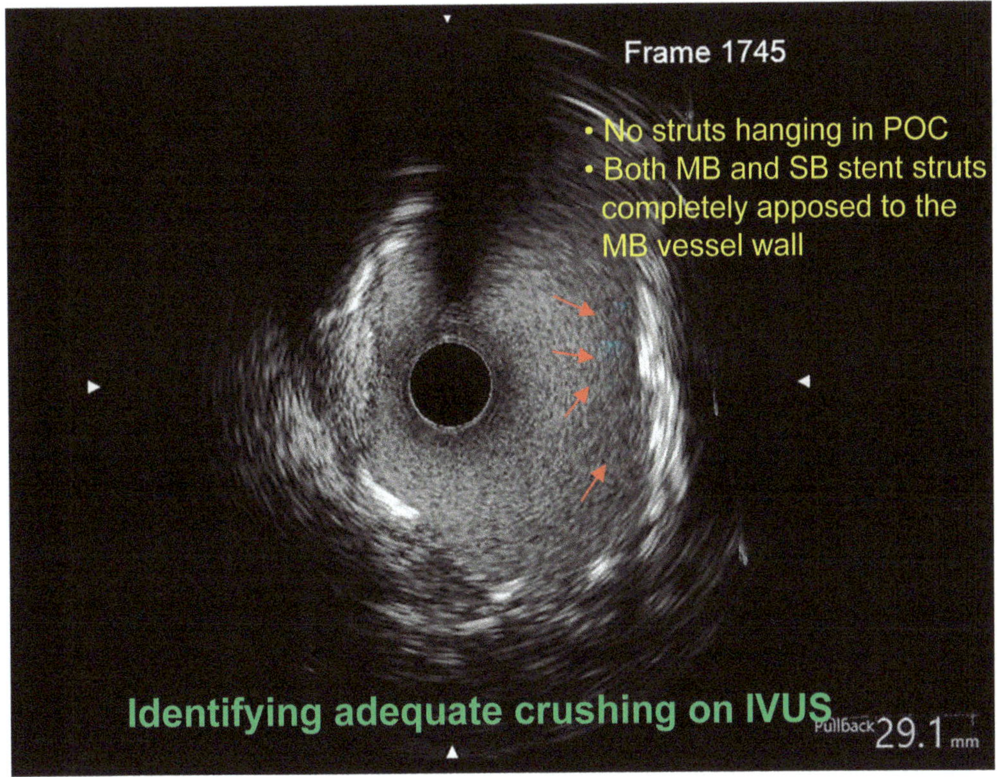

Fig. 3: Identifying adequacy of crush. (IVUS: intravascular ultrasound; MB: main branch; POC: polygon of confluence; SB: side branch)

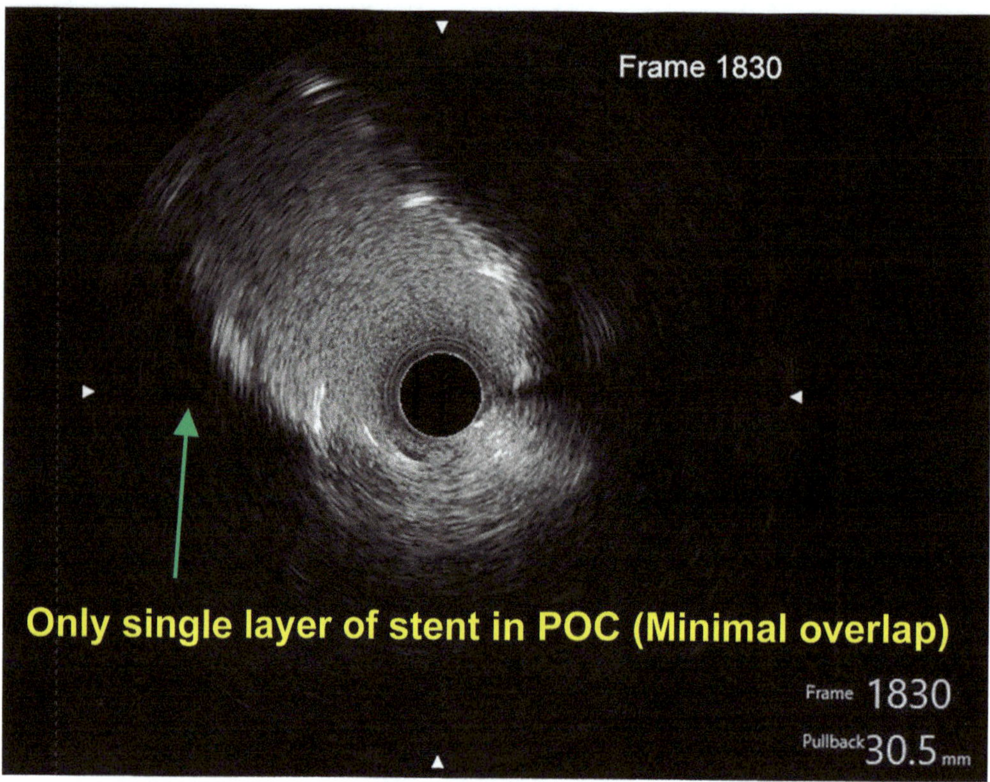

Fig. 4: Ensuring minimal overlap on IVUS. (IVUS: intravascular ultrasound; POC: polygon of confluence)

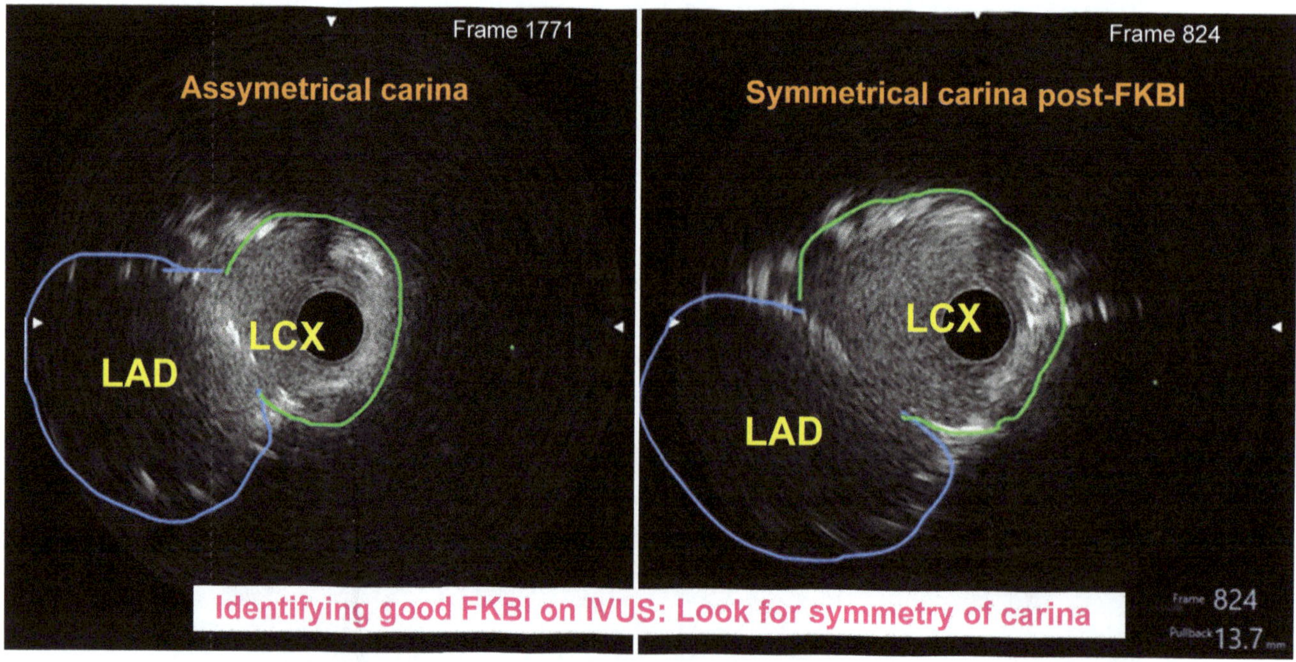

Fig. 5: Identifying good FKB on IVUS. (FKB: final kissing balloon; FKBI: final kissing balloon inflation; IVUS: intravascular ultrasound; LAD: left anterior descending; LCX: left circumflex)

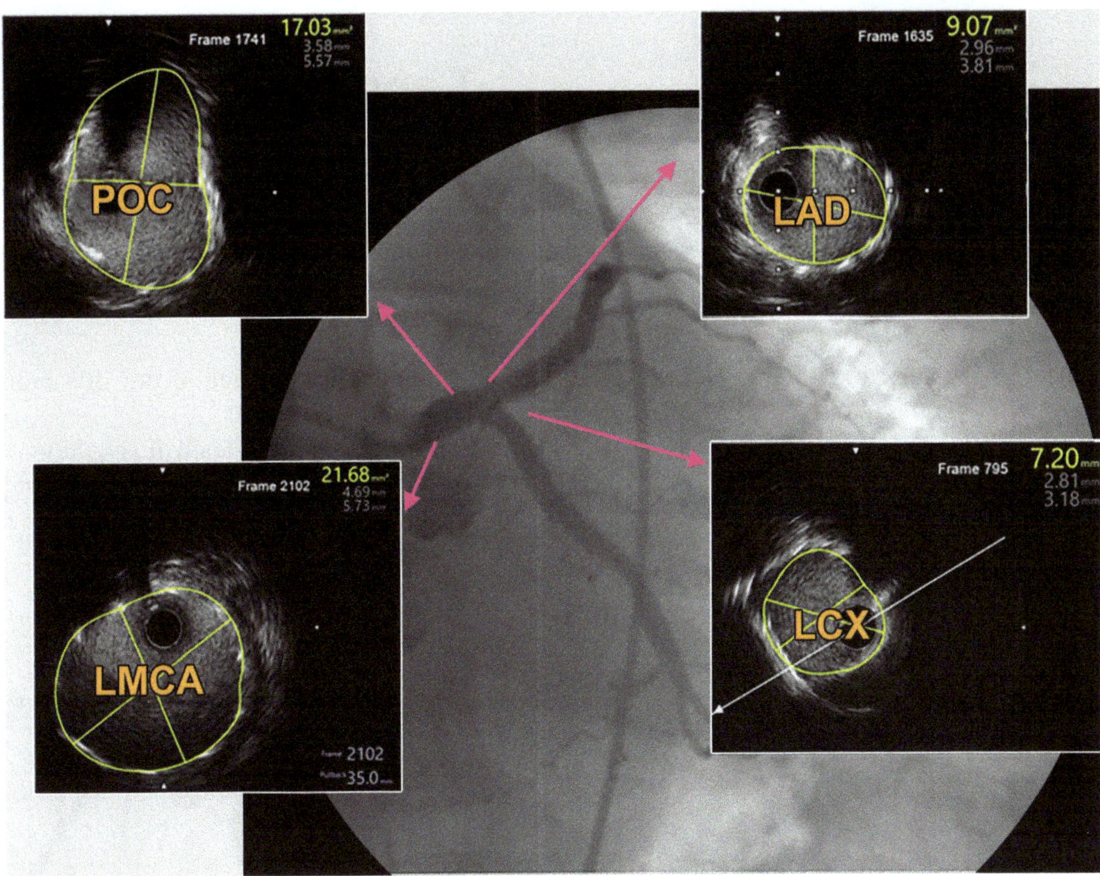

Fig. 6: Calculating the final score after DK Crush on IVUS. The minimum MSAs to aim for are 6, 8, and 10 for LCX, LAD, and LMCA, respectively. Additionally, if possible achieving a score more than 7, 9, and 12 for the respective arteries may be more beneficial like in this case.

"Exploring the unseen: IVUS brings clarity to vascular mysteries."

CHAPTER 34

T and Small Protrusion on Intravascular Ultrasound

Schematic diagram showing how T and small protrusion (TAP) looks on intravascular ultrasound (IVUS) is shown in **Figure 1**.

Besides routine evaluation, three things one should look for in IVUS in a case of TAP:

1. Distal crossing of the side branch **(Fig. 2)**
2. Adequate stent coverage of the side branch ostia (it should not be missed)
3. Length of neocarina (ideally it should be <2.5 mm) **(Fig. 3)**. If it is >2.5 mm then one should convert TAP into culotte or reverse crush for better long term outcome.

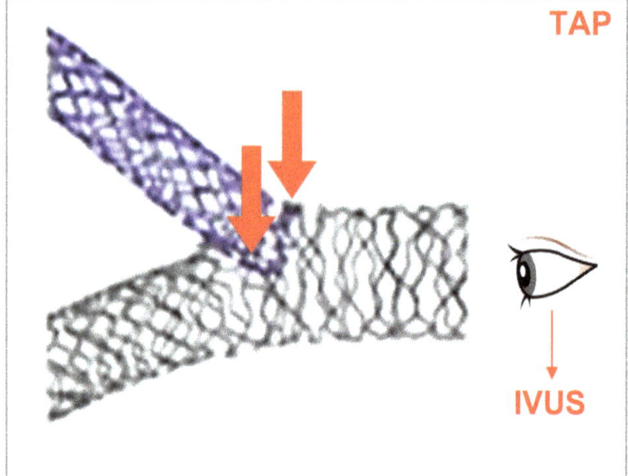

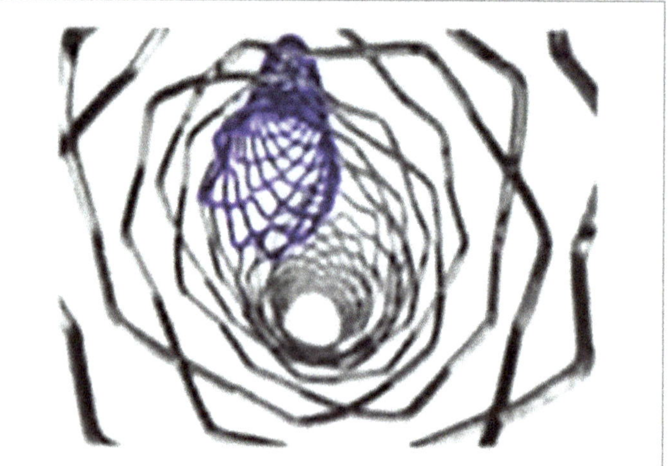

Fig. 1: Schematic diagram showing how T and small protrusion (TAP) looks on intravascular ultrasound (IVUS).

"IVUS is like a third eye of interventional cardiologists"

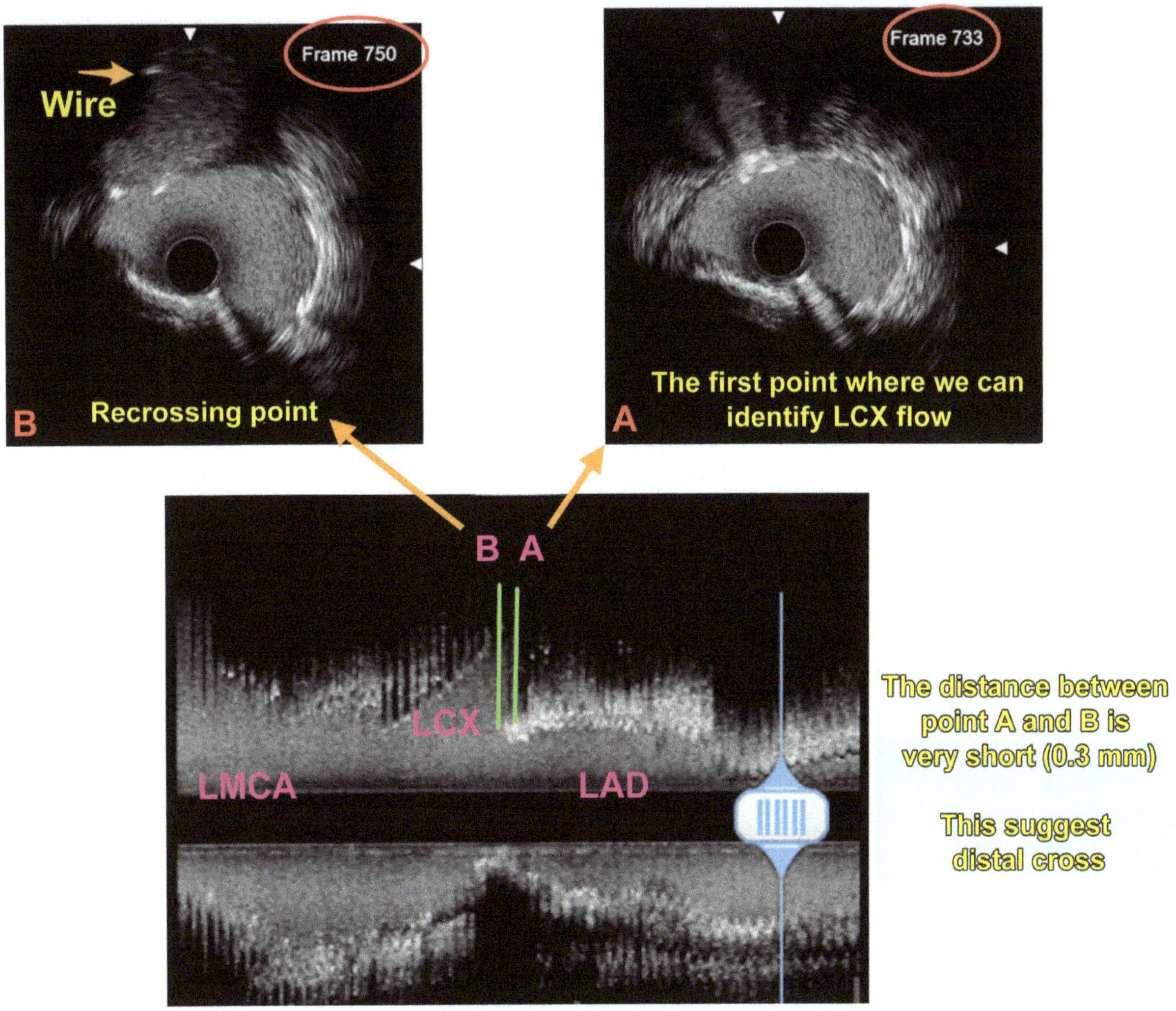

Fig. 2: Identifying distal cross on HD IVUS. (HD IVUS: high-definition intravascular ultrasound; LAD: left anterior descending; LCX: left circumflex; LMCA: left main coronary artery)

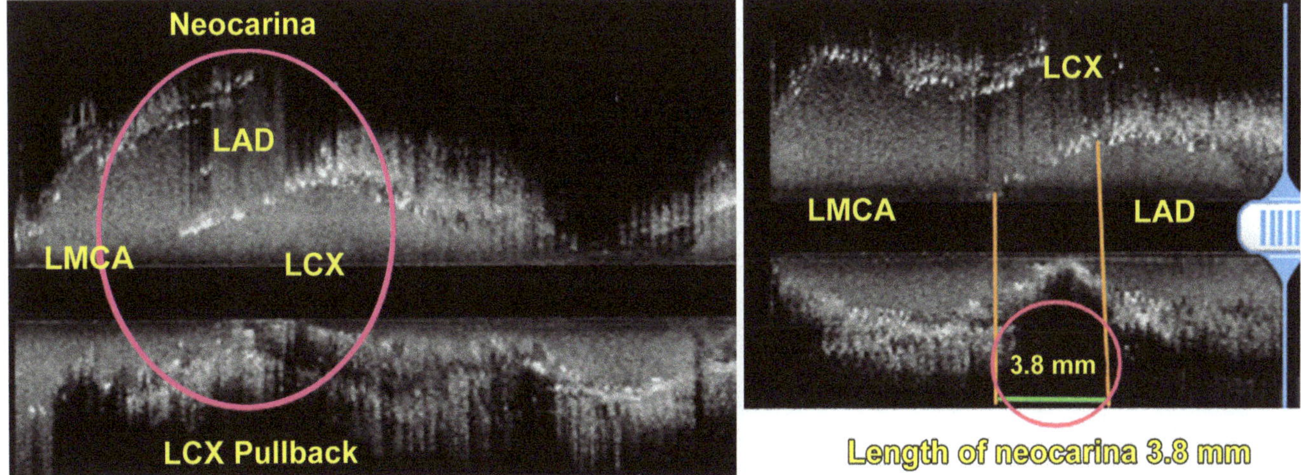

Fig. 3: Measuring length of neocarina. (LAD: left anterior descending; LCX: left circumflex; LMCA: left main coronary artery)

CHAPTER 35

Ostial LAD Dilemma: To Nail the Ostia or LMCA Crossover

In cases of ostial left anterior descending (LAD) lesions, there is a dilemma whether to stent the ostium or perform a crossover from left main coronary artery (LMCA) to LAD. Intravascular ultrasound (IVUS) studies show that in 90% of cases, plaque in the LAD extends into the LMCA **(Fig. 1)** and the decision is based on assessing the plaque burden at the LAD ostium and distal LMCA. Angiography can lie many times in such situations. Even with a PB of 40%, the angio may appear normal. Therefore, it is important to do IVUS in such cases to assess the extent of disease. If the plaque burden is <50%, stenting in the ostioproximal segment is recommended, otherwise, a crossover stenting is preferred **(Flowchart 1)**. IVUS plays a crucial role in this scenario as demonstrated by two examples **(Fig. 2)**, showing the distribution of plaque and the decision-making process for stent placement. Case 1 involved no plaque in the distal LMCA, leading to stent placement in the ostium, while Case 2 with significant plaque burden at LAD ostium and distal LMCA so we preferred crossover stenting.

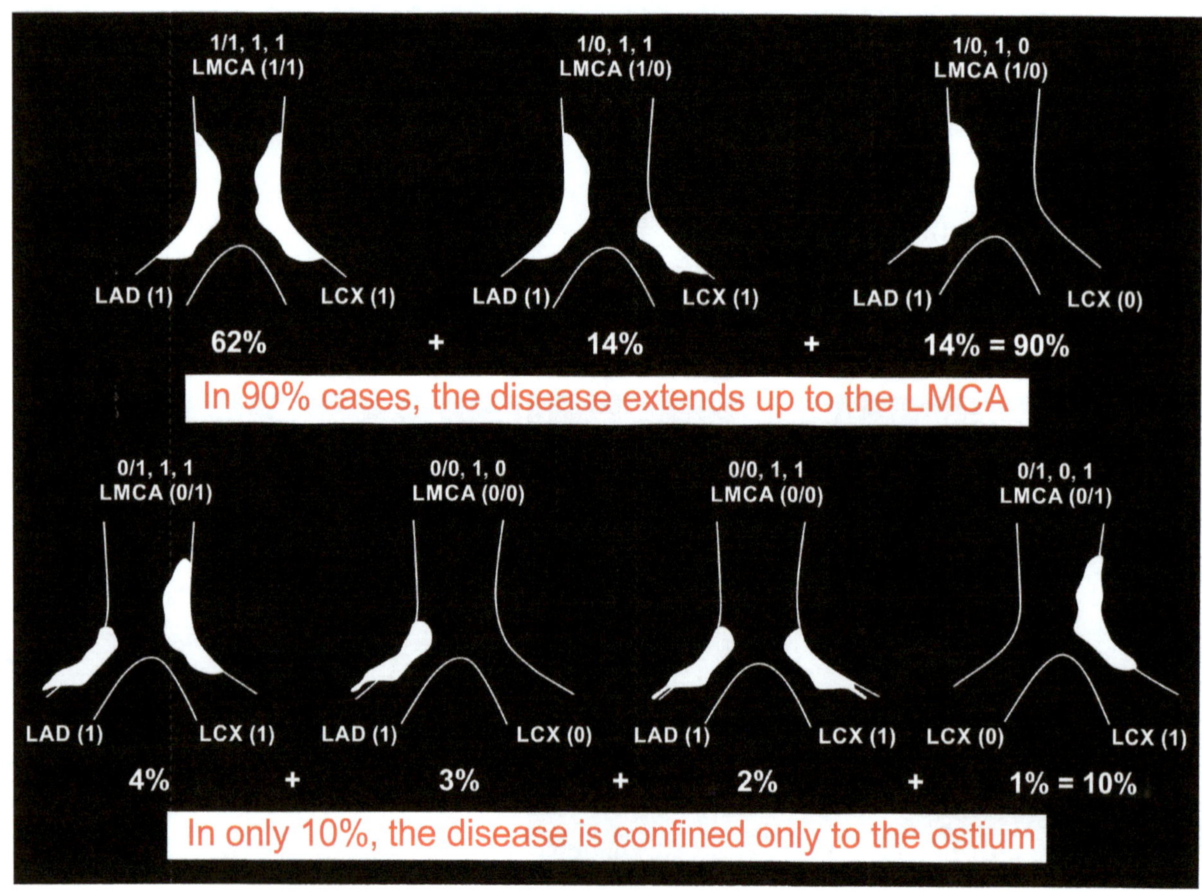

Fig. 1: Distribution of plaque at the left main coronary artery (LMCA) bifurcation.

Flowchart 1: Intravascular ultrasound (IVUS)-based approach in a case of ostioproximal left anterior descending (LAD) lesion.

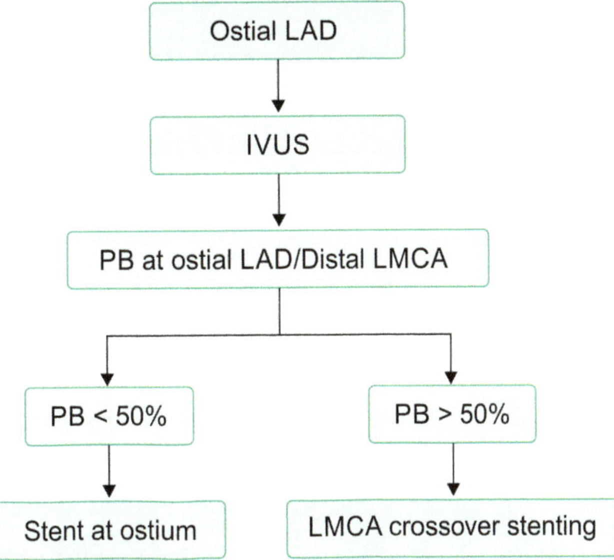

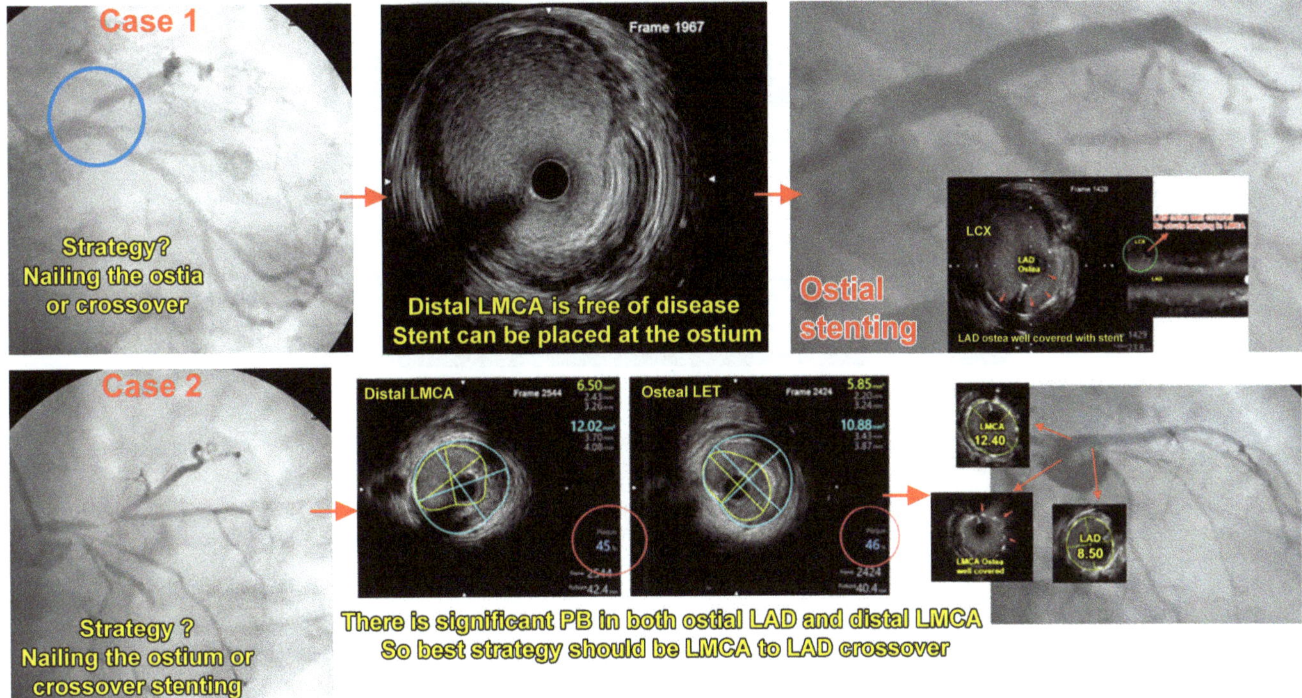

Fig. 2: In Case 1, there was no plaque in the distal left main coronary artery (LMCA), so a stent was placed in the ostia. In Case 2, there was significant plaque buildup at left anterior descending (LAD) ostia and distal LMCA, so a crossover stenting was preferred.

"Exploring the unseen: IVUS brings clarity to vascular mysteries."

CHAPTER 36

Longitudinal Stent Deformation

When multiple layers or crowding of stent struts are visible on intravascular ultrasound (IVUS), it is due to longitudinal stent deformation (LSD) **(Fig. 1)**.

It is important to recognize LSD since its is one of the precursor for future MACE in LMCA stenting **(Fig. 2)**.

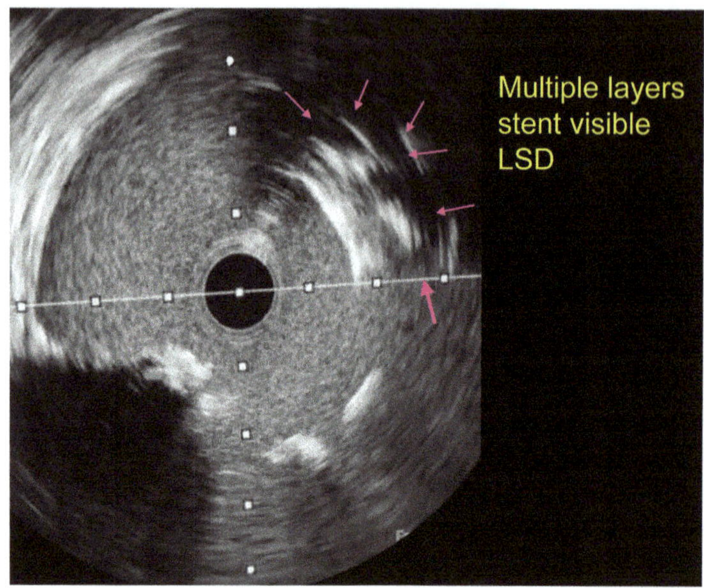

Fig. 1: Longitudinal stent deformation (LSD) in left main coronary artery (LMCA) stent.

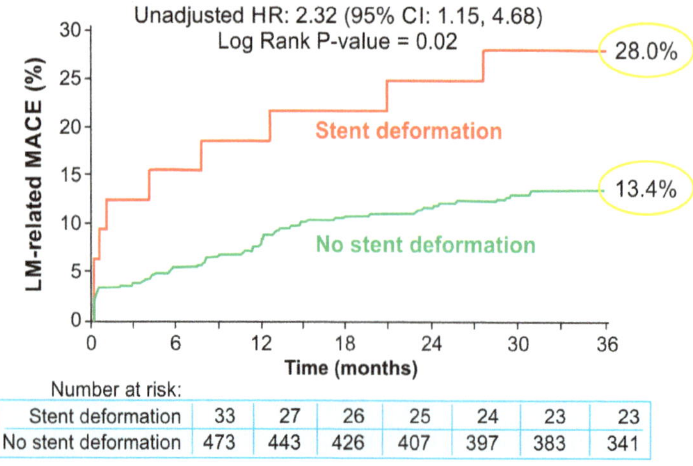

Stent deformation	33	27	26	25	24	23	23
No stent deformation	473	443	426	407	397	383	341

Fig. 2: Date from EXCEL Study showing that any LSD can lead to more than 2 times risk of future MACE.

CHAPTER 37

Confirming Aorto-ostial Coverage of Stent on Intravascular Ultrasound

IDENTIFYING AORTO-OSTIAL COVERAGE OF STENT ON INTRAVASCULAR ULTRASOUND

Start the pullback from the left main coronary artery (LMCA) or proximal right coronary artery (RCA). The moment you see medial discontinuity (stop seeing three layers of vessel), this is the point of aorto-ostial. Now if you are seeing stent struts on the opposite wall at that place, it means ostium is covered **(Figs. 1 and 2)**.

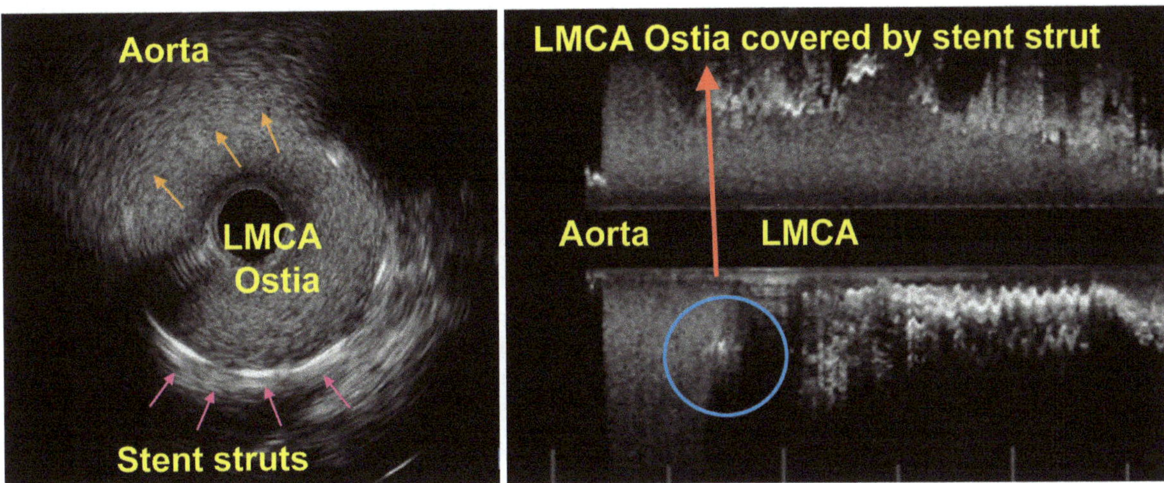

Fig. 1: Adequate aorto-ostial coverage seen in both L and cross-sectional view. (LMCA: left main coronary artery)

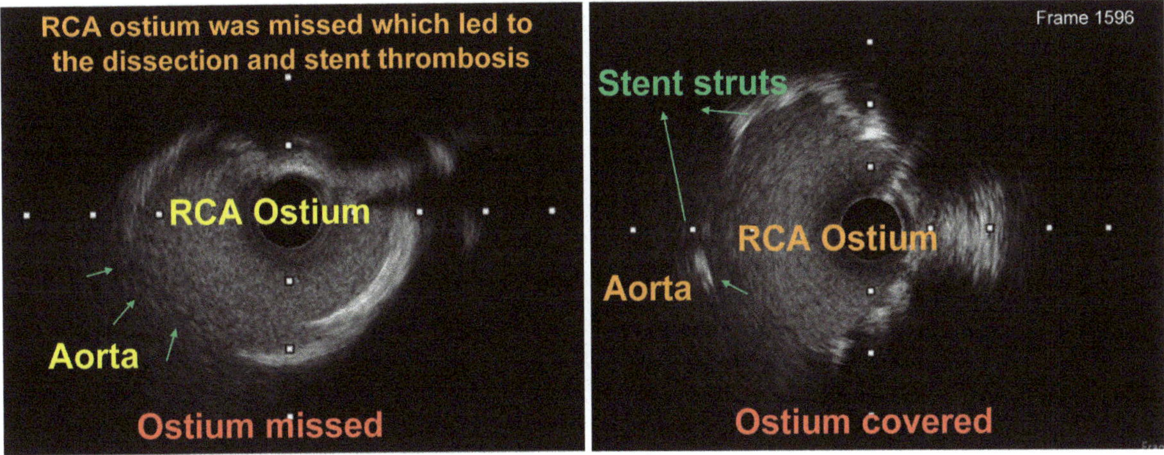

Fig. 2: Ostium was missed initially and then later covered with another stent. (RCA: right coronary artery)

CHAPTER 38

Intravascular Ultrasound in Intermediate Lesions

Fractional flow reserve (FFR) is the preferred method for evaluating intermediate lesions' severity, as there is no specific minimal lumen area (MLA) threshold for revascularization. Also, the cut-off MLA to decide about the need for revascularization in non-left main situations should always be interpreted in context to the reference vessel MLA. For example, a cut-off MLA of 3.75 mm for vessels >3.5 mm, 3.16 mm for vessels 3–3.5 mm, and 2.68 mm for vessels <3 mm has a good correlation with FFR <0.80. The recent trial which has used a cutoff of MLA to decide whether to do percutaneous coronary intervention (PCI) or not was the "FLAVOUR Study".

Criteria for PCI based on intravascular ultrasound (IVUS) in this trial were:

- MLA <3 mm
- MLA between 3 and 4 mm with plaque burden (PB) >70%

Assessing the need for revascularization in intermediate lesions involves considering both MLA and PB, with FFR being a crucial tool for evaluation.

For example, if we see this case in **Figure 1**, the MLA is 3.9 mm^2 but the PB is huge (close to 80%). Considering the very low risk of stent thrombosis in this case with good minimal stent areas (MSAs) achievable, stenting it would be the best option to reduce future major adverse cardiovascular event (MACE) in this patient.

The need for revascularization may not be totally based on functional stenosis but also upon the vulnerability of plaque, as shown in the PREVENT TRIAL. In this trial, those lesions with FFR (≥0.80) and meeting two of the following imaging-defined vulnerable plaque criteria, preventive PCI reduced MACE arising from high-risk vulnerable plaques, compared with optimal medical therapy alone. These criteria for preventive PCI were:

1. Minimal lumen area (MLA) ≤4.0 mm^2
2. Plaque burden >70%
3. Thin-cap fibroatheroma by (OCT) or radiofrequency intravascular ultrasound (IVUS)
4. Lipid-rich plaque by near-infrared spectroscopy (maxLCBI4mm 315)

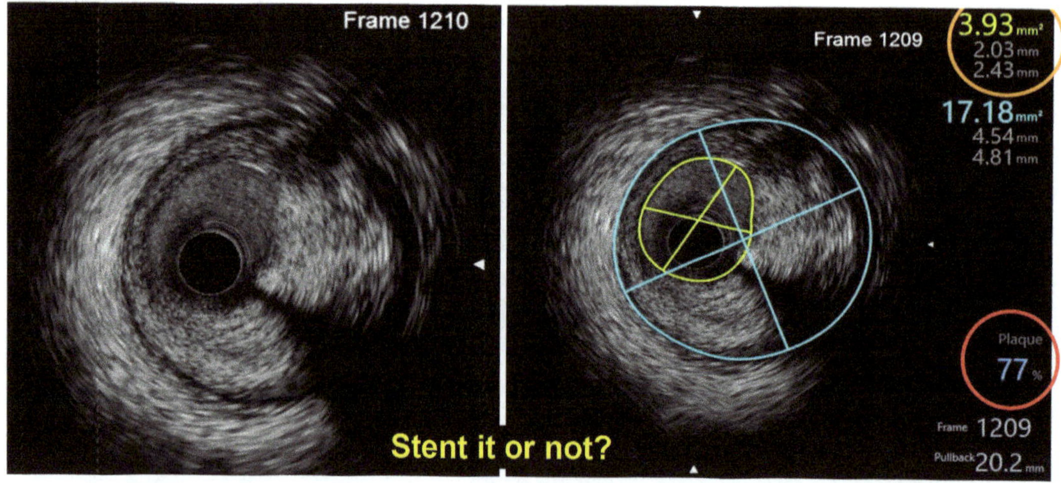

Fig. 1: Intravascular ultrasound (IVUS) to assess the need for revascularization in intermediate lesions.

"Time to commit ourselves to see more and see better when making PCI decisions"

CHAPTER 39

Slow Flow on Intravascular Ultrasound

IDENTIFYING SLOW FLOW ON INTRAVASCULAR ULTRASOUND

During slow flow, the red blood cells (RBCs) aggregate and reflect the sound waves strongly, so the lumen appears white and foggy as compared to a grayish-black appearance of the lumen in a normal flow **(Fig. 1)**.

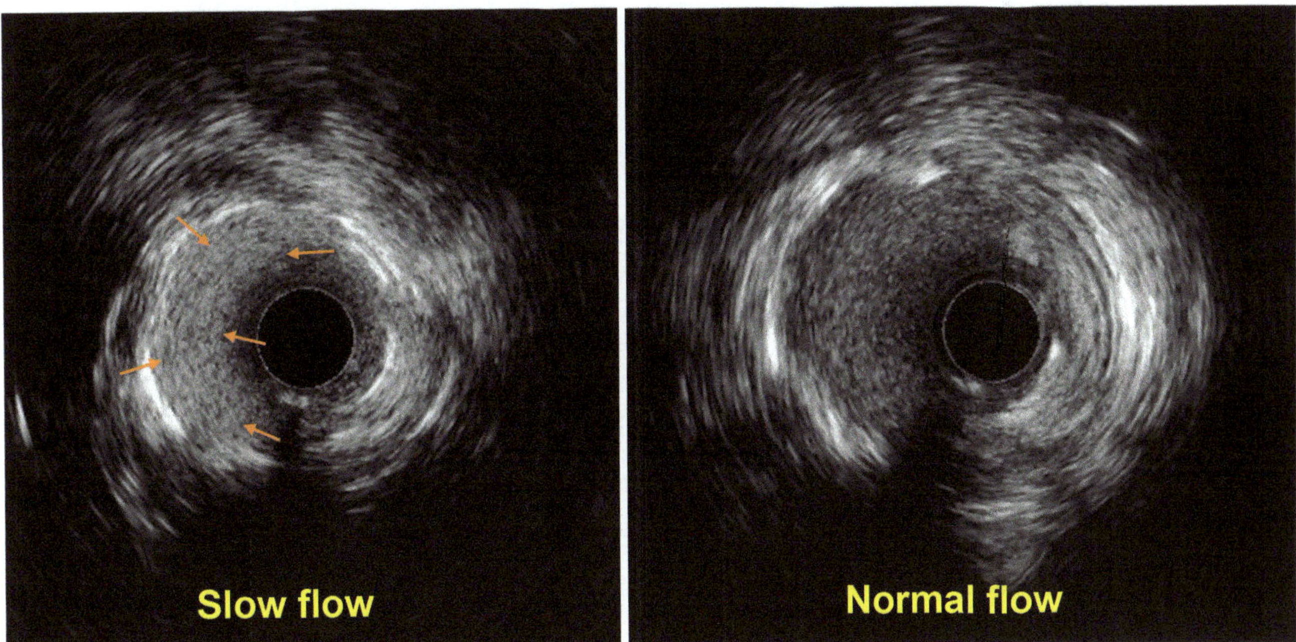

Fig. 1: Identifying slow flow on IVUS.

CHAPTER 40

Differentiating True from False Lumen on Intravascular Ultrasound

Following are the differentiating points on intravascular ultrasound (IVUS) between true and false lumen **(Fig. 1)**:

- Recognition of three-layered appearance (true lumen)
- Identification of side branches taking off (true lumen)
- Slower, more echogenic blood reflectance (false lumen)
- Contrast material injections can aid in distinguishing true and false lumen. Echogenic patterns from contrast "hang-up" in false lumen compared to true lumen.

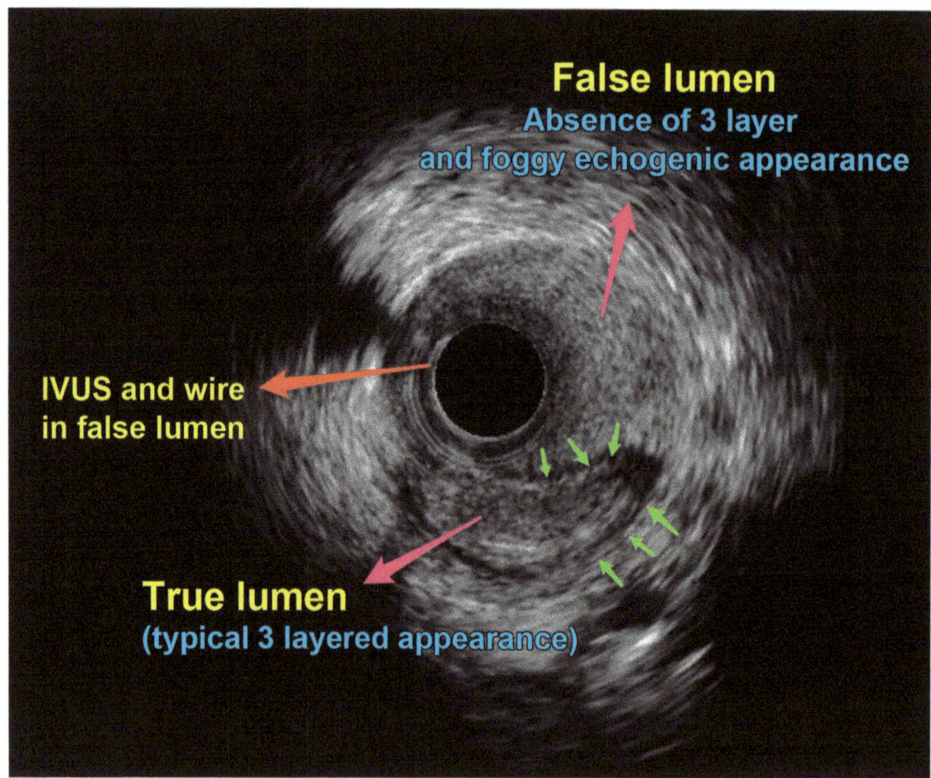

Fig. 1: Differentiating true from false lumen on intravascular ultrasound (IVUS).

"What eyes does not see, IVUS does"

CHAPTER 41

Stent Fracture

It is defined as the absence of stent struts in one-third of the circumference of the artery **(Fig. 1)**. However, with the present generation stents which have less number of connectors, the definition can be relaxed to one half of the circumference. It has to be correlated with stent boost always.

Stent fracture on intravascular ultrasound (IVUS) can be classified into five types as shown in **Figure 2**.

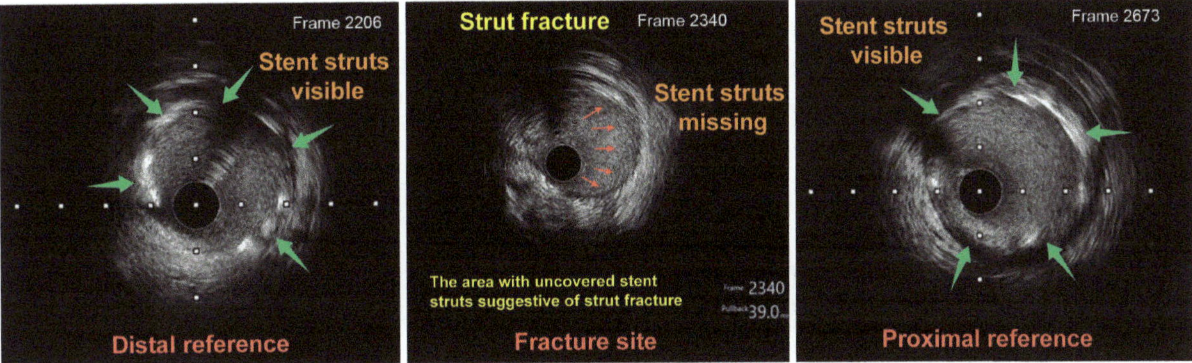

Fig. 1: Stent fracture on intravascular ultrasound (IVUS).

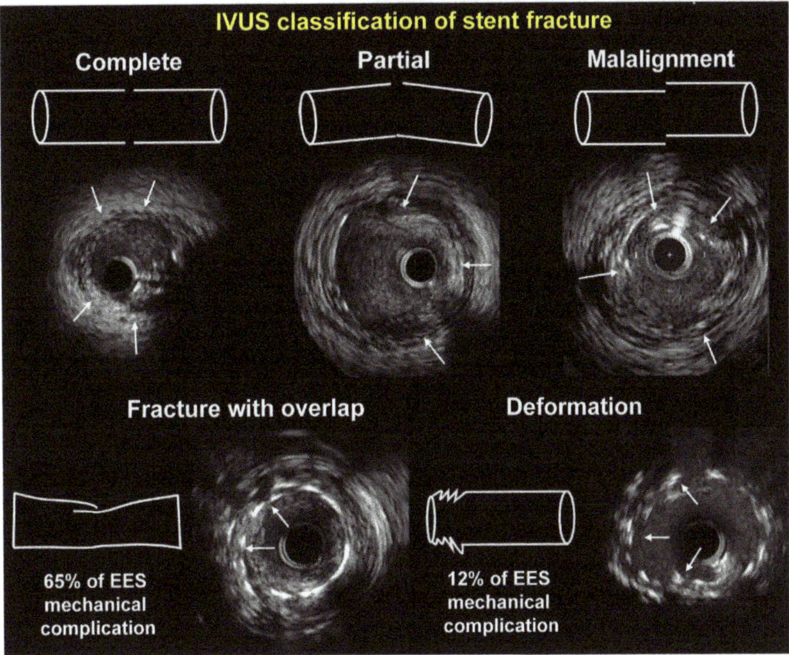

Fig. 2: Intravascular ultrasound (IVUS) classification of stent fracture.

CHAPTER 42

Myocardial Bridge

Myocardial bridge (MB) on intravascular ultrasound (IVUS) is defined as an echolucent area between the epicardial tissue and the compressed vessel, which resembles a *half-moon* **(Fig. 1)**.

Intravascular ultrasound not only helps in diagnosing MB but can also help us in assessing the severity of MB by estimating the following parameters:

- Arterial compression % **(Fig. 2)**
- Hallo thickness **(Fig. 3)**
- MB **(Fig. 3)** index

Though the MB itself is free of disease, you will always see plaque burden proximal to MB.

The higher the MB index and the greater the hallo thickness, the more chance there will be of plaque burden proximal to MB.

Similarly, the more arterial compression, the greater the chance of plaque burden proximal to MB. (A minimum 10% arterial compression is required to make a diagnosis of MB)

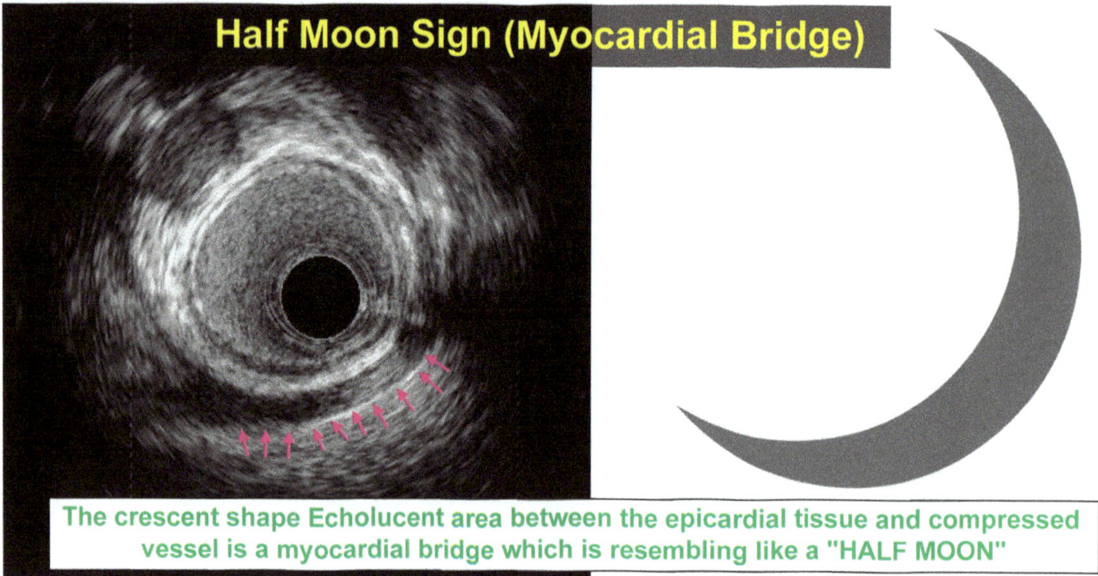

Fig. 1: Myocardial bridge with "half-moon sign".

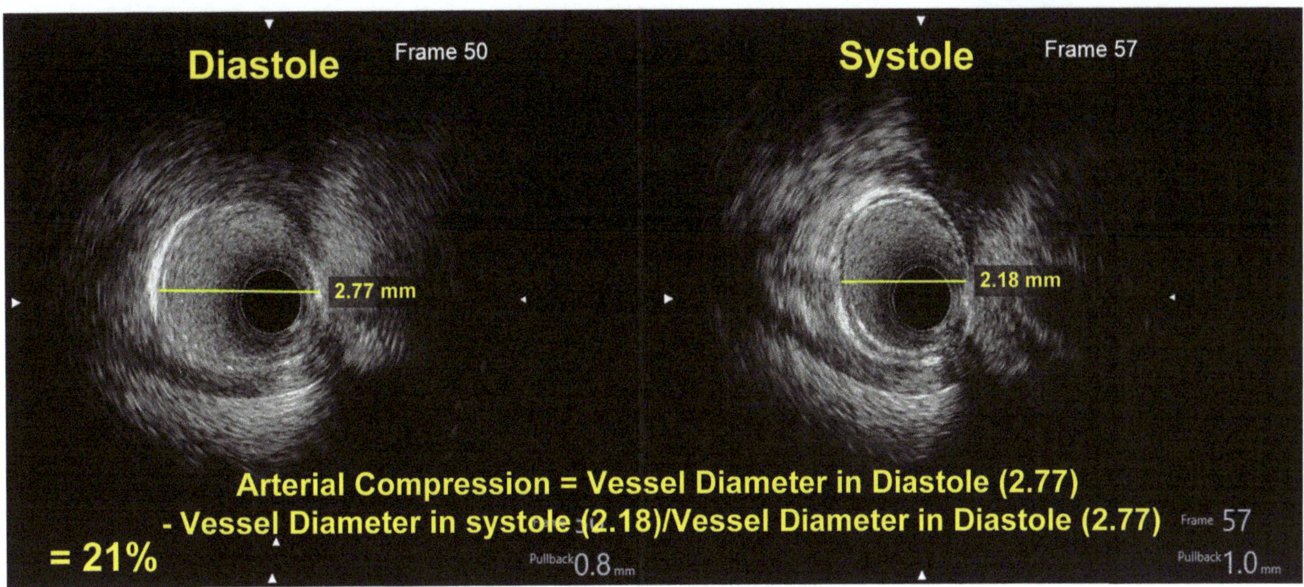

Fig. 2: Arterial compression index.

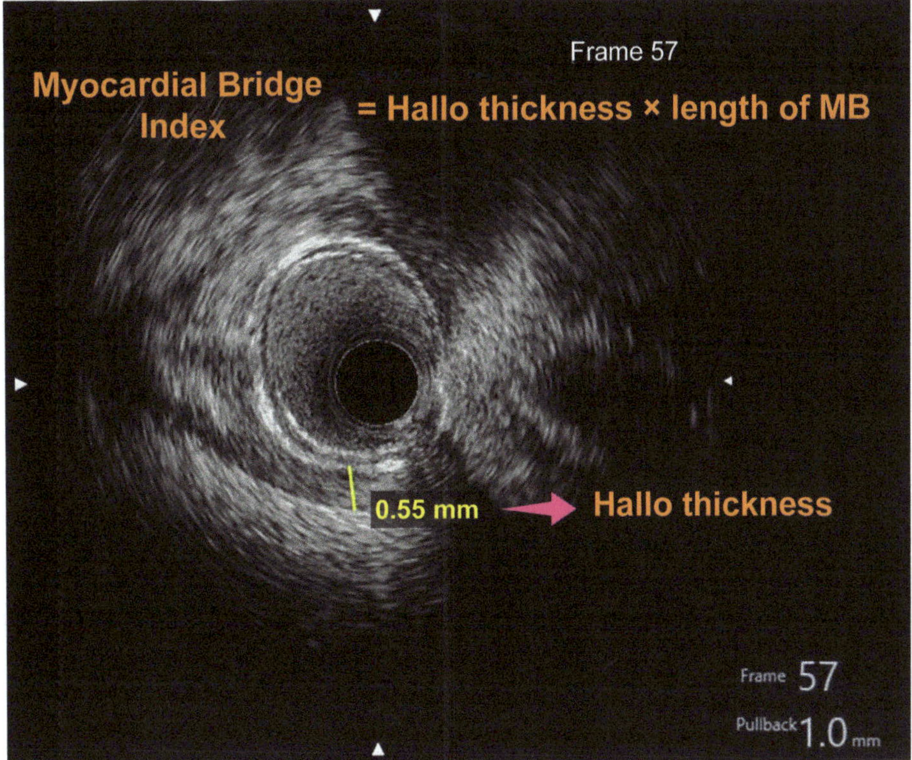

Fig. 3: Myocardial bridge (MB) index and hallo thickness.

The practical importance of identifying myocardial bridge on IVUS is that it helps us in avoiding landing our stents in myocardial bridge which can have poor long-term outcome.

CHAPTER 43

Spontaneous Coronary Artery Dissection

In a normal coronary artery with no atherosclerosis, there is a medial dissection with a collection of blood in the false lumen leading to compression of the true lumen, called spontaneous coronary artery dissection (SCAD) **(Fig. 1)**. The clues to differentiate SCAD from other causes of dissection on intravascular ultrasound (IVUS) are:

- SCAD is free of atherosclerosis.
- Intimal tear is rare in SCAD.
- Usually no communication between true and false lumen in SCAD.

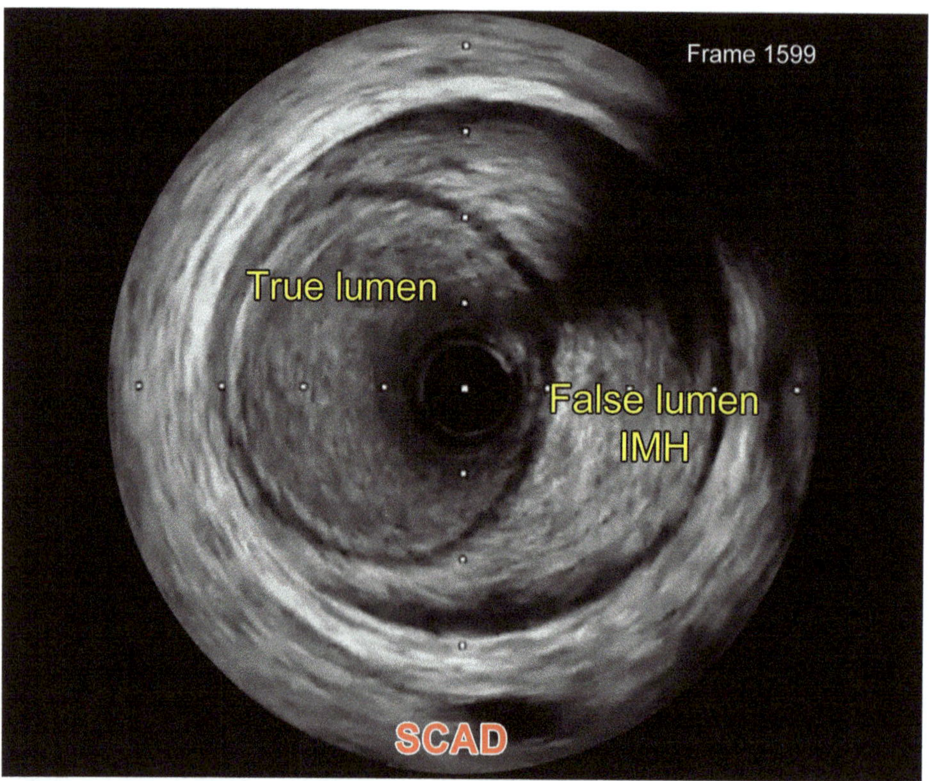

Fig. 1: Appearance of spontaneous coronary artery dissection (SCAD) on intravascular ultrasound (IVUS).

CHAPTER 44

True Aneurysm and Pseudoaneurysm

True aneurysm is defined as having a maximum lumen area >50% larger than the proximal reference area with an intact vessel wall **(Fig. 1)**.

Pseudoaneurysm has a loss of vessel integrity, absence of three-layered structured and damage to the adventitia and perivascular tissue **(Fig. 2)**.

The difference between a true and a false aneurysm is the presence of media. In a true aneurysm, the media is thinned and expanded but fully encompasses the perimeter of the aneurysm. In a false aneurysm, there is absence of three-layered structured with the media been damaged, and the vessel is contained by adventitia and periadventitial stroma.

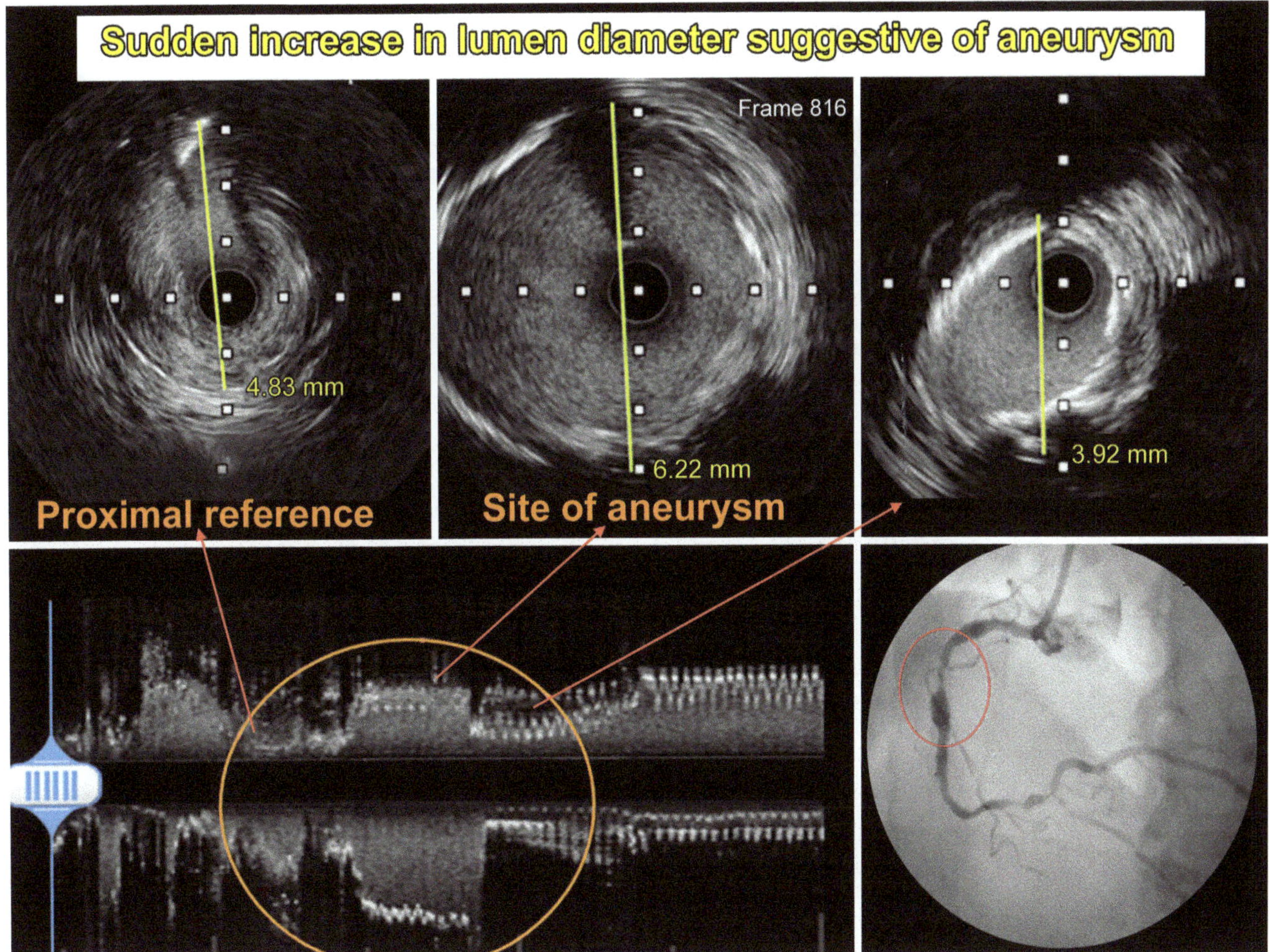

Fig. 1: True aneurysm on intravascular ultrasound (IVUS).

Usually, covered stents are used to treat these aneurysms.

The peculiar feature of a covered stent on intravascular ultrasound (IVUS) is that the IVUS does not penetrate the mesh within the covered stent, so you do not see anything beyond the covered stent (also known as the "eclipse sign") **(Fig. 3)**.

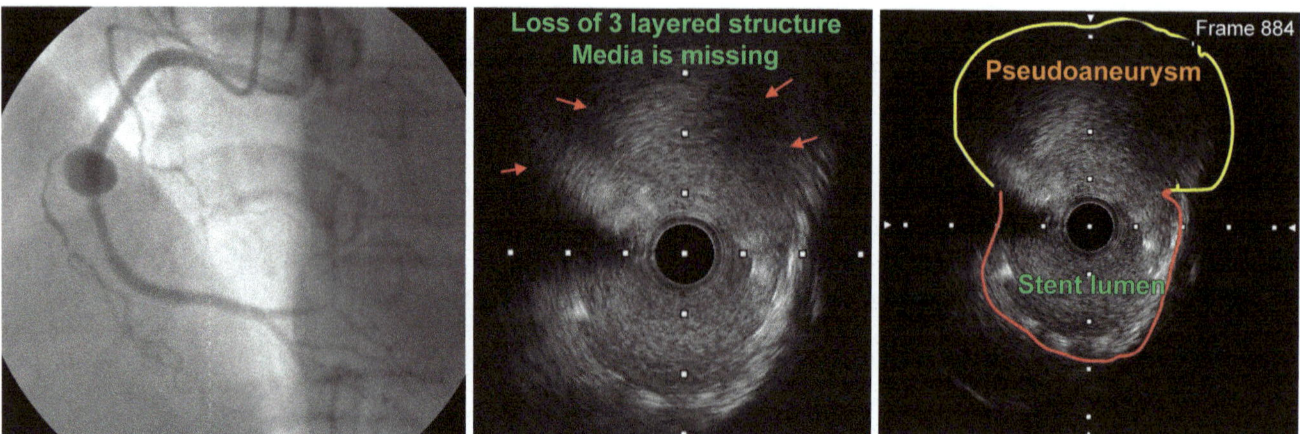

Fig. 2: Pseudoaneurysm on intravascular ultrasound (IVUS).

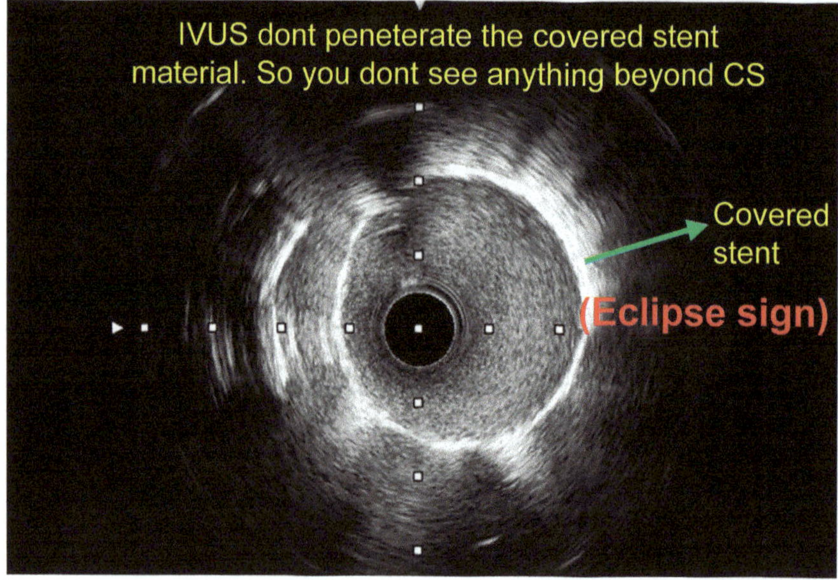

Fig. 3: Covered stent on intravascular ultrasound (IVUS) (eclipse sign).

"Seeing beyond the surface: IVUS unveils the heart's hidden paths."

CHAPTER 45

Intravascular Ultrasound in Saphenous Vein Grafts

Typically, veins have a thin muscular media layer and a thick adventitia layer, whereas coronary arteries have a well-developed media layer and a thinner adventitia. The saphenous veins undergo "arterialization" when placed as a graft in the arterial system, with morphological changes that include intimal fibrous thickening, medial hypertrophy, and lipid deposition **(Figs. 1 and 2)**. Positioned in this new environment, saphenous vein grafts (SVGs) experience hemodynamic stress over the entire length of the conduit. Significantly, graft calcification occurred mainly within the wall and not within the plaque, which suggests that SVG calcification is not just a result of lesion formation but also of wall changes associated with arterialization and (passive or active) degeneration. In support of this, SVG calcium was as common in the reference segments as within the lesion.

In short, the wall morphology and plaque characteristics are different in vein grafts than those in native coronaries **(Box 1)**.

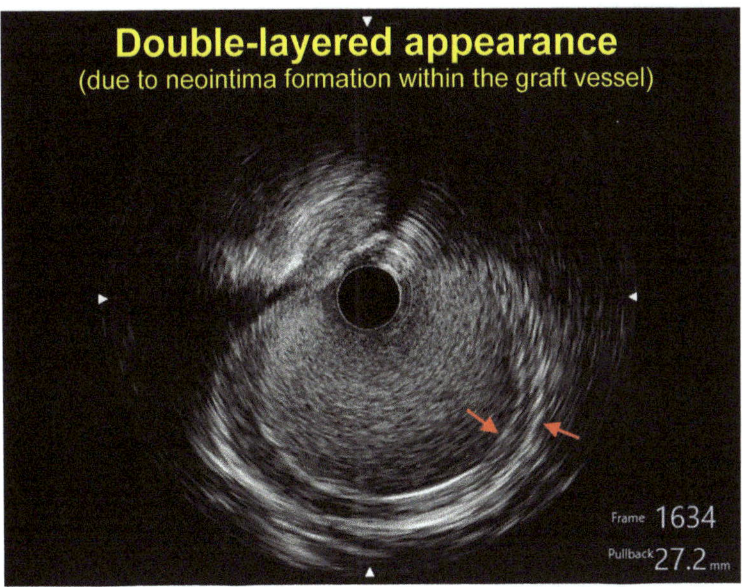

Fig. 1: Saphenous vein graft (SVG) on intravascular ultrasound (IVUS) showing double layered appearance.

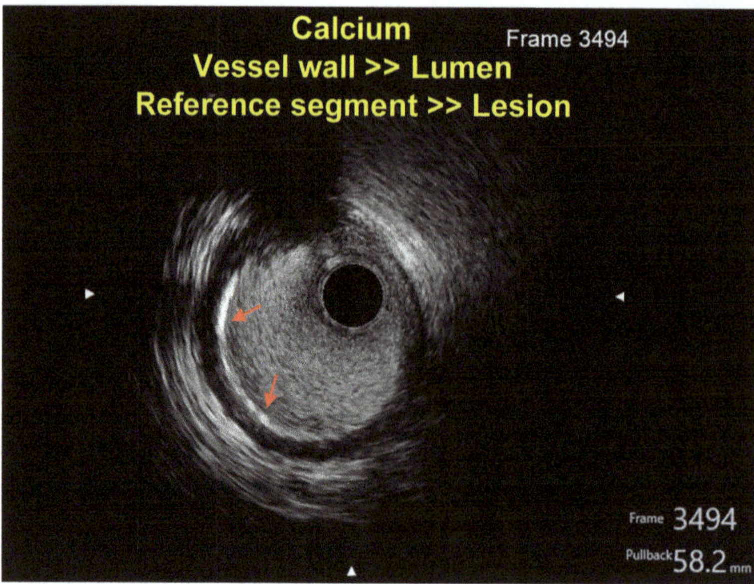

Fig. 2: Saphenous vein graft (SVG) on intravascular ultrasound (IVUS).

Box 1: Clue to diagnose vein graft on intravascular ultrasound (IVUS).

- Long artery
- No branches
- No tapering
- Double-layered appearance **(Fig. 1)**
- Calcium more in wall than lumen **(Fig. 2)**
- Calcium more in the reference segment than lesion
- Presence of calcified venous valves **(Fig. 3)**

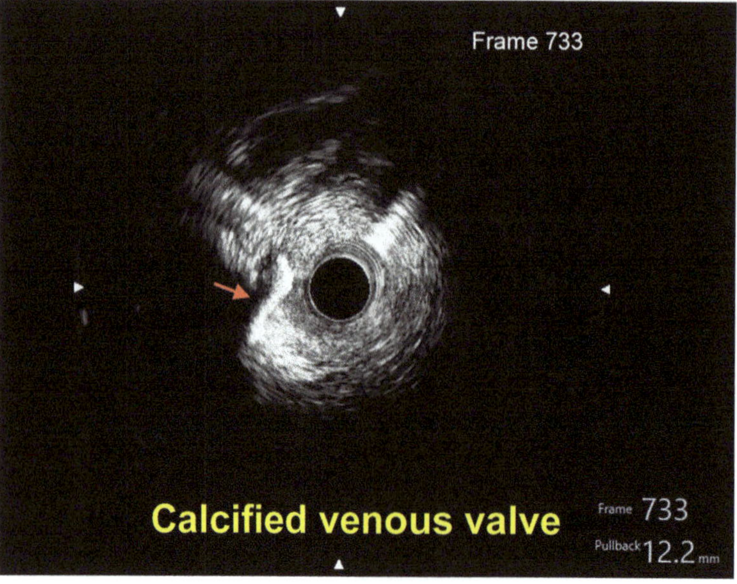

Fig. 3: Calcified venous valves in saphenous vein graft (SVG).

CHAPTER 46

Diagnosing Perforation and Impending Perforation on Intravascular Ultrasound

Clues to the diagnosis of perforation on intravascular ultrasound (IVUS) are:

- **Disruption of vessel architecture:** Notice any signs of disrupted or interrupted vessel wall structure, which may appear as irregular or jagged edges.
- **Presence of extramural hematoma:** It is extravasation of blood or contrast, which may appear as echodense structure outside the vessel wall which happens due to adventitial dissection **(Fig. 1)**.
- **Pseudoaneurysm formation:** Identify any out-pouching adjacent to the vessel wall that may indicate contained perforation **(Fig. 2)**.

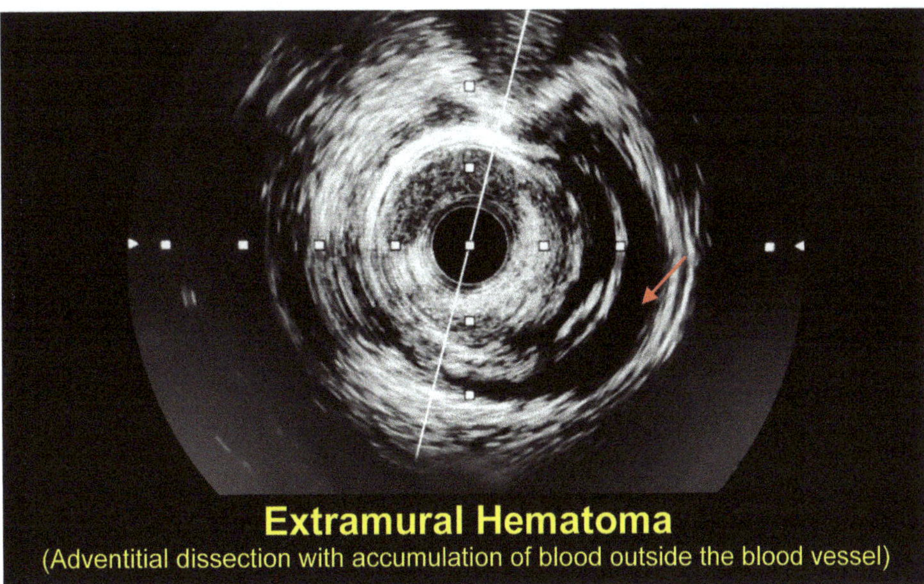

Fig. 1: Extramural hematoma.

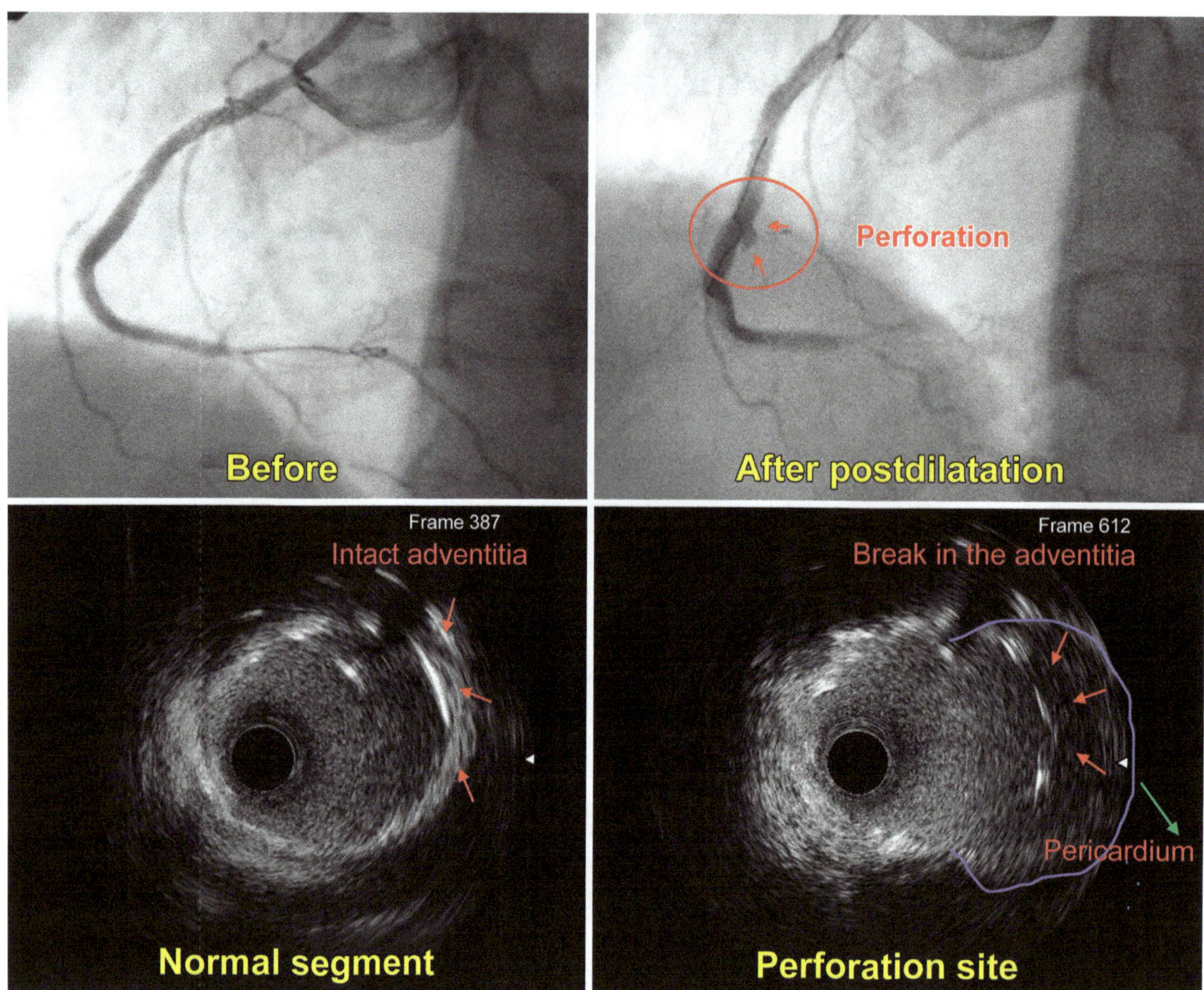

Fig. 2: Contained perforation seen on intravascular ultrasound (IVUS) with corresponding angiography.

HOW TO DIAGNOSE IMPENDING PERFORATION ON IVUS?

Diagnosing impending perforation is even more important than diagnosing perforation after it has happened. If you see the **Figure 3**, you will realize that this artery is on the verge of perforation if it is dilated anymore. This is because this is an eccentric compression with calcified plaque on one side and media on the opposite site completely compressed, and adventitia is stretched. Now, if any more dilation is done, then the entire pressure is going to be transmitted on one side (adventitial side), and since adventitia is a weak structure and it can break off easily, leading to perforation.

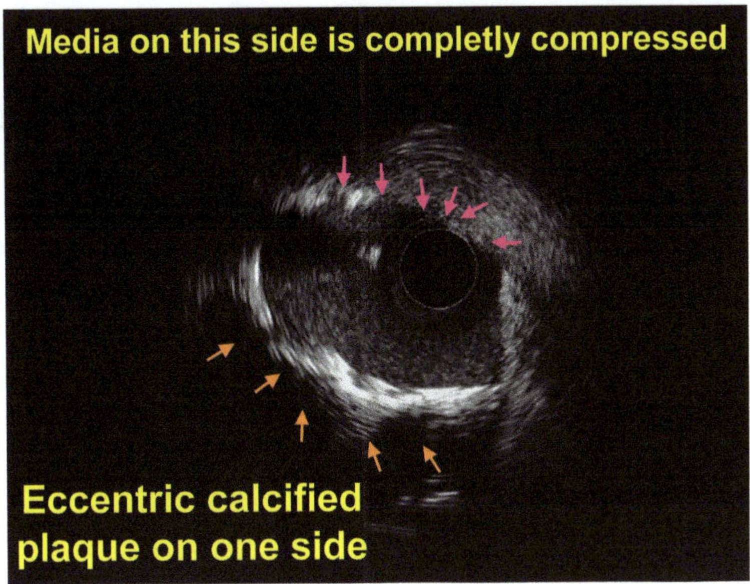

Fig. 3: Eccentric expansion with compressed media on one side.

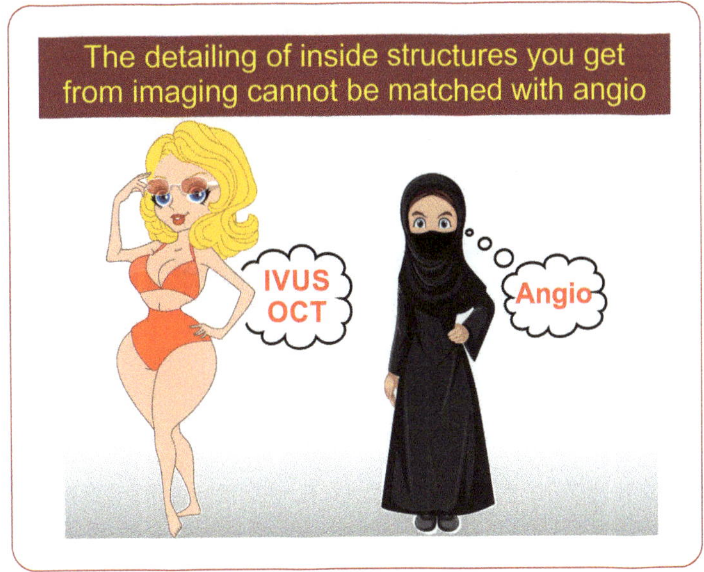

CHAPTER 47

Application of IVUS during ROTA

- **Assessing the need for ROTA ablation:** If in a severely calcified lesion you are not able to cross the intravascular ultrasound (IVUS) catheter, it automatically becomes a case for ROTA. However, if you are able to cross the lesion, then calculate the calcium score. If the score is 2 or >2, then ROTA should be used to modify the calcium **(Fig. 1)**.

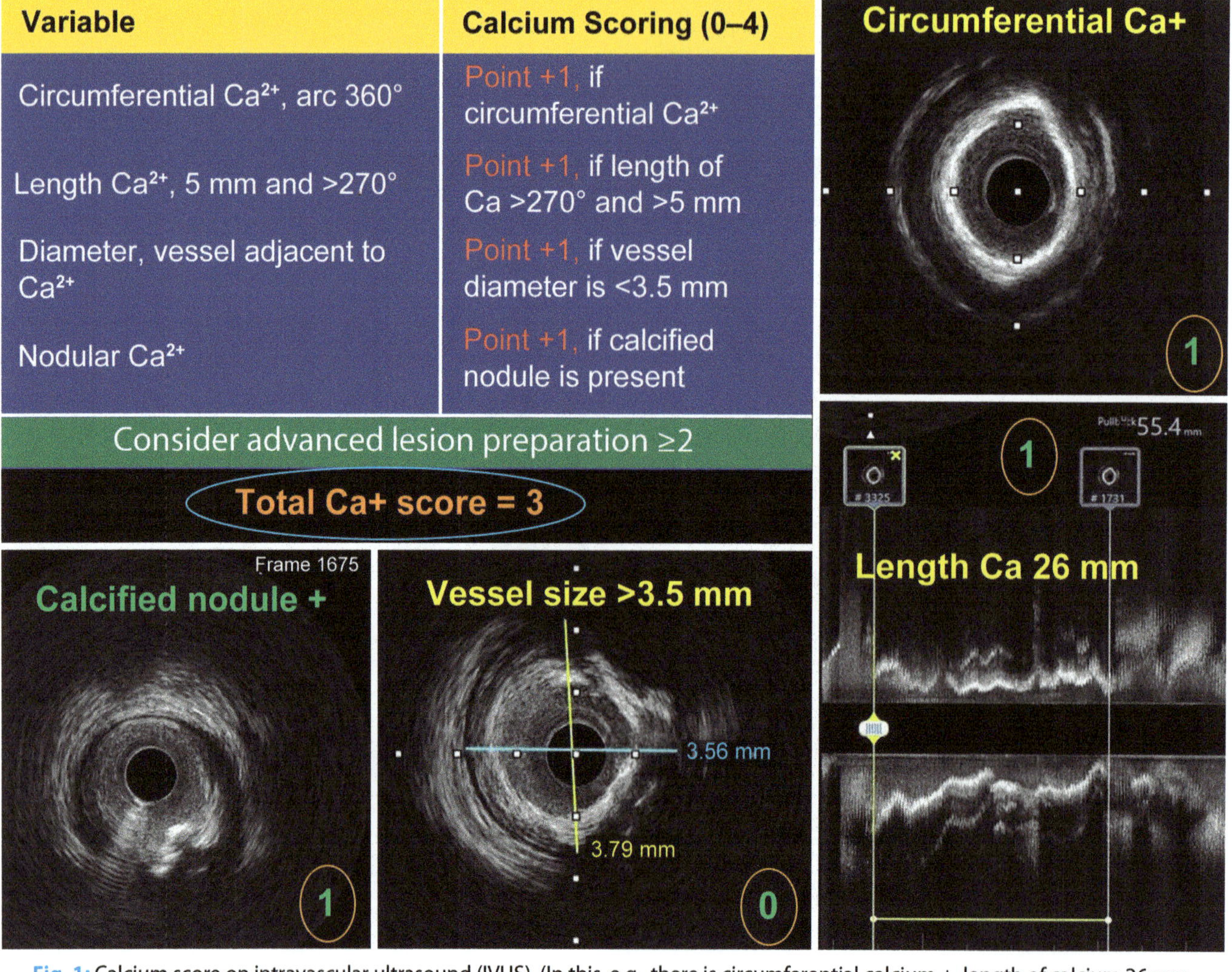

Fig. 1: Calcium score on intravascular ultrasound (IVUS). (In this, e.g., there is circumferential calcium +, length of calcium 26 mm, calcified nodule seen but vessel size is >3.5 mm so the calcium score is 3, which suggests that it requires rotablation).

- **Selecting burr size:** For effective rotablation, the size of the burr should be greater than the minimal lumen area (MLA) at the tightest calcified segment **(Fig. 2)**. Also, it should not be <0.5 of the vessel size.
- **Identifying guidewire bias:** Favorable wire bias is the key to successful rotablation, and this can be easily identified by IVUS **(Fig. 3)**. If on IVUS you do not see a favorable wire bias, then various standard techniques can be applied to change the wire bias.

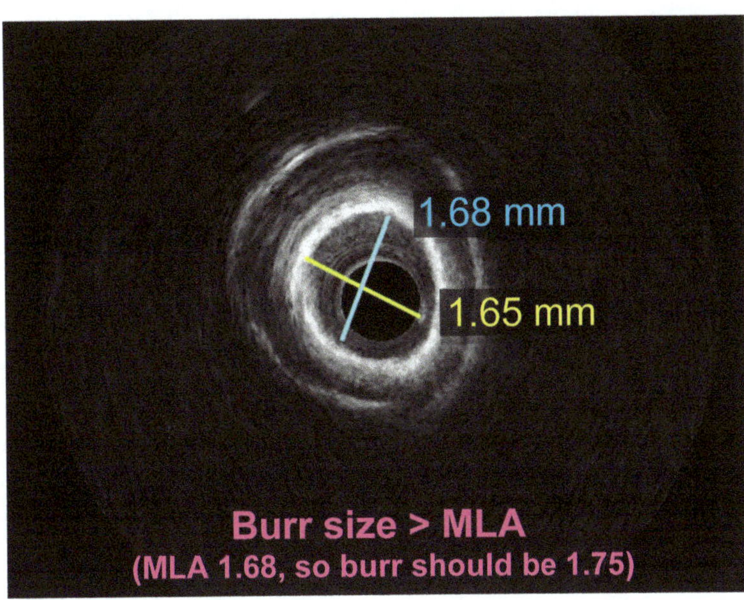

Fig. 2: Calculating burr size on IVUS. (IVUS: intravascular ultrasound; MLA: minimal lumen area)

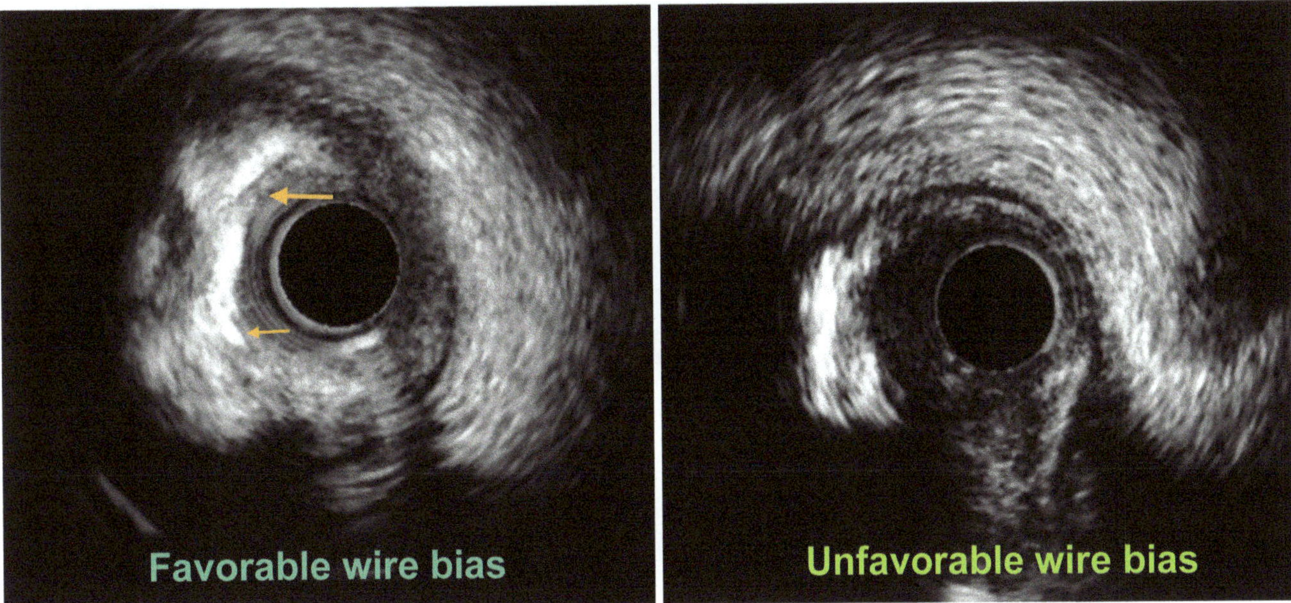

Fig. 3: Identifying wire bias on intravascular ultrasound (IVUS).

- **Ensuring safe rotablation in eccentric calcium in tortuous anatomy:** Rotablation is relatively safer if calcium is present on the smaller curvature side than on the larger curvature side because the ROTA floppy wire always follows the lesser curvature side. This differentiation can be easily done by IVUS **(Figs. 4A and B)**.

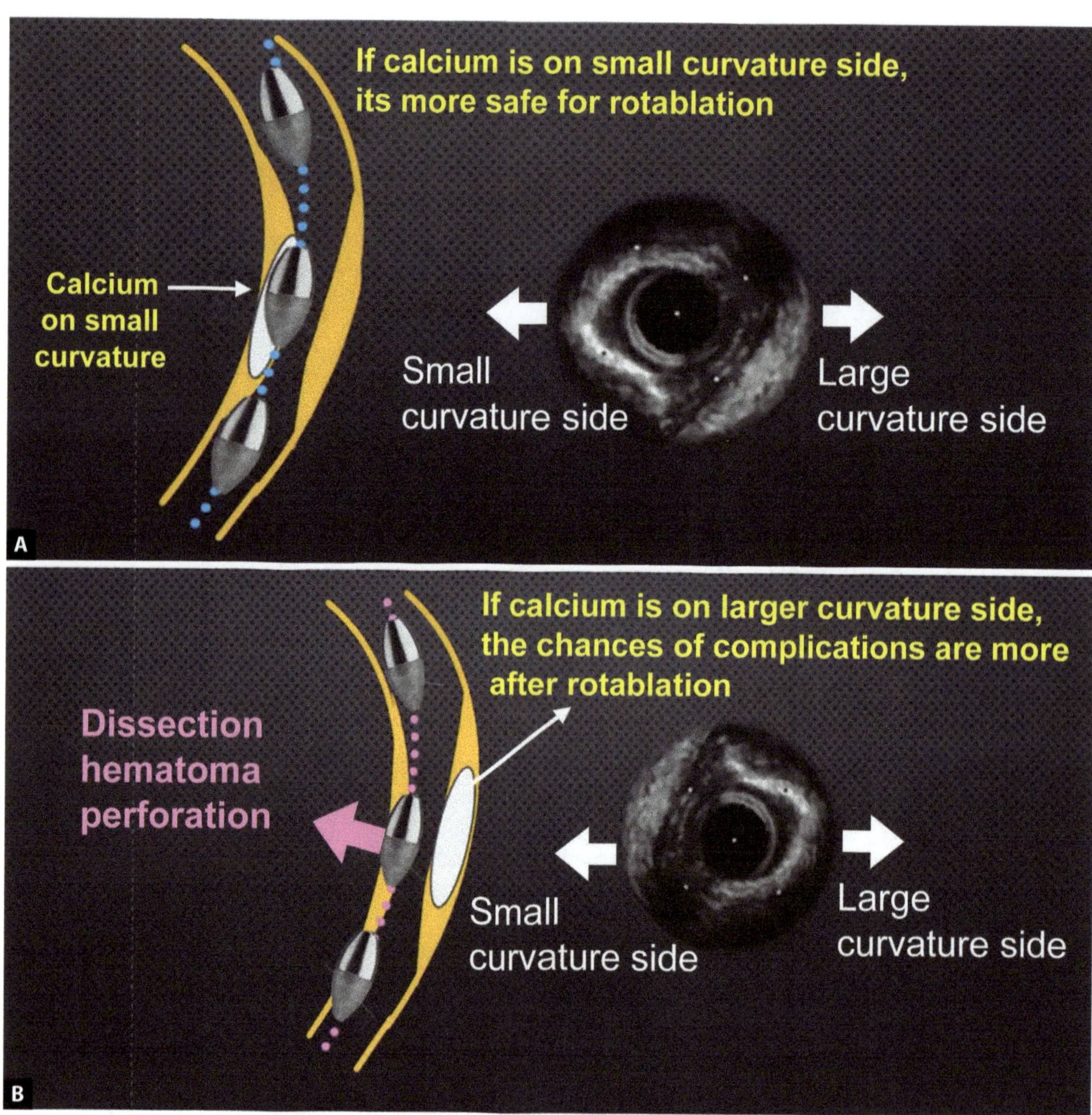

Figs. 4A and B: Effect of the presence of calcium on lesser or greater curvature on rotablation.

- **Confirming adequate rotablation:** Two ways to confirm it—
    1. *Reverberation:* If we see reverberations post-ROTA, it means we have shaved off the superficial calcium and converted thick calcium into thin **(Figs. 5 and 6)**.
    2. *Luminal gain:* A significant difference in the MLA pre- and postindicates good luminal gain, which confirms adequate rotablation **(Fig. 7)**. If we do not see any of these, then we need to upgrade the size of the burr or change the wire bias.
- **Deciding further calcium modification strategy post-ROTA ablation:** On IVUS, assess the residual calcium burden post-ROTA ablation. If the arc of the residual calcium is >270°, then the preferred modality may be an intravascular lithotripsy (IVL) or OPN. However, if the arc is <270°, then a cutting balloon or a noncompliant (NC) balloon can be used to achieve calcium fractures **(Fig. 8)**.
- **Optimizing stent expansion in calcified lesions:** Look for absolute minimal stent area (MSA) >5.5 mm^2 or 80% of the distal reference lumen area as criteria for optimal stent expansion. Eccentric expansion is acceptable if absolute MSAs are good **(Fig. 9)**.

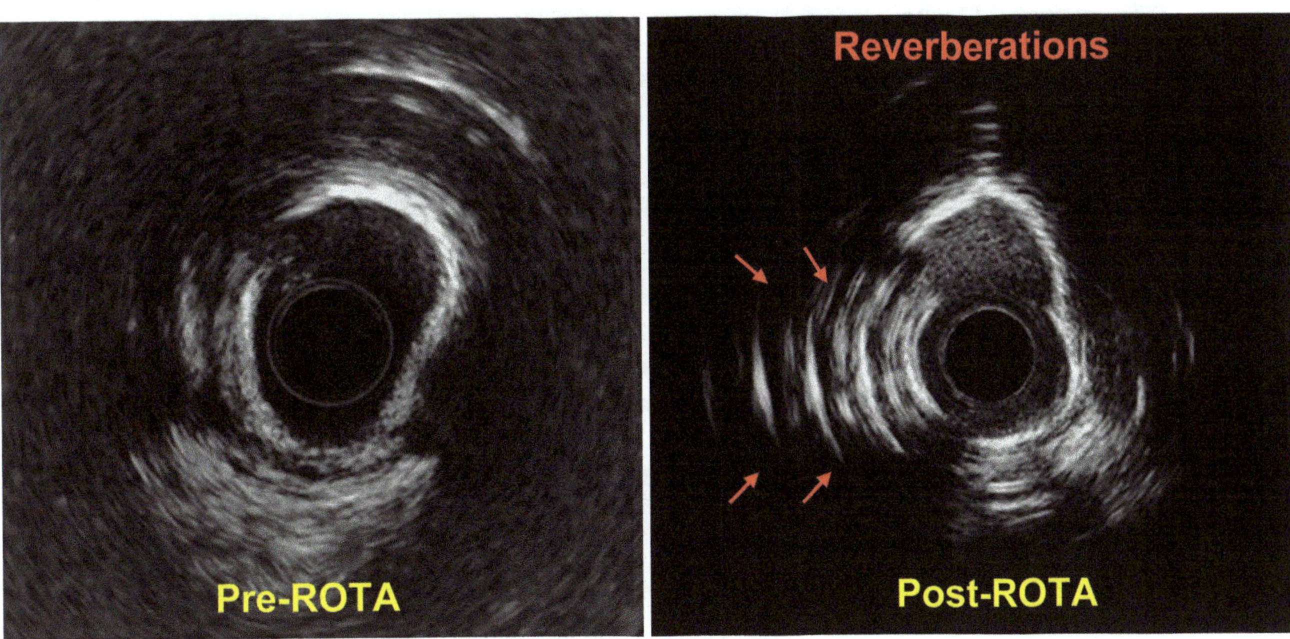

Fig. 5: Reverberations post-ROTA.

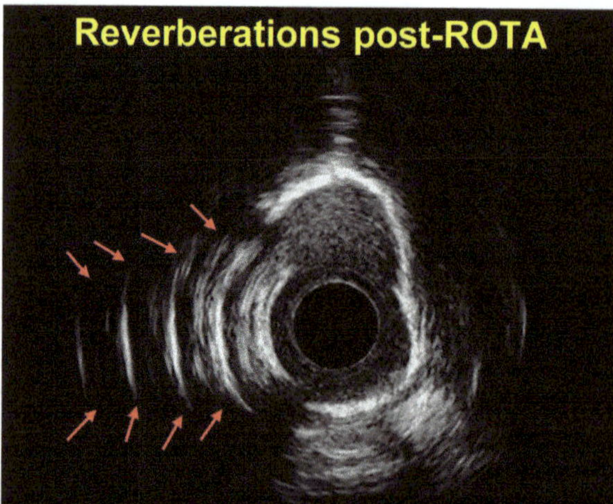

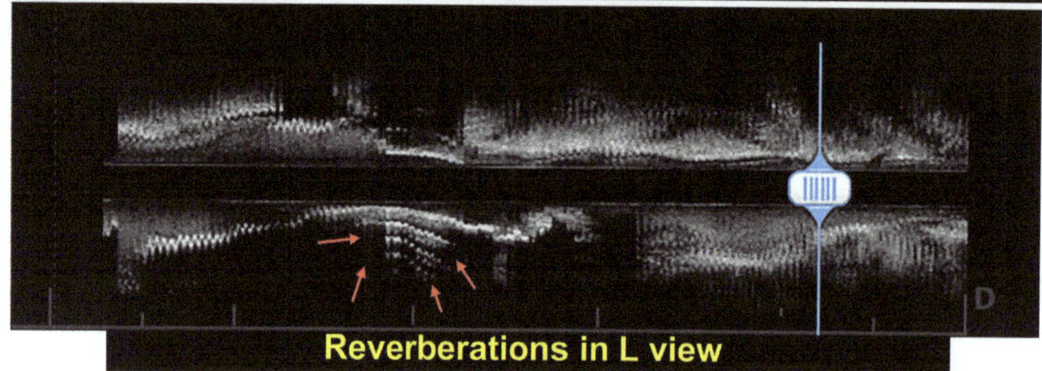

Fig. 6: Reverberations seen on both cross sectional and L view indicating adequate rotablation.

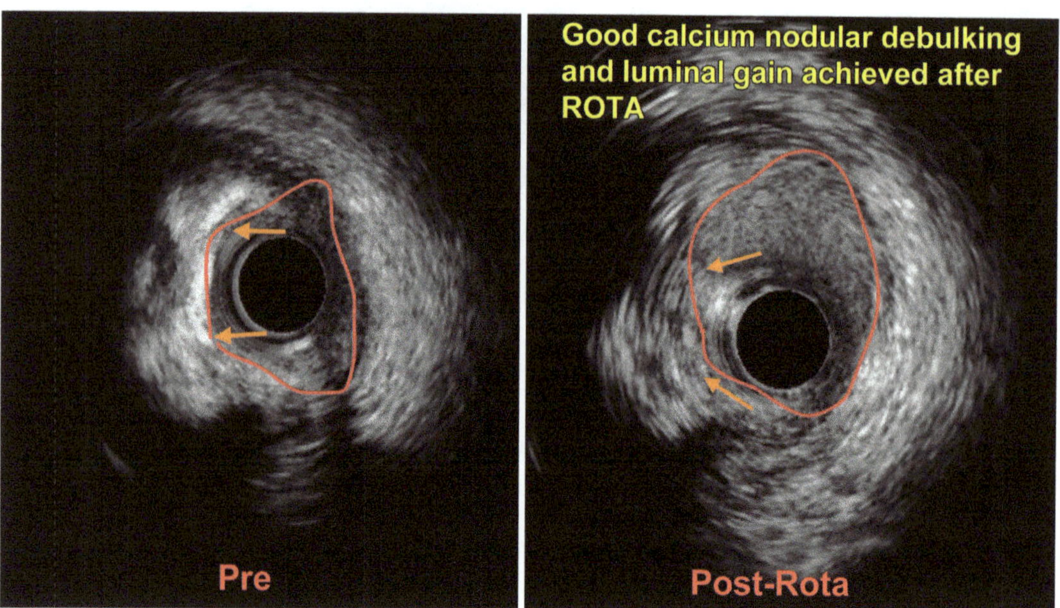

Fig. 7: Luminal gain post-ROTA.

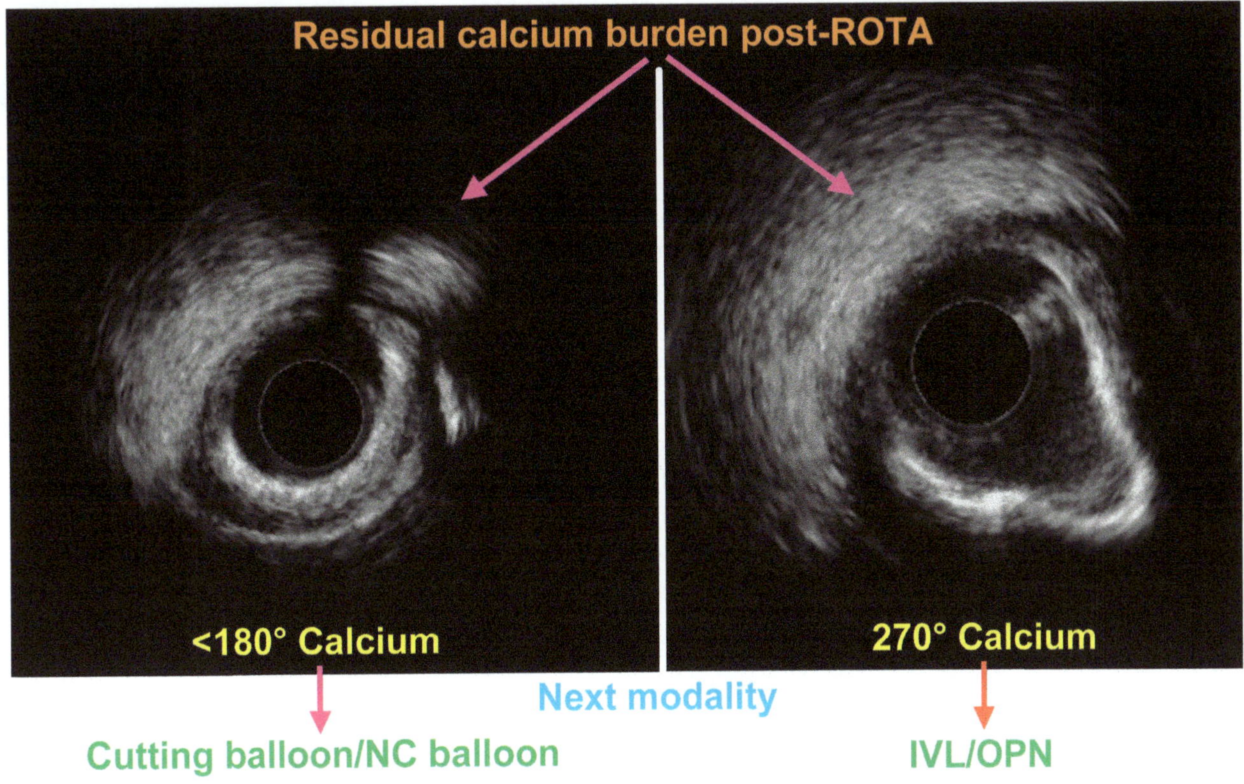

Fig. 8: Calcium modification strategy post-ROTA. (IVL: intravascular lithotripsy; NC: noncompliant)

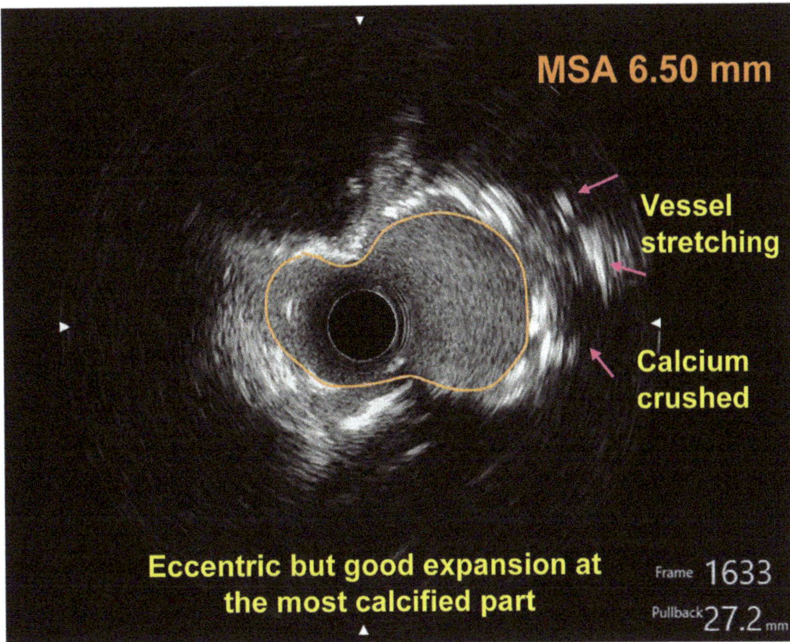

Fig. 9: Ensuring optimal stent expansion. (MSA: minimal stent area)

"Why worry about calcified arteries when you have ROVUS (Rota + IVUS)"

CHAPTER 48

IVUS-guided Puncture of an Ambiguous Proximal Cap

Intravascular ultrasound (IVUS)-guided puncture of an ambiguous proximal cap can be done in two ways:

1. Live IVUS using 8-F guide
2. IVUS marking technique using cine while using IVUS

STEPS FOR IVUS MARKING OF AMBIGUOUS CAP

Step 1: Start the IVUS pullback from the nearby side branch

Step 2: The moment you identify the proximal cap, stop the pullback

Step 3: Take a cine with IVUS parked right at the proximal cap

Step 4: Make this a reference image

Step 5: Remove the IVUS

Step 6: Take the penetrating wire and try to negotiate it exactly at the same spot marked by the IVUS using the reference image (do not change the view and angle of the cine)

Step 7: Do the IVUS again to confirm the entry into the true lumen

IMPORTANT POINTS DURING IVUS MARKING OF AMBIGUOUS CAP

- **Selection of side branch for IVUS pullback for ambiguous cap identification:** The branch should be parallel to the occluded artery and not perpendicular. Because IVUS pullback from a parallel artery will give you a better profile of the proximal cap and also will give you more time to identify as compared to a perpendicular branch which will just come and go. For example, in a case of occluded ostial left anterior descending (LAD), the success of identification of the proximal cap will be more if pullback is done from the ramus rather than left circumflex (LCX). Also, the dimensions of the side branch should be such to accommodate the IVUS catheter; e.g., length should be at least >20 mm since the tip to transducer length is 20 mm and the width should be wide enough to accommodate a 5-F catheter.
- **Identification of proximal cap:** This can be done in multiple ways
  - Identify the point where there is a sudden increase in the size of the vessel. The cap will be just somewhere distal to that
  - Try to identify blood speckles
  - Look for the absence of media
- **Frequency of transducer:** Lower frequency catheters such as 20 or 40 MHz should be preferred over higher frequency 60 MHz (the lower the frequency of the transducer, the more will be its penetrating power). Here we need more far-field penetration rather than near-field resolution.

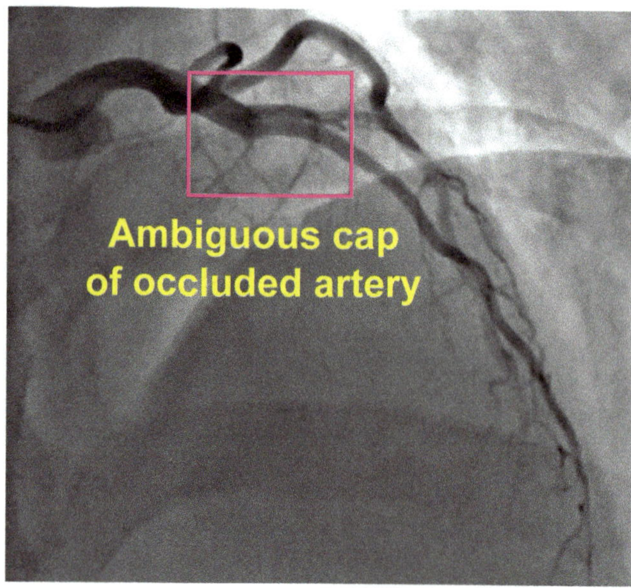

Fig. 1: Ambiguous proximal cap in an occluded mid left anterior descending (LAD).

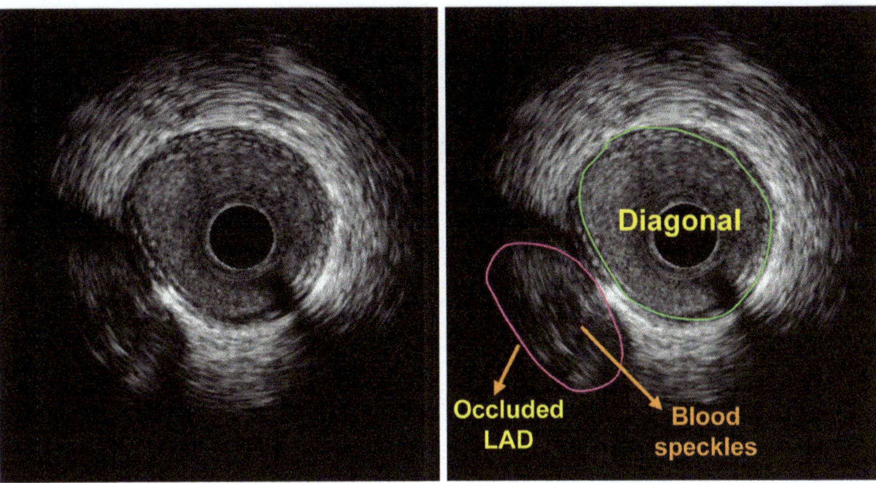

Fig. 2: Identification of the proximal cap on IVUS. (IVUS: intravascular ultrasound; LAD: left anterior descending)

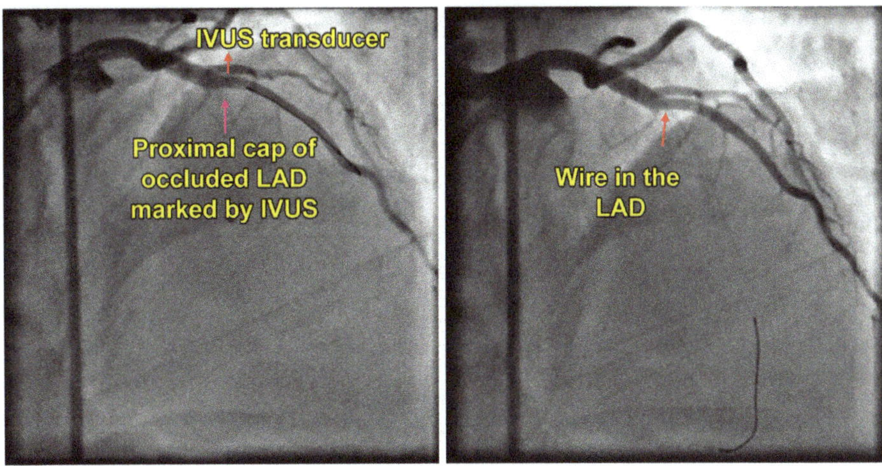

Fig. 3: IVUS angio-coregistration done. (IVUS: intravascular ultrasound; LAD: left anterior descending)

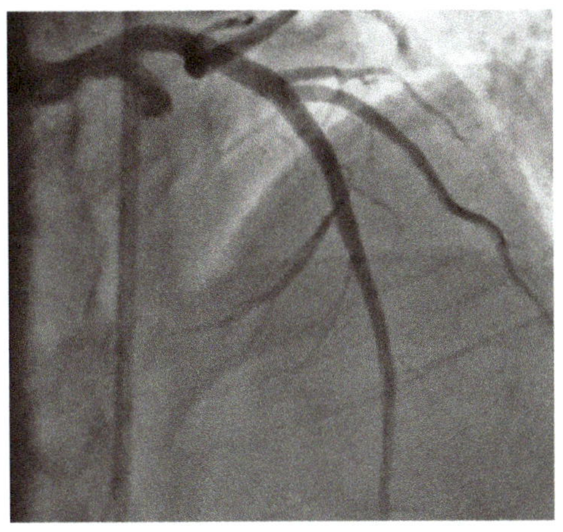

Fig. 4: Good final result in the end.

- **Setting of the machine:** The depth scale can be increased so that we are able to see the structures beyond the vessel.

A case of IVUS-guided puncture of an ambiguous cap of an occluded mid LAD is demonstrated here **(Fig. 1)**. IVUS pullback was done from the diagonal and the moment the proximal cap was identified **(Fig. 2)**, the pullback was stopped and a cine was taken. Using this as a reference image and as a landmark, puncturing of the proximal cap was done **(Fig. 3)** and a good final result was achieved **(Fig. 4)**.

"Why to take blind decisions when you have the IVUS"

CHAPTER 49

Absolute Zero-contrast Percutaneous Coronary Intervention

Here is the step-by-step demonstration of how to do zero-contrast percutaneous coronary intervention (PCI) in a case of calcified mid left anterior descending (LAD) lesion **(Fig. 1)**.

Step 1: Confirm catheter engagement without contrast puff by either injecting saline and observing for ST changes or feeling the dance motion of the guide catheter with the vessel or by wire entry confirmation **(Fig. 2)**.

Step 2: No contrast puffing for wiring. Use reference image as a roadmap for wiring **(Fig. 3)**.

Step 3: Do predilatation based on reference angiography.

Step 4: Do the intravascular ultrasound (IVUS) and assess the morphology, length, and diameter of the lesion **(Fig. 4)**. If calcium is present as in this case, make sure that adequate plaque modification has been done or not **(Fig. 5)**.

Step 5: IVUS-angiography co-registration using MARKER WIRE technique.

Step 5a: Take the marker wire from separate Y connector and park somewhere in distal LAD **(Fig. 6)**.

Step 5b: Take IVUS on the operating wire and stop the pullback when you see the proximal landing zone and take a dry cine.

Step 5c: Pull the marker wire and place its radiopaque end exactly at the distal landing zone marked by the IVUS catheter **(Fig. 7)**.

Step 5d: Close the toue tightly and remove the IVUS. Now, I have the marker wire in place exactly at the proximal landing zone. I just have to park my stent at the radiopaque tip of the marker wire **(Fig. 8)**.

Step 5e: Take stent on operating wire and place it exactly at the radiopaque tip of marker wire **(Fig. 9)**. (Here we are not worried about the distal landing zone since we have made the measurements about the stent length already on IVUS. So if we place our stent correctly at the proximal landing zone then automatically the stent is going to land correctly distally.)

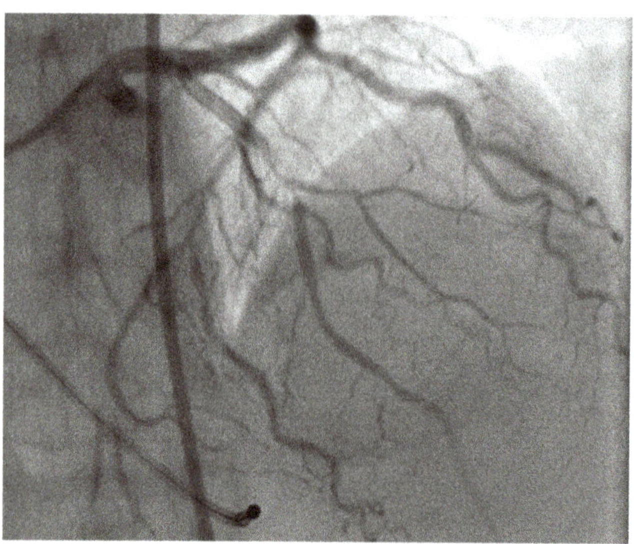

Fig. 1: Baseline angiography showing calcified mid left anterior descending (LAD) lesion.

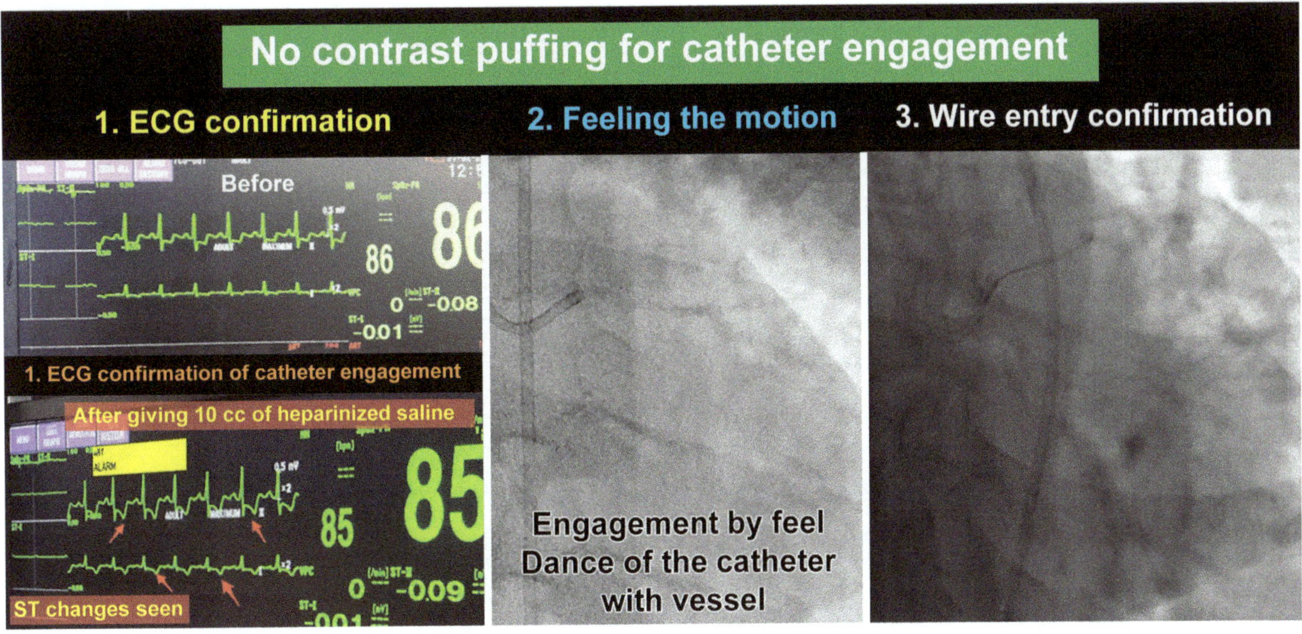

Fig. 2: Confirming catheter engagement without contrast puffing. (EEG: electroencephalogram)

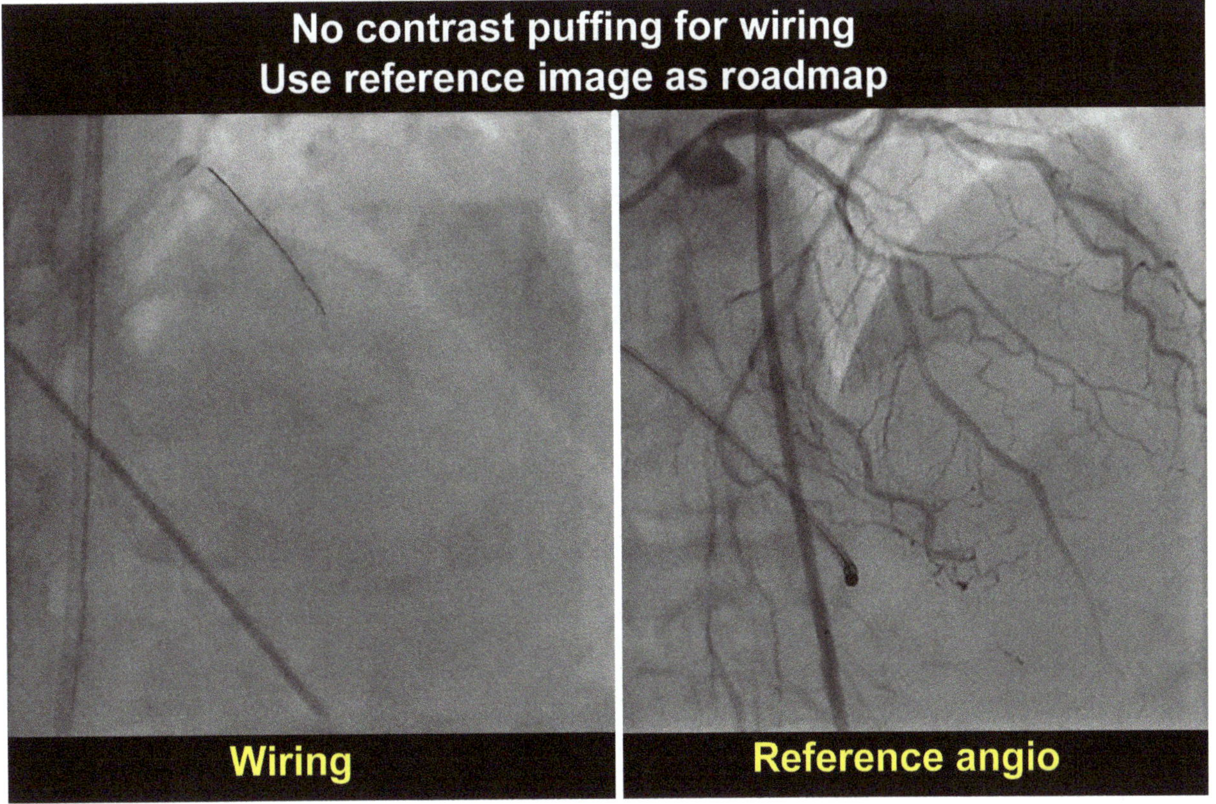

Fig. 3: Wiring without contrast using reference image.

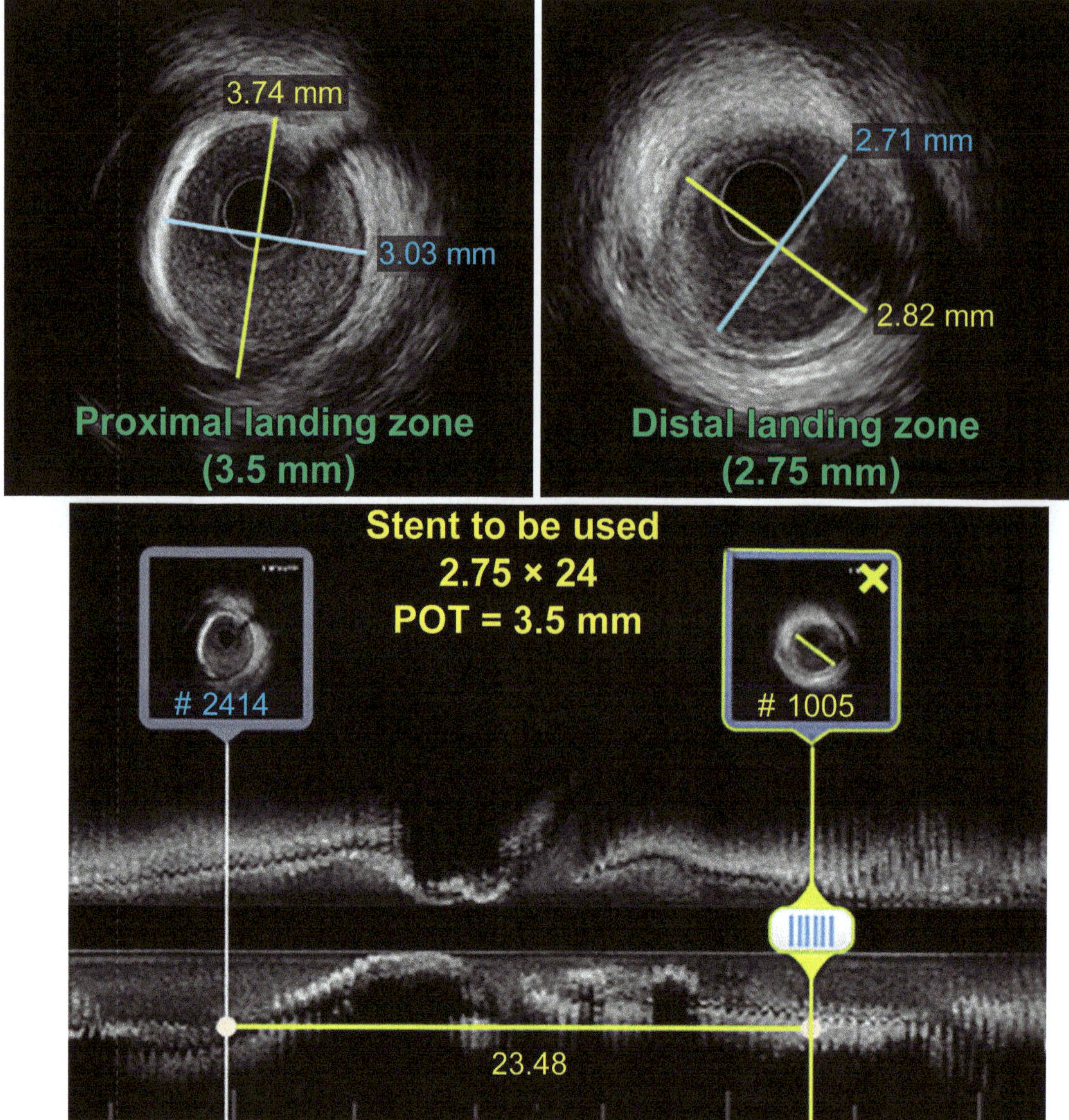

Fig. 4: Pre PCI measurements on IVUS.

Step 5f: Inflate the stent and remove the marker wire.

Step 6: Do the proximal optimization technique (POT) and postdilation as planned.

Step 7: Do the postprocessing IVUS **(Fig. 10)**. Besides the routine MLD-MAX algorithm (stent expansion, malapposition, and dissection), one must also look for the following things:

- Exclude slow flow
- Exclude major perforation
- Exclude luminal thrombus
- Exclude plaque prolapse
- Exclude left main coronary artery (LMCA) dissection

Step 8: Do the physiology testing fractional flow reserve (FFR). If the post PCI FFR is >0.92, it gives us an assurance that everything is ok below, within, and above the stent **(Fig. 11)**.

Step 9: Do a bedside echo to rule out distal small artery perforation.

Step 10: Take the final cine with 3 mL dye in the end **(Fig. 12)**.

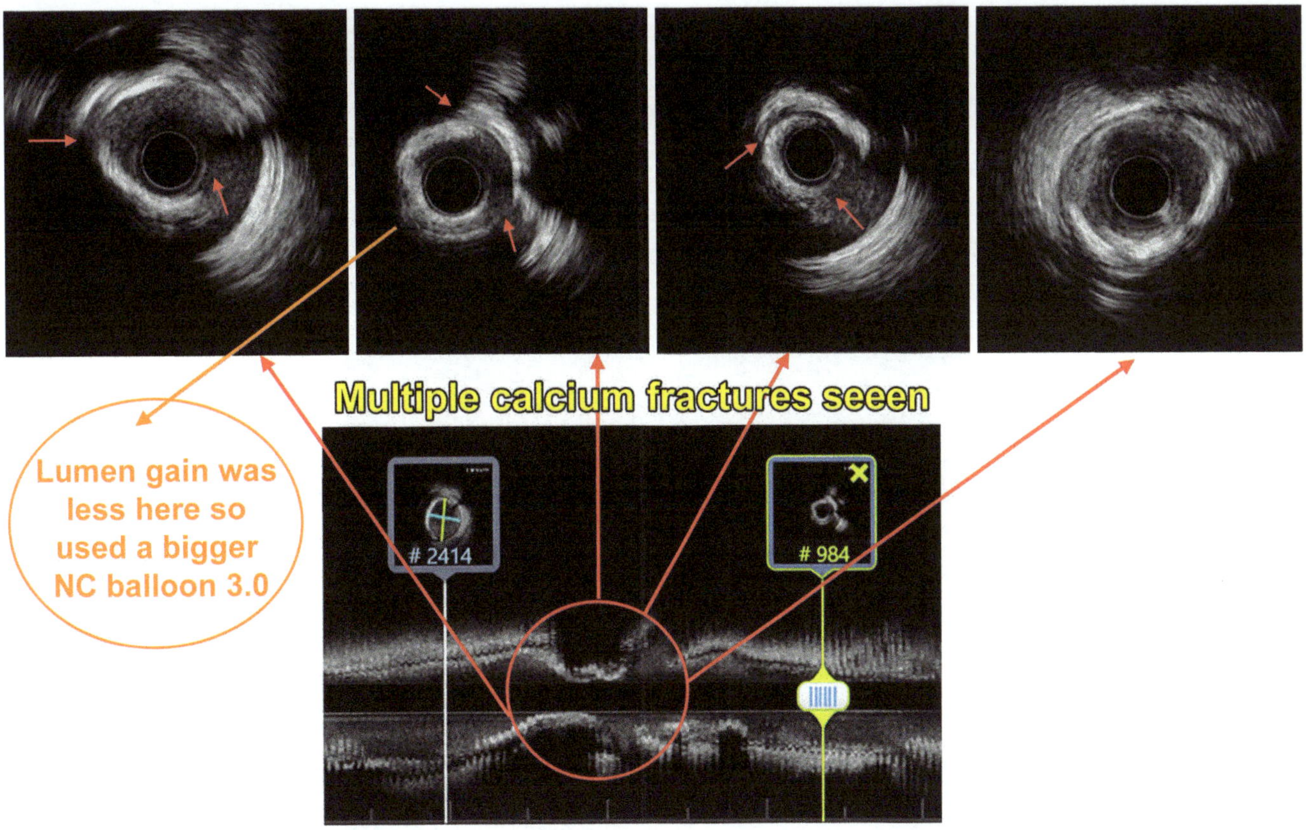

Fig. 5: Assessment of plaque morphology and plaque modification.

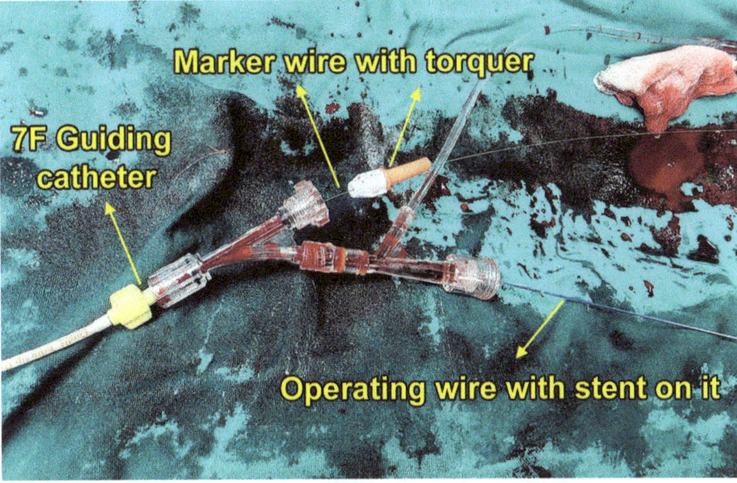

Fig. 6: Marker wire through a separate Y connector.

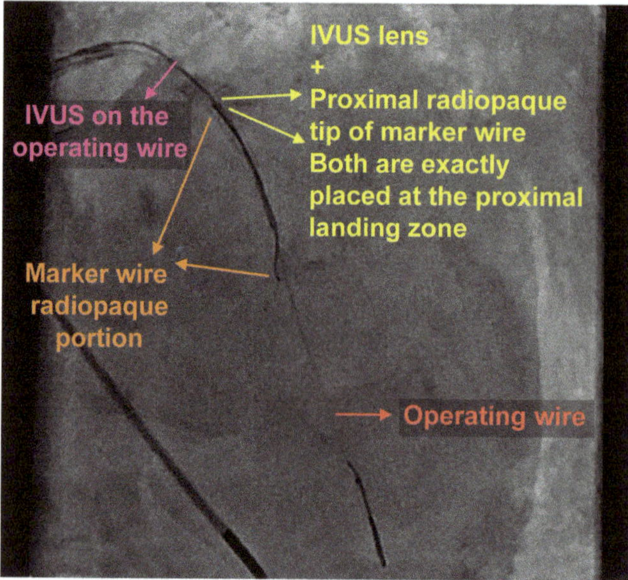

Fig. 7: IVUS-angiography co-registration.

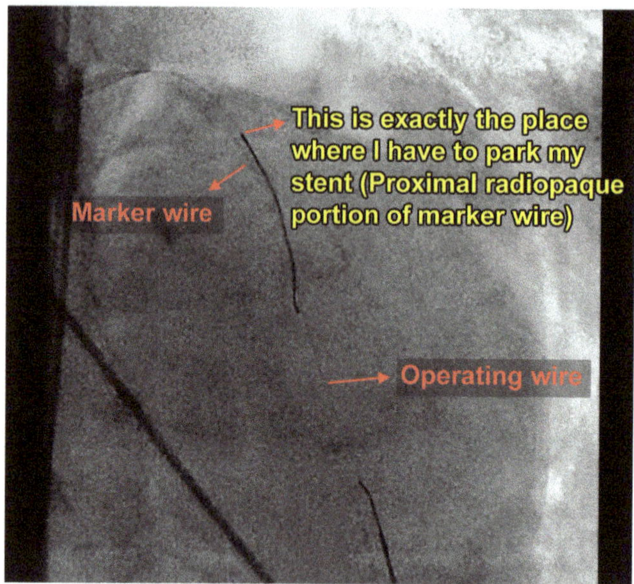

Fig. 8: Marker wire placed exactly at the stent landing zone.

Precautions to be taken to prevent displacement of marker wire when using MARKER WIRE technique for stent placement:

- MW to be inserted through a separate Y connector
- The Y connector should be rotating types
- Tighten the toue firmly and put torquer
- The guiding catheter should not move much

Advantages of MARKER WIRE technique over metallic silhouette for stent placement:

- More accurate than the metallic silhouette
- Do not need multiple wires (only 1 is sufficient)
- Less time-consuming

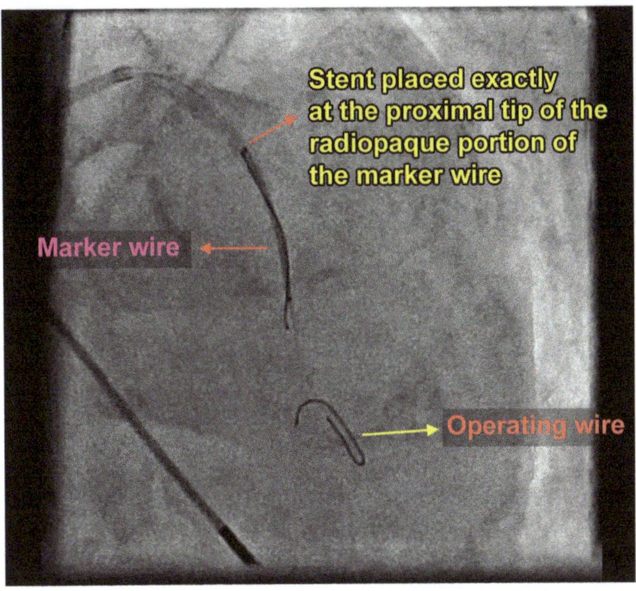

Fig. 9: Stent being placed at the radiopaque tip of the marker wire (MW).

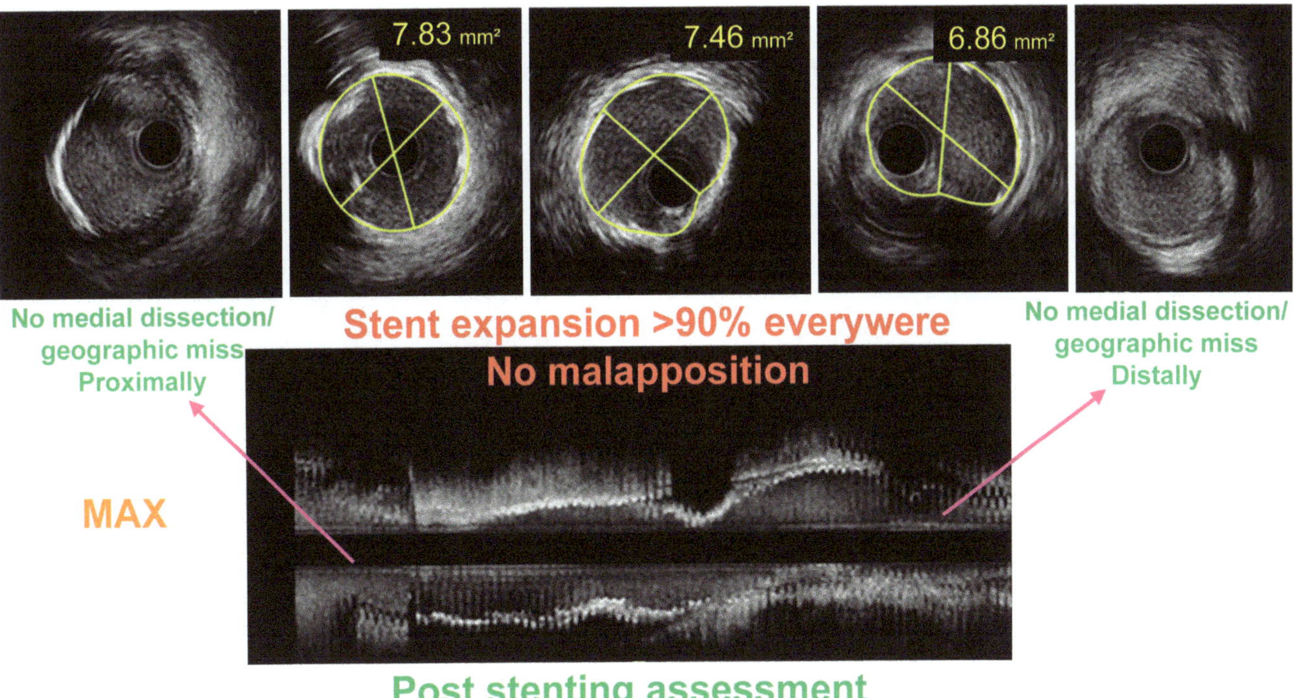

Fig. 10: Post stenting IVUS assessment.

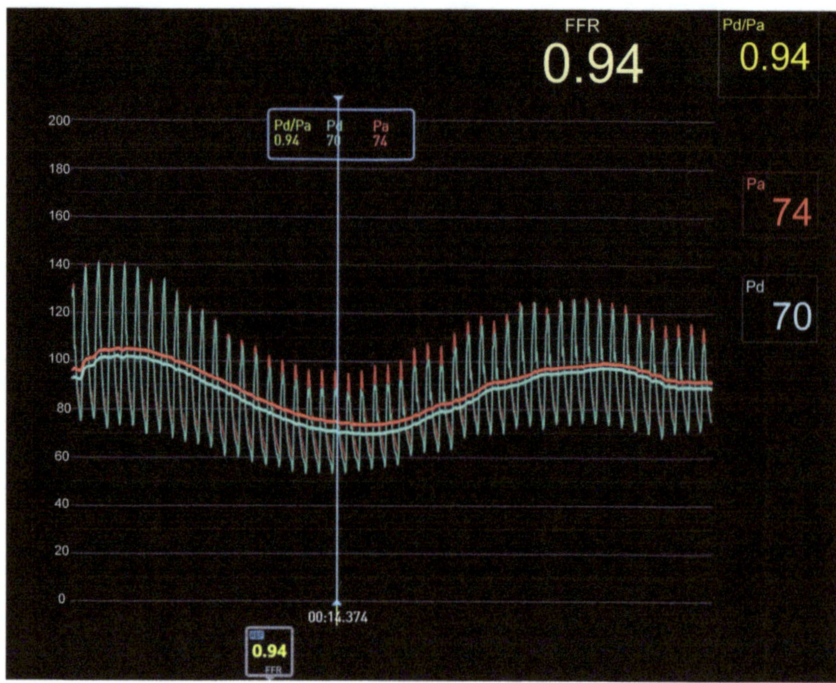

Fig. 11: Post PCI FFR.

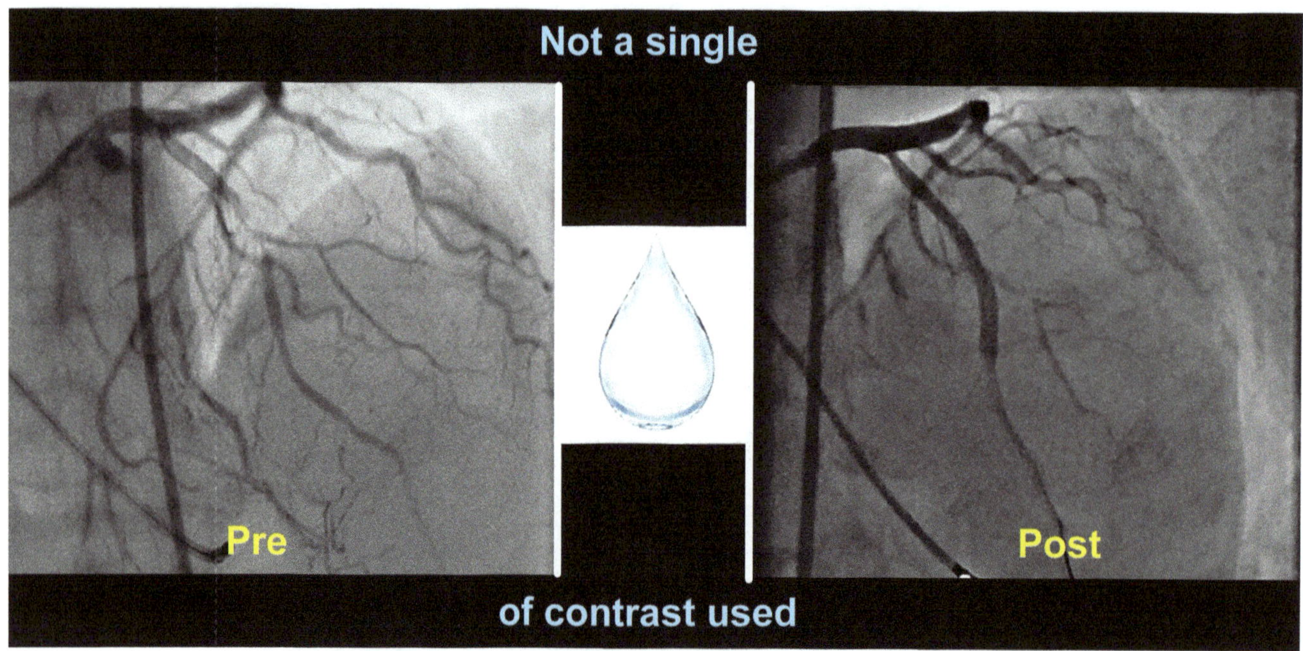

Fig. 12: Final angiography (the only time where dye was used).

"The only thing worse than being blind is having sight but no vision.
Yes! WE were BLIND throughout the procedure
But we had the vision to use this great tool (HD IVUS)
to make life of kidney patient better.!"

CHAPTER 50

Possible Intravascular Ultrasound Complications and Troubleshooting

Though not very common, intravascular ultrasound (IVUS) examination may lead to some complications such as:

- **Transient ischemia:** When IVUS is inserted into a tight stenosis and the examination time is prolonged, chest pain with electrocardiogram (ECG) changes can occur sometimes. However, this is transient and it resolves with removal of the IVUS catheter. A fast automated pullback may reduce the chance of ischemia caused by the IVUS catheter.
- **Coronary spasm:** Coronary spasm can sometimes occur with IVUS catheter insertion. The clue to diagnose spasm is a thickened media with wrinkled intima. However, the spasm can be easily removed by intracoronary nitroglycerin (NTG) **(Fig. 1)**. To avoid spasms,

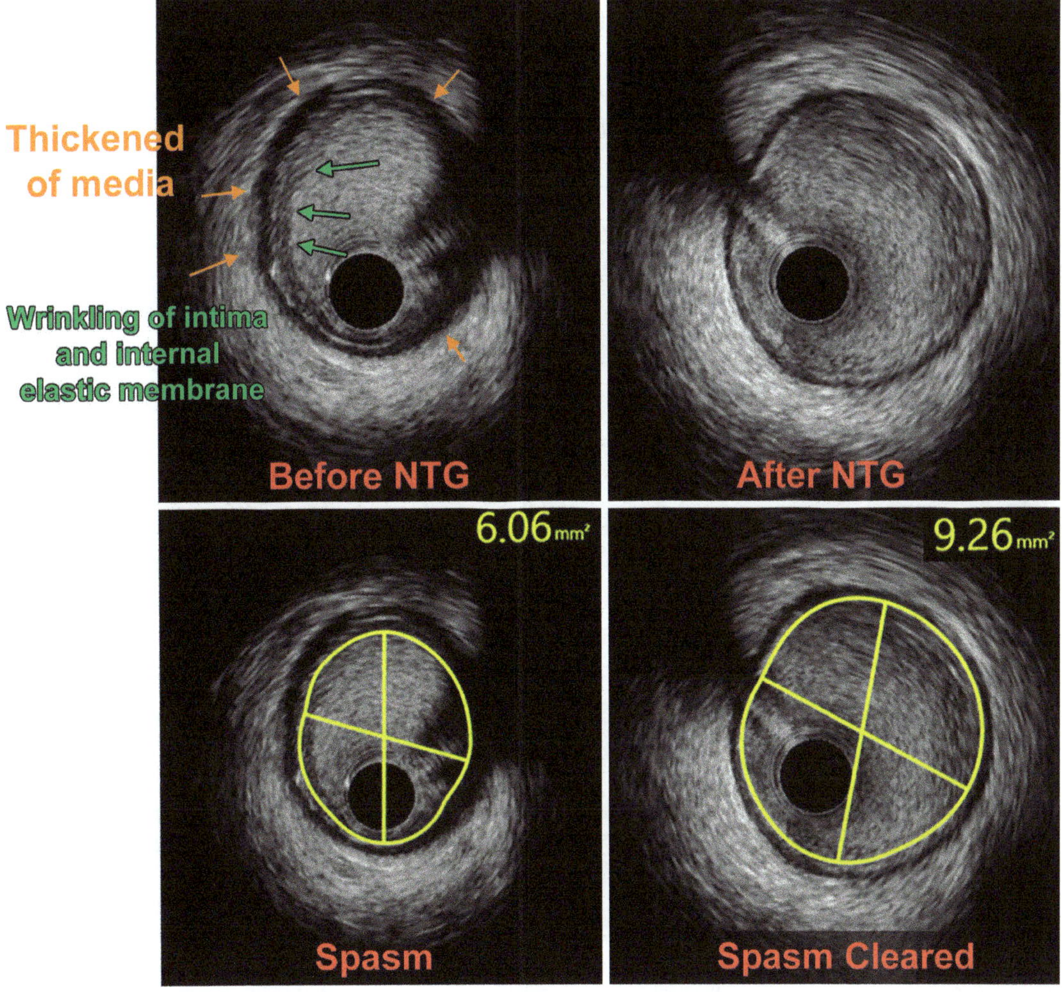

Fig. 1: Coronary spasm caused by intravascular ultrasound (IVUS) catheter, which was later relieved by nitroglycerin (NTG).

intracoronary NTG should be administered before the IVUS catheter insertion.

- **Air embolism:** Inadequate air evacuation during IVUS catheter preparation can lead to dark and blurred images **(Fig. 2)**. If we do multiple flushes in the coronary artery during this time, it may cause air embolization and chest pain with ST-segment elevation. It is necessary to perform flushing while rotating the imaging core outside the body to remove air bubbles before inserting the IVUS catheter.
- **Entanglement of IVUS catheter and guidewire:** The IVUS catheter has a short monorail system. Sometimes in angulated lesions, withdrawal of the IVUS catheter results in misalignment of the trajectory between the catheter and the guidewire. If you continue to pull out with a misaligned trajectory, the guidewire will be kinked at the tip of the guiding catheter, resulting in entwining of the IVUS catheter with the guidewire or IVUS getting stuck in the distal portion of the stent **(Fig. 3)**. If such a thing happens, then the best strategy is to remove the IVUS catheter and guidewire as a single unit. This usually works most of the time, but if this fails, then standard bailout retrieval methods of the entrapped imaging catheter should be attempted.
- **Inability to cross the IVUS catheter beyond the lesion:** When the IVUS catheter does not cross the lesion, the first dictum is to not force the lesion because it is a short monorail system and any force will bend the tip of the catheter and will damage the transducer. The solution to this problem will depend upon its cause. If the reason for uncrossing is tight stenosis or calcium, then do good lesion preparation with a balloon or ROTA and then do imaging. But if the mechanism of uncrossability of the IVUS catheter is angulation or bends, then two things can be done:
    1. Use a guide extension catheter to insert the IVUS catheter **(Fig. 4)**
    2. *Advancement of the sheath first than the imaging core:* In a sheath-type catheter, the protective sheath follows the vessel while the rigid imaging core tries to go straight. The tip of the imaging core is near the exit port of the guidewire, making it vulnerable to bending. To prevent bending, it is recommended to retract the imaging core 2–3 cm, advance the entire catheter, and then advance the imaging core after crossing the lesion **(Fig. 5)**.

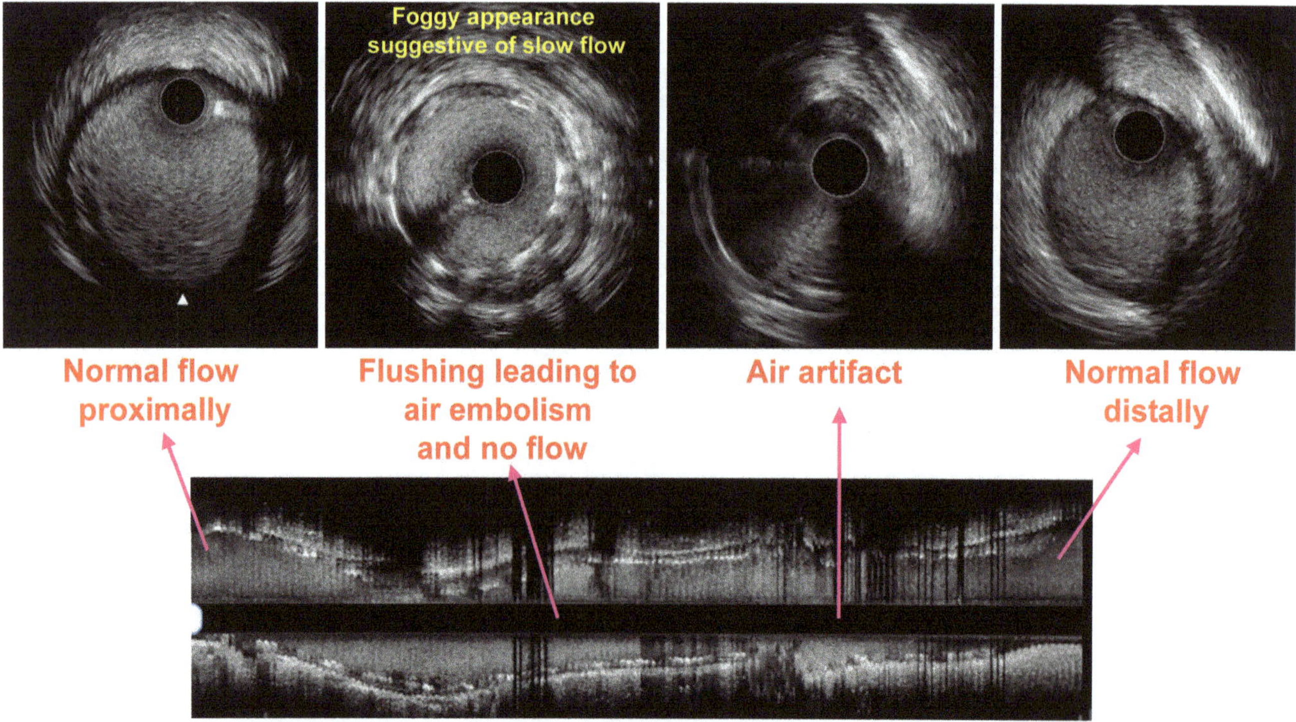

Fig. 2: During the pullback, a blurry image was observed due to an air artifact. Multiple flushes were performed inside the coronary artery to remove the air artifact, resulting in air embolism and transient no flow. This was revealed by the presence of a white foggy lumen.

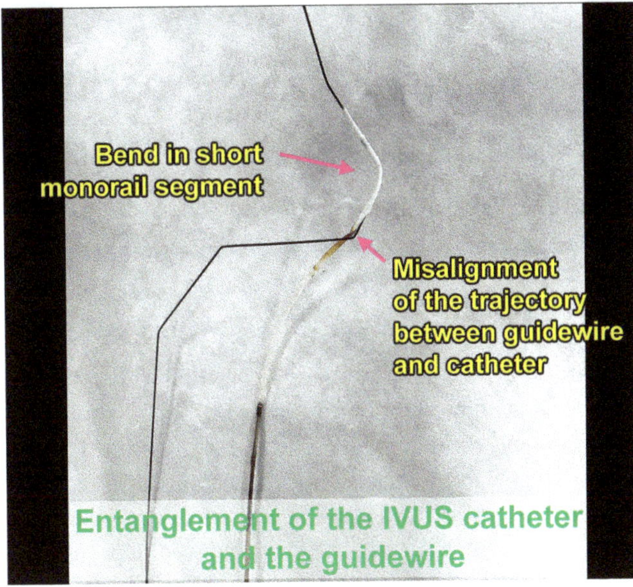

Fig. 3: Entanglement of intravascular ultrasound (IVUS) catheter and guidewire.

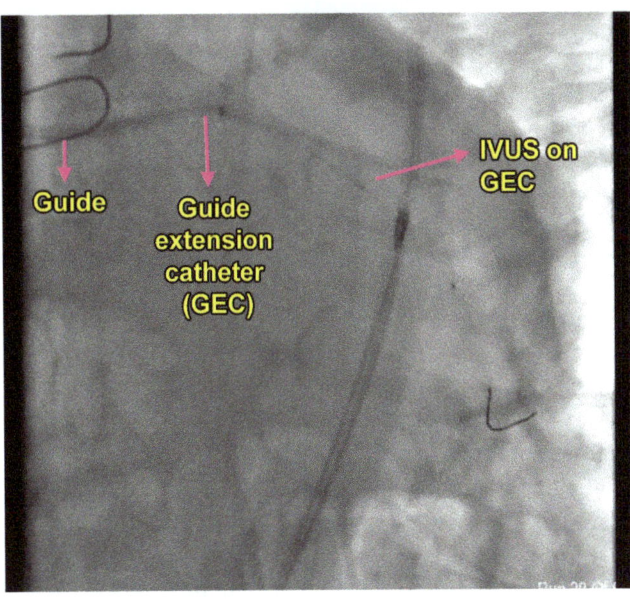

Fig. 4: Guide extension catheter used to deliver the intravascular ultrasound (IVUS) catheter.

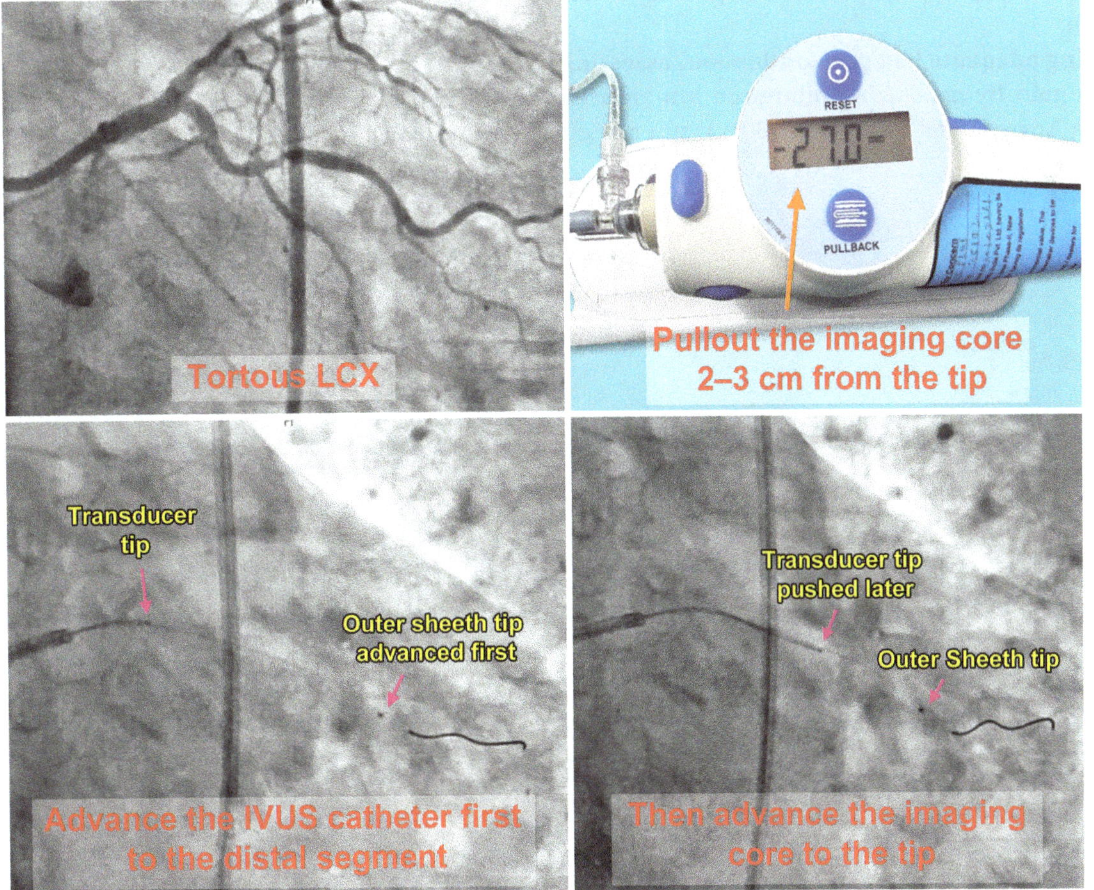

Fig. 5: Tips to advance IVUS catheter in tortuous lesion: Pull out the imaging core 2–3 cm from the tip, then advance the IVUS catheter into the distal segment of the lesion, and finally advance the imaging core to the tip. (IVUS: intravascular ultrasound; LCX: left circumflex)

CHAPTER 51

Role of Intravascular Ultrasound in Drug-eluting Balloon

1. **Determining the correct size of predilation balloon and drug-eluting balloon (DEB)** based on the distal reference with a ratio of 0.8 to the media diameter or 1:1 to the lumen diameter **(Fig. 1)**.
2. **Selecting the right device for plaque modification before DEB:** If the plaque is fibrotic with minimal calcium, then a cutting balloon can be used to achieve lumen gain **(Fig. 2)**. However, if there is severe calcium, then an intravascular lithotripsy (IVL) or atherectomy can be used depending upon the morphology of the calcium.
3. **Ensuring adequate bed preparation and assessing lumen gain by measuring minimum lumen area (MLA):** Any residual stenosis of >30% is not a good candidate for going ahead with DEB, which can be easily calculated by measuring MLA at the site of the lesion and comparing it with the distal reference lumen area, e.g., in this case the MLA achieved after bed preparation is 5 mm and the distal reference diameter is 7 mm which means lumen gain is >70% or in other words the residual stenosis is <30% **(Fig. 3)**.
4. **Risk assessment for acute vessel closure in the end:** Because of the risk of acute coronary occlusion with stentless percutaneous coronary intervention (PCI), endpoint determination with intravascular ultrasound (IVUS) is much safer than angiography. This can be done by differentiating ugly from healthy dissections. Any dissection extending up to the media with an arc

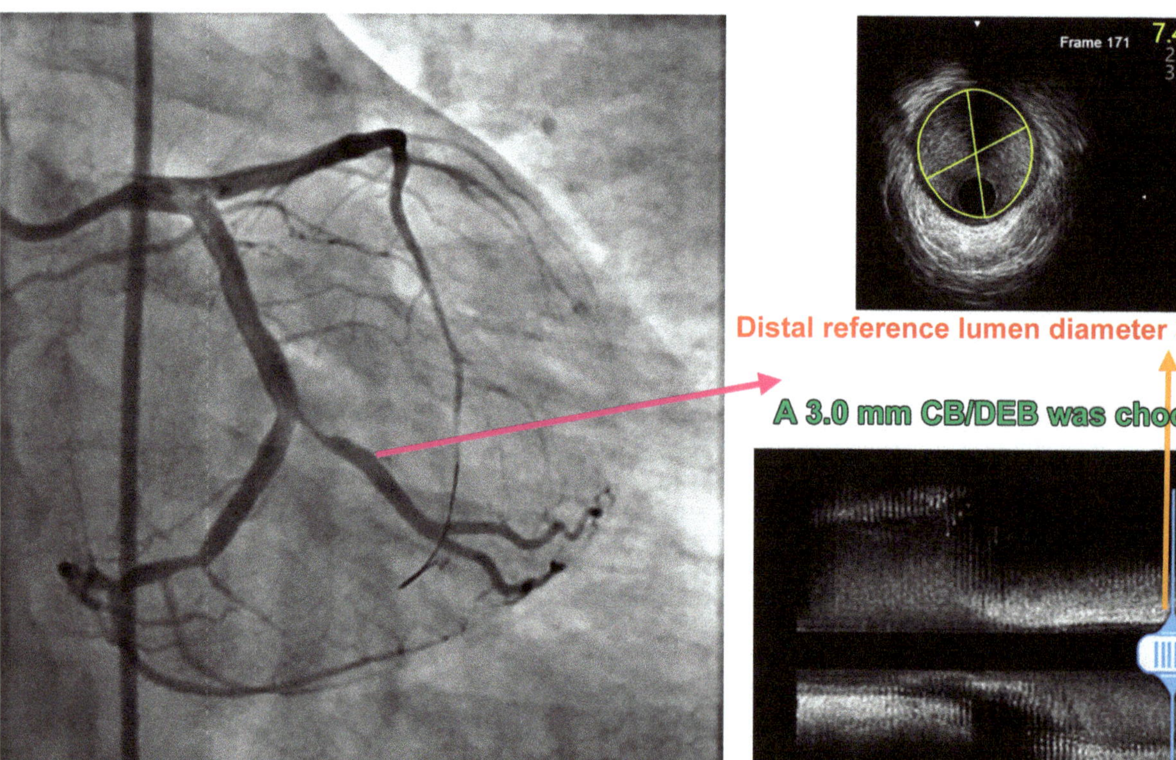

Fig. 1: Correct size of predilation balloon and drug-eluting balloon (DEB) calculated by intravascular ultrasound (IVUS).

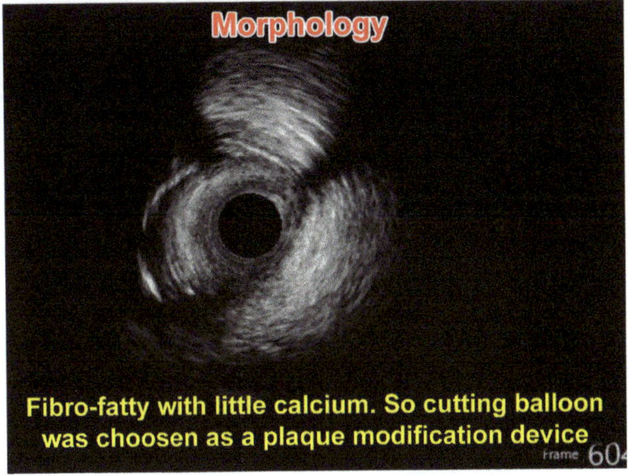

Fig. 2: Device selection based on morphology as detected by intravascular ultrasound (IVUS).

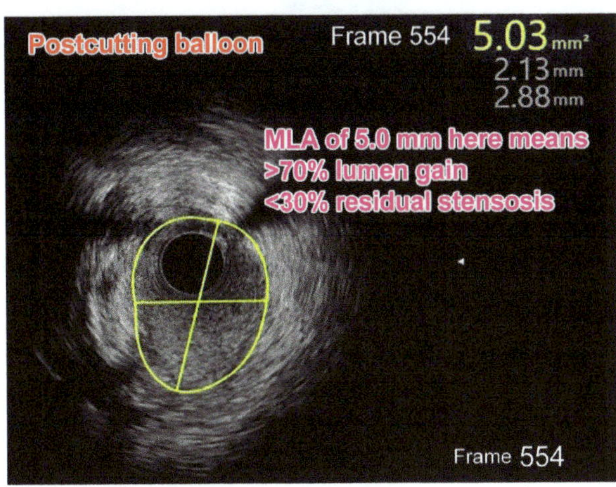

Fig. 3: Ensuring adequate bed preparation and assessing lumen gain by measuring minimum lumen area (MLA).

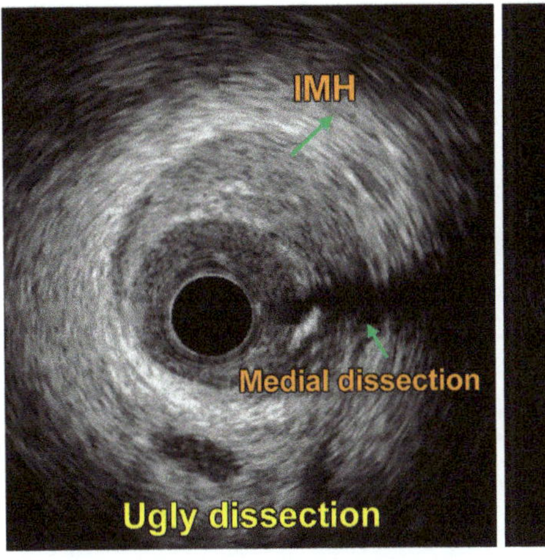

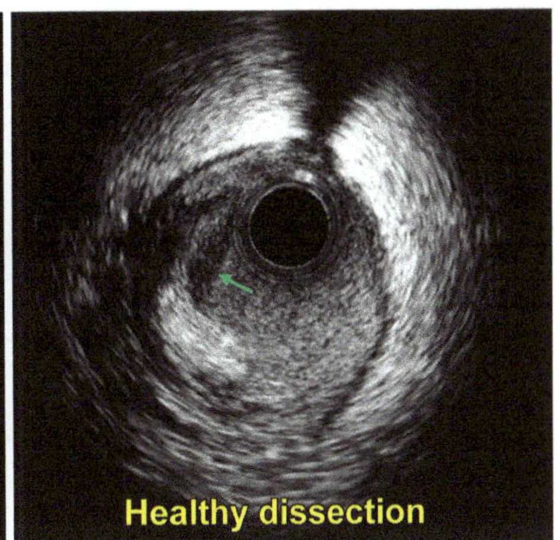

Fig. 4: Differentiating ugly from healthy dissections. (IMH: intramural hematoma)

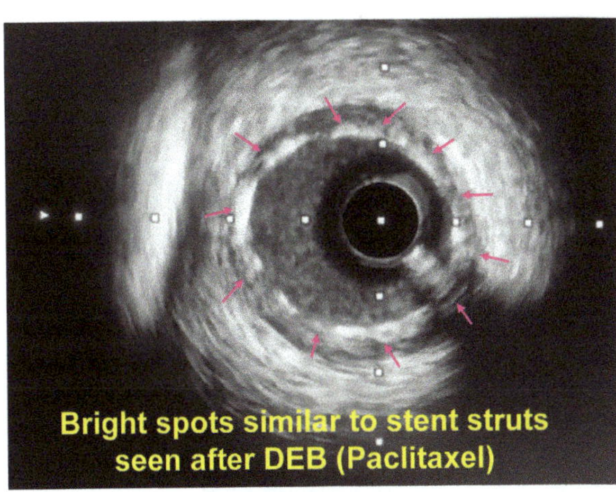

Fig. 5: Bright spots similar to stent struts seen after drug-eluting balloon (DEB).

>60° and length > 5 mm, and with associated intramural hematoma (IMH), is an ugly dissection **(Fig. 4)**.

5. **Ensuring drug delivery:** Sometimes bright spots similar to stent struts are visible after DEB, especially after paclitaxel DEB **(Fig. 5)**. However, whether their visualization is associated with better drug response and lower risk of restenosis is not known.

"In DEB: Don't over do, don't under do. Do it just on the line with the help of IVUS."

CHAPTER 52

Ostium Marking Technique by Intravascular Ultrasound

The purpose of the marking technique with intravascular ultrasound (IVUS) is to reduce geographic miss through accurate stenting. The marking technique is particularly important in the left main coronary artery (LMCA) ostium, ostial left anterior descending (LAD), and ostial right coronary artery (RCA), where the shift of a stent can result in significant protrusion into the aorta and risk of side branch occlusion.

There are a number of ways by which it can be done using IVUS:

1. Live IVUS using 8-F guide.
2. Using a marker wire technique through using 2 Y connectors (*see Chapter 49*).
3. IVUS marking technique using cine while using IVUS.

Here we will be discussing the steps for the third technique (IVUS ostium marking technique using cine while using IVUS) **(Fig. 1)**.

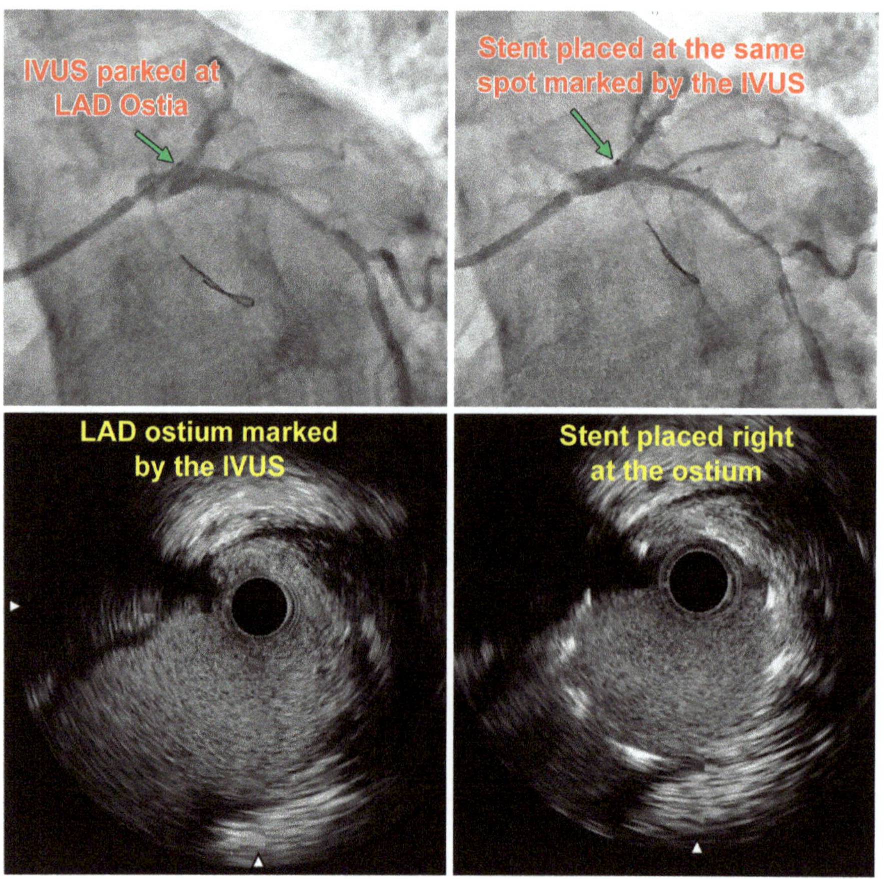

Fig. 1: Left anterior descending (LAD) ostium marking technique using intravascular ultrasound (IVUS).

"IVUS: Where technology meets the art of precision."

Step 1: Determine the length and diameter of the stent by marking the distal and proximal landing zone (the proximal landing zone is the ostium).

Step 2: Once you have marked the ostium by IVUS, take a cine with IVUS parked at the ostium.

Step 3: Make this a reference image.

Step 4: Remove the IVUS.

Step 5: Take the stent and park it exactly at the same spot marked by the IVUS using the reference image (do not change the view and angle of the cine).

Step 6: Again take the IVUS to confirm your ostial stent positioning.

SOME IMPORTANT CAVEATS DURING IVUS-GUIDED OSTIAL STENTING

- Be careful of stent elongation.
- Different stents have different overhanging balloon edges.
- If you miss the ostium by 1 mm, we can use the stent elongation technique by doing proximal optimization technique (POT) at high pressure from distal to proximal.

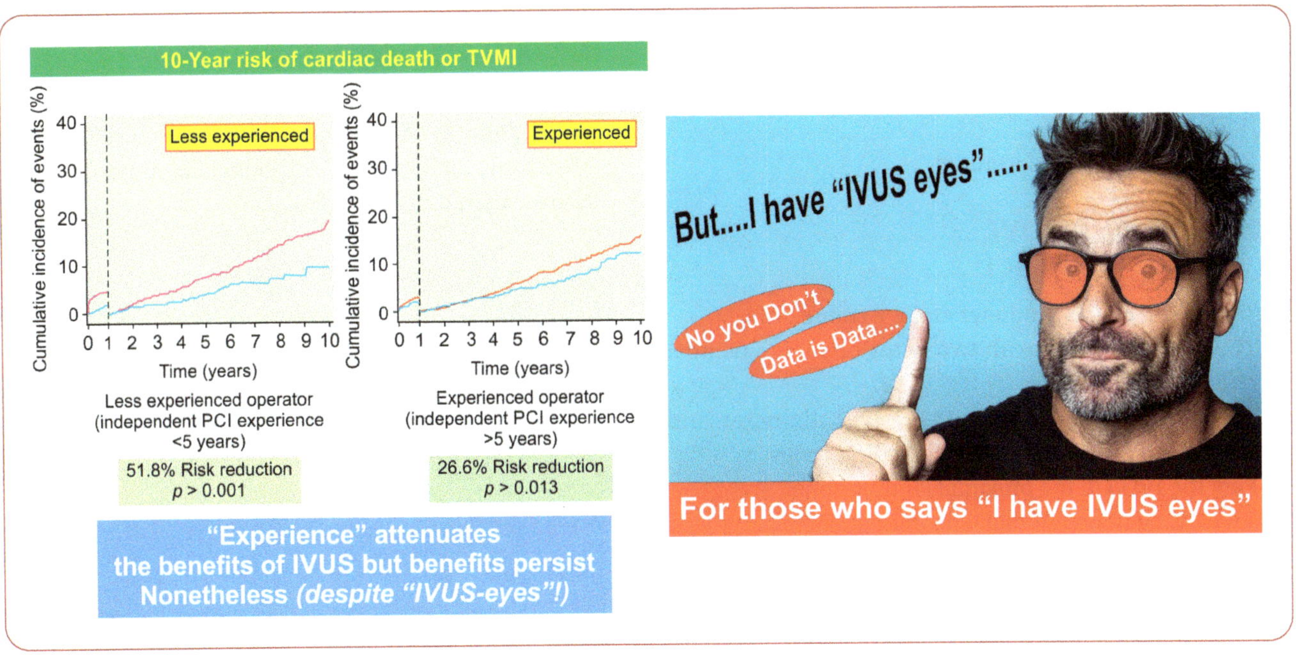

CHAPTER 53

Real-time Intravascular Ultrasound Guidance (Live-IVUS)

This technique involves positioning coronary stents under the live guidance of an intravascular ultrasound (IVUS) catheter which is positioned simultaneously either side by side to a stent or in a nearby side branch.

INDICATIONS OF LIVE INTRAVASCULAR ULTRASOUND

- Zero-contrast percutaneous coronary intervention (PCI)
- Precise ostial stent placement

TECHNIQUE OF LIVE IVUS GUIDANCE PCI

- Take an 8F guiding catheter and 2 Y connectors.
- The lesion is wired with two wires of choice using a reference image.
- Do the IVUS to determine the stent diameter and length and proximal and distal landing zones.
- Park the IVUS in the proximal landing zone.
- Take the stent on another wire and place it exactly side by side to the IVUS (which is the proximal landing zone already marked by the IVUS) **(Fig. 1)**.
- Confirm the landing zone again by doing live IVUS with the stent side by side (**Figure 2** to find out how stent and the delivery system looks on live IVUS).
- Pull the IVUS and its wire.
- Deploy the stent.
- Do the postdilation or proximal optimization technique (POT) as planned.
- Repeat the final IVUS to assess stent expansion, dissection, etc.

Note: In the live IVUS technique with IVUS catheter in the side branch, there is no need to remove the IVUS before stent deployment. You may deploy the stent during live streaming of IVUS.

SOME CAVEATS DURING LIVE INTRAVASCULAR ULTRASOUND

- 8F guide preferably; otherwise, there may be difficulty in the passage of hardware. (If 7F is used than prefer Medtronic guide over Cordis since its inner diameter is more than that of Cordis)

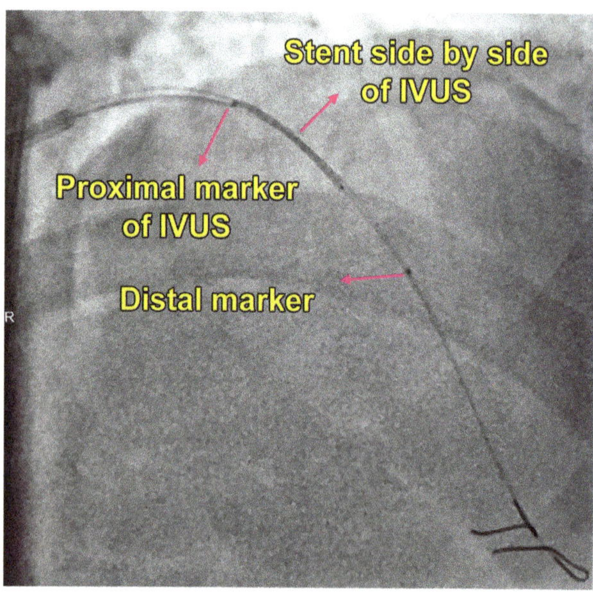

Fig. 1: Intravascular ultrasound (IVUS) verifying adequacy of stent proximal landing zone with IVUS catheter and stent side by side.

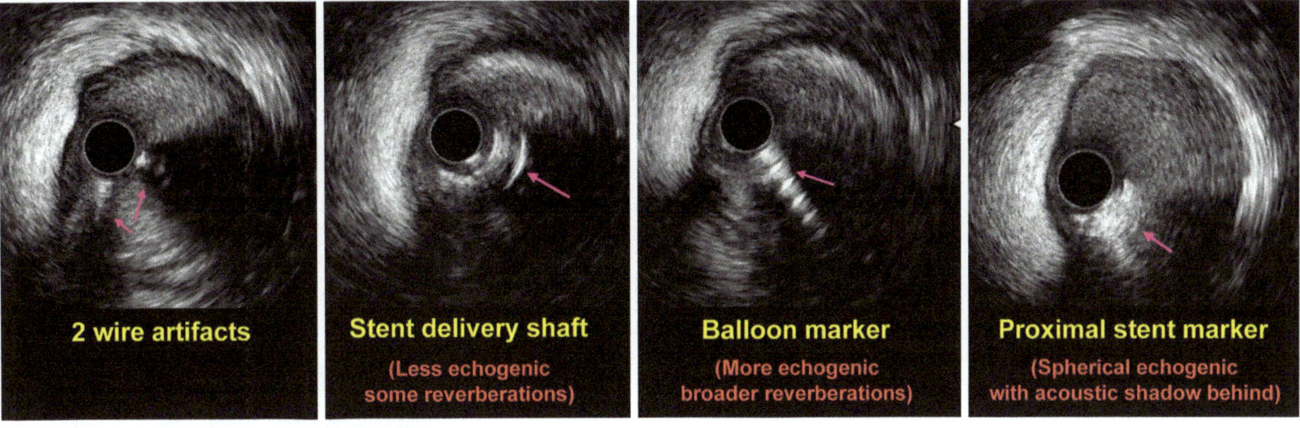

Fig. 2: How stent and the delivery system looks on live intravascular ultrasound (IVUS).

- Excessive friction between the stent and the IVUS catheter may raise the potential for stent degloving (so be careful).
- The bed should be aggressively prepared for simultaneous crossing of both devices.
- The IVUS catheter should never be jailed. Always remove it before stent implantation.
- Take the IVUS first and then the stent, since the crossing profile of the IVUS is poorer than that of the stent due to the short monorail.
- Do not try this technique in small arteries <2.5 mm and in severely tortuous calcified vessels.

PTCA with angio alone is like driving in dark with headlights off, you can met with an accient anytime

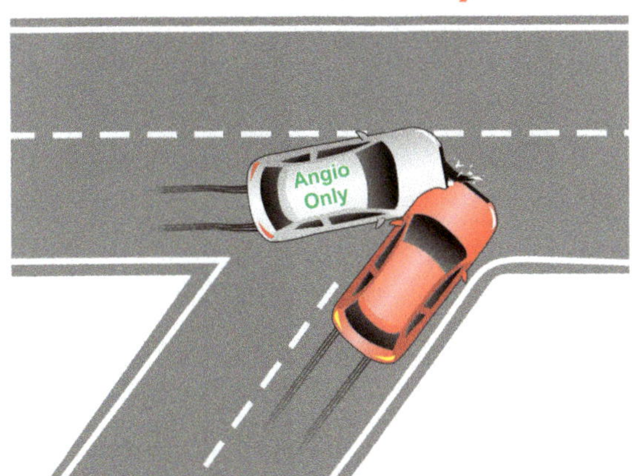

PTCA with IVUS is like driving in dark with headlights on, you can easily avoid accidents

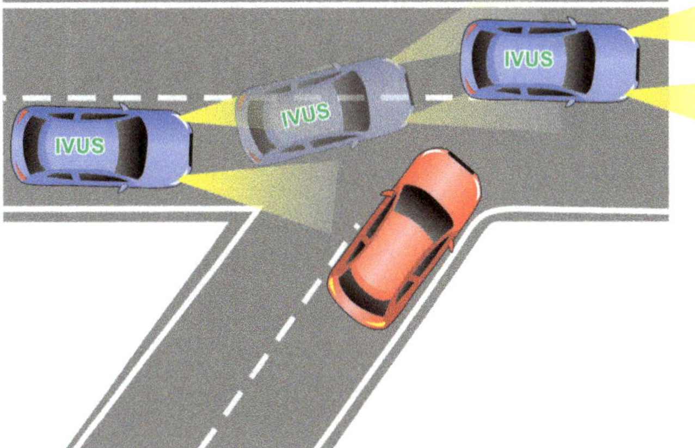

what a day... i'm exhausted

finally...

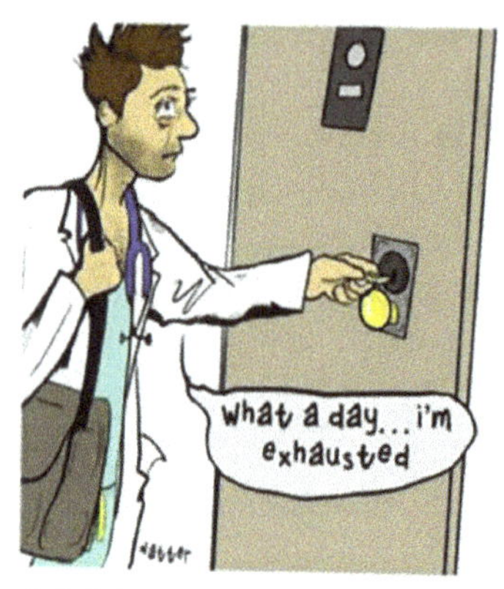

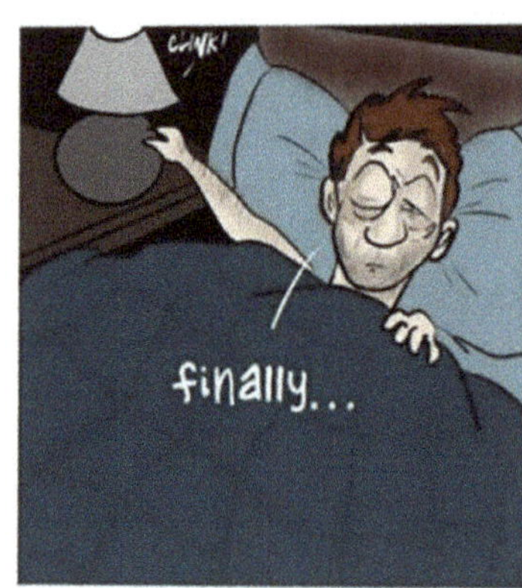

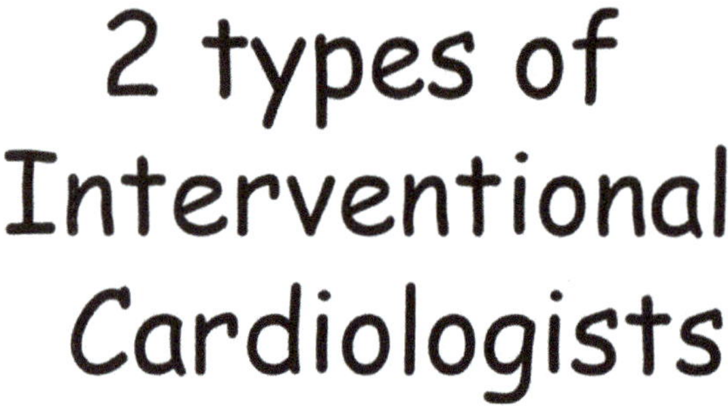
2 types of
Interventional
Cardiologists

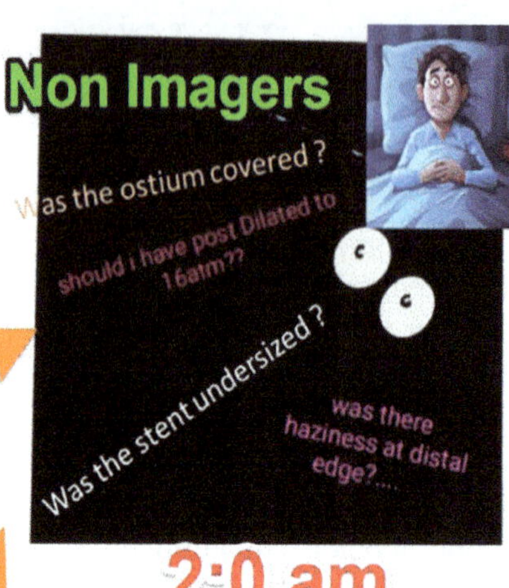
Non Imagers
Was the ostium covered ?
should i have post Dilated to 16atm??
Was the stent undersized ?
was there haziness at distal edge?....

2:0 am

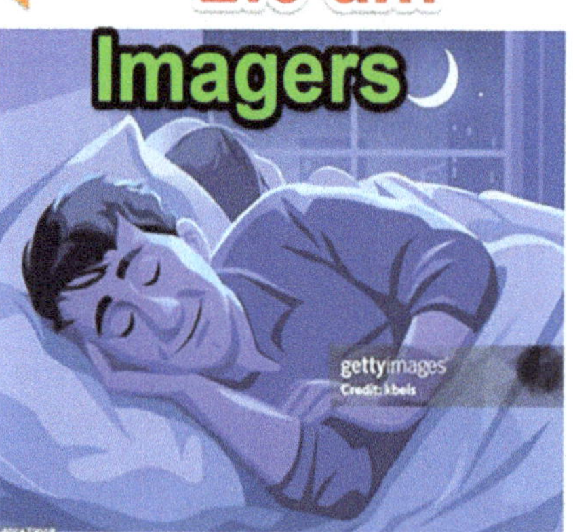
Imagers
gettyimages

Index

Page number followed by *f* refer to figure, and *t* refer to table.

EU GSPR Authorised Reprsentative
Logos Europe, 9 rue Nicolas Poussin
1700, La Rochelle, France
Phone: +33 (0) 6 67 93 73 78
E-mail: contact@logoseurope.eu

www.ingramcontent.com/pod-product-compliance
Ingram Content Group UK Ltd.
Pitfield, Milton Keynes, MK11 3LW, UK
UKHW052208180626
472359UK00005B/144

* 9 7 8 9 3 6 6 1 6 6 5 2 0 *